PSYCHIATRY
IN THE
NEW MILLENNIUM

PSYCHIATRY
IN THE
NEW MILLENNIUM

EDITED BY

Sidney Weissman, M.D.
Melvin Sabshin, M.D.
Harold Eist, M.D.

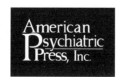

American
Psychiatric
Press, Inc.

Washington, DC
London, England

6-23-99

Note: The authors have worked to ensure that all information in this book concerning drug dosages, schedules, and routes of administration is accurate as of the time of publication and consistent with standards set by the U.S. Food and Drug Administration and the general medical community. As medical research and practice advance, however, therapeutic standards may change. For this reason and because human and mechanical errors sometimes occur, we recommend that readers follow the advice of a physician who is directly involved in their care or the care of a member of their family.

Books published by the American Psychiatric Press, Inc., represent the views and opinions of the individual authors and do not necessarily represent the policies and opinions of the Press or the American Psychiatric Association.

Copyright © 1999 American Psychiatric Press, Inc.
ALL RIGHTS RESERVED
Manufactured in the United States of America on acid-free paper
02 01 00 99   4 3 2 1
First Edition

American Psychiatric Press, Inc.
1400 K Street, N.W., Washington, DC   20005
www.appi.org

Library of Congress Cataloging-in-Publication Data
Psychiatry in the new millennium / edited by Sidney Weissman, Melvin Sabshin, and Harold Eist.   —   1st ed.
      p.   cm.
    Includes bibliographical references and index.
    ISBN 0-88048-938-3 (alk. paper)
    1. Psychiatry—Forecasting. 2. Clinical psychology—Forecasting.   I. Weissman, Sidney H.   II. Sabshin, Melvin, 1925- . III. Eist, Harold.
    [DNLM: 1. Psychiatry—trends. 2. Forecasting. 3. Psychology, Clinical—trends.   WM 100T971   1999]
    RC455.2F67T94   1999
    616.89—dc21
    DNLM/DLC   98-30132
    for Library of Congress   CIP

British Library Cataloguing in Publication Data
A CIP record is available from the British Library.

Cover design by Anne Friedman
Cover photograph copyright © PHOTODISC 1999

In memory of my wife,
Julie Weissman,
in honor of her courage and decency

CONTENTS

SECTION I

The Discipline of Psychiatry, Part I

The Impact of Changing Conceptual, Organizational, and Philosophical Issues on the Shape of Psychiatry

CHAPTER 1

CHAPTER 2

CHAPTER 3

CHAPTER 4

Psychiatric Diagnosis
Sidney Weissman, M.D.

CHAPTER 5

Normality and the Boundaries of Psychiatry
Daniel Offer, M.D.

CHAPTER 6

The Evolution of Psychiatric Subspecialties.
Lois T. Flaherty, M.D.

The Discipline of Psychiatry, Part II
The Impact of Research Findings on the Shape of Psychiatry

Introduction

CHAPTER 7

Looking to the Future: The Role of Genetics and Molecular Biology in Research on Mental Illness
Steven E. Hyman, M.D.

CHAPTER 12

A Clinical Model for Selecting

Mark Levey, M.D.

CHAPTER 13

Studying the Respective Contributions of
Pharmacotherapy and Psychotherapy:

Donald F. Klein, M.D.

CHAPTER 14

Less Is More: Financing Mental Health

Steven S. Sharfstein, M.D.

CHAPTER 15

Jeremy A. Lazarus, M.D.

SECTION III

The Psychiatric Workforce and Its Education

CHAPTER 16

James H. Scully Jr., M.D.

CHAPTER 17

CHAPTER 18

SECTION IV

The Future

CHAPTER 19

CHAPTER 20

CONTRIBUTORS

Boris M. Astrachan, M.D.
Distinguished Professor of Psychiatry, University of Illinois at Chicago

Richard Balon, M.D., F.A.P.A.
Professor of Psychiatry, Director of Medical Student Education in Psychiatry, Wayne State University School of Medicine, Detroit, Michigan

Joseph H. Callicott, M.D.
Research Fellow, Clinical Brain Disorders Branch, National Institute of Mental Health, National Institutes of Health, Bethesda, DC

Joseph T. Coyle, M.D.
Eben S. Draper Professor of Psychiatry and Neuroscience; Chairman of the Consolidated Department of Psychiatry, Harvard Medical School, Cambridge, Massachusetts

Harold Eist, M.D.
Past President, American Psychiatric Association; Medical Director, Montgomery Child and Family Health Services, Inc., Bethesda, Maryland

Joseph A. Flaherty, M.D.
Professor and Head, Department of Psychiatry, University of Illinois at Chicago

Lois T. Flaherty, M.D.
Adjunct Associate Professor, University of Maryland School of Medicine, Baltimore, Maryland

Glen O. Gabbard, M.D.
Bessie Walker Callaway Distinguished Professor of Psychoanalysis and Education in the Karl Menninger School of Psychiatry and Mental Health Sciences, The Menninger Clinic; Clinical Professor of Psychiatry, University of Kansas School of Medicine, Wichita, Kansas

Steven E. Hyman, M.D.
Director, National Institute of Mental Health, Bethesda, Maryland

Donald F. Klein, M.D.
Professor of Psychiatry, Columbia University College of Physicians and Surgeons; Director of Research and Director of Department of Therapeutics, New York State Psychiatric Institute, New York, New York

Jeremy A. Lazarus, M.D.
Associate Clinical Professor of Psychiatry, University of Colorado Health Sciences Center, Englewood, Colorado

Mark Levey, M.D.
Training and Supervising Analyst, Chicago Institute for Psychoanalysis, Chicago, Illinois; Clinical Assistant Professor of Psychiatry, Department of Psychiatry, University of Illinois at Chicago

John S. McIntyre, M.D.
Chair, Department of Psychiatry and Behavioral Health, Unity Health System, Rochester, New York; Chair, Steering Committee on Practice Guidelines, American Psychiatric Association, Washington, DC

Steven M. Mirin, M.D.
Medical Director, American Psychiatric Association, Washington, DC; Professor of Psychiatry, Harvard Medical School, Cambridge, Massachusetts

Rodrigo A. Muñoz, M.D., F.A.P.A.
Clinical Professor of Psychiatry, University of California, San Diego, San Diego, California

Daniel Offer, M.D.
Professor of Psychiatry, Northwestern University Medical School, Chicago, Illinois

Harold A. Pincus, M.D.
Deputy Medical Director, Director of Office of Research, American Psychiatric Association, Washington, DC

Nyapati R. Rao, M.D.
Associate Professor, Director of Residency Training, Brookdale Hospital Medical Center, Brooklyn, New York

Carolyn B. Robinowitz, M.D.
Professor of Psychiatry and Dean for Students, Georgetown University
School of Medicine, Washington, DC

Melvin Sabshin, M.D.
Medical Director Emeritus, American Psychiatric Association, Washington,
DC

Alan F. Schatzberg, M.D.
Kenneth T. Norris Jr. Professor in Psychiatry and Behavioral Sciences;
Chairman, Department of Psychiatry and Behavioral Sciences, Stanford
University School of Medicine, Stanford, California

James H. Scully Jr., M.D.
Professor and Chairman, Department of Neuropsychiatry and Behavioral
Science, University of South Carolina School of Medicine, Columbia, South
Carolina

Steven S. Sharfstein, M.D.
Clinical Professor of Psychiatry, University of Maryland; President, Medical
Director, and Chief Executive Officer, Sheppard Pratt Health System, Balti-
more, Maryland

Daniel R. Weinberger, M.D.
Chief, Clinical Brain Disorders Branch, Division of Intramural Research,
National Institute of Mental Health (NIMH) Neuroscience Center at St.
Elizabeth's, Washington, DC

Sidney Weissman, M.D.
Professor of Psychiatry, Department of Psychiatry and Behavioral
Neurosciences, Stritch School of Medicine, Loyola University, Chicago,
Illinois; Faculty, Chicago Institute for Psychoanalysis, Chicago, Illinois

Deborah A. Zarin, M.D.
Deputy Medical Director, Director of Office of Quality Improvement and
Psychiatric Services, American Psychiatric Association, Washington, DC

SENIOR EDITOR'S SPECIAL ACKNOWLEDGMENT

In conceiving the idea to produce a volume that would serve as the conceptual framework for psychiatry at the dawn of the new millennium, Dr. Harold Eist, then President of the American Psychiatric Association, and I sought to honor Dr. Melvin Sabshin, who was completing more than two decades of service as Medical Director of the American Psychiatric Association, and to acknowledge his contribution to world psychiatry. Although we thought of this volume as a tribute to Dr. Sabshin, we also wanted to signal his ongoing active role in the intellectual life of world psychiatry. We therefore asked Dr. Sabshin to join us in this enterprise. Because this volume is published by the American Psychiatric Press, Inc. (APPI), whose growth was nurtured by Melvin Sabshin's vision, we felt that a specific view of this element of Sabshin's work was required. APPI's growth serves as a model for Dr. Sabshin's courage, creativity, and vision. To provide this closeup of Melvin Sabshin's effort, we have invited Carol Nadelson, President, CEO, and Editor-in-Chief of APPI, to write a special Foreword.

FOREWORD

Carol C. Nadelson, M.D.

For the past three decades, the creative influence of Dr. Melvin Sabshin has permeated the American Psychiatric Association (APA) and the field of psychiatry worldwide. His vision and leadership have taken psychiatry in new directions. He has inspired innovative developments in a wide variety of areas, as you will see in this volume. Among Dr. Sabshin's major contributions to psychiatry has been American Psychiatric Press, Inc. (APPI).

The story of APPI is unique and Dr. Sabshin's role has been pivotal. For more than a decade, I have had the opportunity to work closely with Dr. Sabshin and share in the maturation of a truly unique publishing enterprise. The APA has had a successful publications program since the 1940s, and much before that, if one considers the *American Journal of Psychiatry*, which began in 1844, and the other successful early publications of the association, which included the *Psychiatric Glossary* and DSM-I (1952) and DSM-II (1968), as well as many task force reports. It was not until the late 1970s, however, that the development of DSM-III signaled an opportunity for a more sophisticated and comprehensive APA publishing arm.

In 1979, the APA Resource Development Committee, chaired by Dr. Charles B. Wilkinson, recommended that the APA explore the feasibility of establishing a publishing company to further the education of APA members, other health care and mental health professionals, and the public. Dr. Shervert H. Frazier was appointed as the first editor-in-chief, and APPI was incorporated in the District of Columbia in March 1981 as a subsidiary of the APA. APPI held its first board of directors' meeting in May 1981, with Dr. Sabshin presiding as president and chairman of the board. Shortly thereafter, an editorial board was also appointed, and seven titles were approved for publication. In addition, DSM-III (1980) translations were authorized in six languages. In 1982, APPI was approved as a nonprofit educational publisher by the Internal Revenue Service. Five new titles were published in this year, including the first volume of *The American Psychiatric Association Annual Review*. Also, an APPI bookstore made its first appearance at the APA annual meeting.

Over the course of the next few years, APPI continued to grow, having sold its millionth book and published its first book for the general reader in 1984. By 1985, APPI books became available throughout many parts of the world.

My own formal role with APPI began in 1986 when I was appointed editor-in-chief and joined with Dr. Sabshin to continue to expand APPI and facilitate its evolution into the foremost psychiatric publisher in the world. Over the next few years, Dr. Sabshin helped guide us through the launching of our textbooks, the establishment of a journals division, and the publication of DSM-III-R (1987). Our success was enhanced by our ability to use emerging technology to augment all aspects of our publication program. We also launched two of our own journals, the *Journal of Neuropsychiatry and Clinical Neurosciences* and the *Journal of Psychotherapy Practice and Research*, and we contracted to publish several others for allied psychiatric organizations. These other journals include *Psychosomatics*, *Academic Psychiatry*, the *American Journal of Addictions*, and the *American Journal of Geriatric Psychiatry*. Annual meeting bookstore revenues continued to climb, we formed a new international distribution network that brought APPI to all parts of the world, and we continued to forge publishing partnerships with a variety of psychiatric organizations and publishers.

In 1993, by virtue of our editorial independence, our rigorous peer review process, and our attention to quality, we were accepted for membership in the prestigious Association of American University Presses. That year also saw the launching of the American Psychiatric Electronic Library on CD-ROM and our entry into the world of the exploding technology that will change the face of publishing in the next century. DSM-IV, published in 1994, was made available electronically, and we continued to develop electronic products. Healthsource, the APPI retail bookstore, an innovative endeavor to bring health-related materials to the professions and the public, successfully opened in 1994. Since that time, APPI has gone online, has continued to expand its book list to meet the comprehensive needs of the field, and has been able to attract increasing interest from our colleagues worldwide. APPI books have been translated into 27 languages, and more than half the psychiatric titles published in the world are APPI titles.

Recently, to allow for full-time attention to APPI, Dr. Sabshin relinquished his role as president and chair of the APPI board, and a restructuring of senior positions took place. We are fortunate that Dr. Sabshin's indispensable contributions continue. In my new role as president and chief executive officer, in addition to my responsibilities as editor-in-chief of APPI, I am grateful to have the opportunity to continue to work closely with such an imaginative person as Dr. Melvin Sabshin. He has guided, and continues to guide, us to new heights. This volume is a tribute to him and a way of thanking him with lasting documentation for his gifts to us.

INTRODUCTION

We live in an era in which scientific advances frequently make the most recent scientific or medical journals obsolete or dated by the time of publication or shortly thereafter. Why then, in light of these realities, one might ask, would anyone attempt to produce a multiauthored volume on the foundations of contemporary psychiatry? Perhaps the endeavor relates to the human desire to celebrate special events, in this case, the birth of a new century and a new millennium. Would the authors have attempted a volume titled, *1998 Psychiatry: The Foundations*? The answer is of course not. A historic event, however, allows contributors in a field to use that event as a marker for progress in that field. The new millennium simply allows us to examine psychiatry and use a universal date as our marker. But, the question remains: Is such a volume necessary at a time of rapid change—with no shortage of journals, specialized volumes, or texts, as well as with the information exchange on the Internet—to keep psychiatrists apprised of advances? One of the risks of this massive information explosion is the possibility that psychiatrists can lose the ability to effectively comprehend or use the vast new areas of knowledge. For example, basic elements of our knowledge base, as well as many of the scientific questions of today, did not exist when most practitioners trained.

This volume is designed to provide the practitioner with the conceptual tools that will enable him or her to assess and use psychiatry's vast professional literature base. Further, it provides the practitioner a basis on which to effectively assess the presentations at scientific meetings. It accomplishes these goals with a mix of chapters. Key chapters present the core concepts in our expanding understanding of neuroscience and behavior. These presentations not only provide the current state of our art and science but also offer the reader a context to understand evolving areas of research and their likely future directions. Other chapters explore similarly the role of an in-depth psychology in understanding behavior. An array of supporting chapters fills in the depth and breadth of our field. These chapters include a discussion of the implication of how society's use of its resources for mental health will affect our field as well as our patients.

Although the authors of this volume are based in the United States, the ideas presented and discussed are of universal concern. Even though specific chapters deal with economics, migration of physicians, nosology, and social psychiatry from an American perspective, the knowledge and insight they offer are equally applicable around the world.

If the new century and millennium were not upon us, we would not have a book with "millennium" in its title, but we would still need a volume to reformulate the foundations of our discipline.

SECTION I

The Discipline of Psychiatry, Part I

The Impact of Changing Conceptual, Organizational, and Philosophical Issues on the Shape of Psychiatry

INTRODUCTION

Perhaps the most obvious starting point in addressing the discipline of psychiatry is to recall that it is a subcomponent of the discipline of medicine. At times in the twentieth century, this seemingly obvious reality was forgotten. Models of the discipline based on ideological points of view periodically dominated psychiatric thinking. Today, the core medical constructs of nosology, etiology, epidemiology, pathology, and therapeutics shape our discipline. In this section we will explore some of these core elements of psychiatry.

Our journey begins with Chapter 1, The Neuroscience Revolution and Psychiatry, with Joseph Coyle as our guide. Coyle alerts us to the brain's remarkable plasticity in its neuronal connectivity and function. He warns us against reducing behavior to what occurs at the synapse. He reviews the history and science that have fueled the psychopharmacological revolution of the past quarter-century. He argues that the next pharmacological advances will be guided by our findings from molecular biology and introduces a framework to understand this rapidly evolving field. Coyle then presents an overview of the impact of brain imaging in our unraveling the mysteries of major psychiatric disorders, again providing us with a conceptual framework.

In Chapter 2, Psychoanalysis, Sidney Weissman elaborates on what seems to some a troubled core component of psychiatry. Weissman first addresses the critics of psychoanalysis who assume that it is either unscientific or based on faulty scientific or philosophical principles. He reviews models of the mind from the time of Aristotle to the present, examining the assumptions that have been made in our concept of the mind. Finally, he concludes that our knowledge of the physical components of the mind "brain functions," although it adds to our understanding of behavior, does not remove the necessity to have an understanding of the mind, which psychoanalysis provides.

Having established the contemporary relevance of psychoanalysis, Weissman reviews 10 psychoanalytic concepts that will be essential to the practice of psychiatry in the twenty-first century. Weissman does not restrict himself to contributions by Freud but also includes the recent contributions of self psychology, with additional reference to the role of empathy and the self-object.

Next, in Chapter 3, Social Psychiatry, Joseph Flaherty and Boris Astrachan argue for a revived and reformulated social psychiatry to serve as a translator, developer, and bridge between the social and behavioral sciences and the worlds of treatment, practice, and public policy.

The authors identify for discussion three areas in which social psychiatry can or must have a critical role in societal problems. These areas include substance use and abuse; violence, aggression, and trauma; and the breakdown of family bonds. The authors discuss each area and present models of how social psychiatry can assist in addressing these major problems. Although both authors write from the perspective of the United States, they demonstrate that their proposals are universal in scope. The specific tactics that contend with the issues they address will vary from country to country, but the underlying theory and its premises remain. Social psychiatry is both alive and well and is again a critical element of the psychiatric foundation.

In Chapter 4, Psychiatric Diagnosis, Sidney Weissman reviews the complex questions a diagnostic system must address if it is to be useful both in informing the therapy of a patient and concurrently expanding the knowledge of a discipline. Weissman reviews problems that have existed in diagnostic systems when theoretical models of diseases—not empirical data—were used in their construction. An effective diagnostic system is informed by theory and built around observable data.

Weissman, in examining our current nosology, argues that the American Psychiatric Association's DSM-IV serves as an effective diagnostic system when focused on major psychotic and affective disorders, but it is of limited utility for disorders in which the meaning of the illness to the patient is critical or where intrapsychic issues have a significant role. Weissman argues for the development of a new multiaxial system that will include axes that address motive and meaning and biological and genetic contributions to behavior. Furthermore, an additional axis would be included that addresses therapeutic planning.

Weissman likens the DSM-IV to Americus Vespucius' maps of the New World. By providing a sharp outline of the dimensions of the New World, they facilitated exploration of its borders. Yet, his maps did not help with the exploration of the interior of the New World. A twenty-first-century diagnostic system must do both, argues Weissman.

Daniel Offer, in Chapter 5, Normality and the Boundaries of Psychiatry, addresses psychiatry's apparent ambivalence toward addressing what is meant by normality. This ambivalence at times has led to the obscuring of the discipline's boundaries. He reviews his earlier work with Melvin Sabshin describing four distinct definitions of normality. The core of this chapter, however, is to argue that the study of normality is important for psychiatrists. Three reasons or specific benefits to the field are presented: 1) it will allow psychiatrists to better understand the totality of behaviors on the continuum from extreme psychopathology to superior functioning; 2) it will help psychiatrists to better understand the factors that help some individuals contend with life experiences and stay symptom free while others with seemingly comparable experiences develop symptoms they are unable to change; and 3) it will help psychiatrists establish a realistic end point of psychiatric treatment. All of these reasons are critical to the field of psychiatry and the care of our patients, but probably the last point, in this era of cost containment, may have the greatest impact.

Next, in Chapter 6, The Evolution of Psychiatric Subspecialties, Lois Flaherty reviews how the growth of psychiatry has paralleled the growth of medicine with a surge in subspecialization. The chapter is written from a U.S. perspective and refers at times to the particular organizational or structural issues in American medicine. Yet the thrust of the chapter is to address how the surge of knowledge—particularly in the neurosciences and psychopharmacology—has had an impact on psychiatry and fueled its development of subspecialties. Flaherty observes that the paradigm of this current knowledge expansion encourages subspecialization, whereas the post–World War II emphasis on psychoanalysis in the United States fostered a generalist perspective. The borders of specialties or subspecialties we observe are not fixed. The identity of the specialist treating patients with syphilis during the past 100 years is an example: One hundred years ago, the patient was treated by psychiatrists; 50 years ago, by dermatologists; and now, by experts in infectious disease. The effects of subspecialization on academic medicine, as well as on the varied economics of medical practice, are further explored.

CHAPTER 1

The Neuroscience Revolution and Psychiatry

Joseph T. Coyle, M.D.

The paradox of contemporary psychiatry is the extraordinary mismatch between the realities of clinical practice in a managed care environment and the impressive advances in research that inform psychiatry. The rapidly spreading managed behavioral health care industry often relies on the least expert of mental health professionals to provide services and penalizes technological and pharmacological innovation. In contrast, the accelerating rate of scientific discovery is providing powerful insights into the causes of serious mental illness that are improving diagnosis and treatment. It is the contention of this chapter that scientific advances will reverse this trivialization of mental illness as the public and policy makers appreciate that these disorders are as "real" as cancer and are subject to rational treatment.

As we pass through the Decade of the Brain and into the twenty-first century, it is clear that the explosion of neuroscience research is both transforming conceptual approaches toward mental illness as well as providing a unifying perspective on psychopathology. The debate between mind and brain or between "nature" and "nurture" has reached endgame. It is abundantly clear that the brain is the organ of the mind and that the Cartesian separation of mind from brain is no longer tenable. This statement, however, is the obverse of reductionism because the defining characteristic of the brain is the remarkable plasticity of its neuronal connectivity and function (Katz and

Shatz 1996; Singer 1995). Thus, neuroscientific perspective can not only recognize the salience of experience in providing meaning at a personal level but can acknowledge that such meaning could not be reduced to the chemistry of the single synapse. In this regard, the neuroscientific foundation of psychiatry represents the leading edge of biomedical research and infuses the field with a zeitgeist similar to that of psychoanalysis in the past as a rapidly expanding cadre of physicians, scientists, and even philosophers confront the interface between mind and brain.

Past Is Prologue

It is worthwhile to briefly take stock of the evolution of pharmacological treatment of mental disorders over the past 30 years. After the serendipitous burst of discovery of effective psychotropic medications in the early 1960s—neuroleptics, tricyclic antidepressants, benzodiazepines, and lithium—no truly novel drugs appeared for three decades. The discovery of psychotropic drugs in the pharmaceutical industry at that time was generally dominated by chemists, who synthesized novel compounds that were then subjected to behavioral screens to identify potential therapeutic targets. Given that the diagnostic categories for mental disorders were poorly defined and that there was an absence of any identifiable brain pathology for psychiatric disorders, it was remarkable that any psychotropic drugs were discovered during this time. Although pharmacological therapy was recognized as an effective intervention in certain disorders, it was generally viewed as ancillary to insight-oriented psychotherapy.

The second wave of psychotropic drug discovery was based on the attempt to understand the molecular sites of action of existing efficacious psychotropic medications. Thus, a focus on biological mechanism began to dictate the pharmacological targets for medicinal chemists. The demonstration by Axelrod that tricyclic antidepressants were potent inhibitors of the neuronal uptake process for norepinephrine on noradrenergic neurons represented an impressive leap forward that focused research attention on the aminergic systems in the pathophysiology of affective disorders (Axelrod et al. 1961). Indirect evidence developed by Carlsson (for a review, see Carlsson 1978) that antipsychotic medications might block dopamine receptors was conclusively affirmed with the demonstration of a compelling correlation between antipsychotic potency and affinity for the dopamine D_2 receptor (Creese et al. 1973). These findings were also critically important in organizing research thinking around the issue of how these sites of therapeutic action of antidepressants and antipsychotics might relate to the pathophysiology of affective disorders and schizophrenia. Thus, these discoveries catalyzed an ever-broadening field of investigation to understand the role of aminergic systems in regulating mood, cognition, and neuroendocrine function and how these processes interdigitated with the physiology of cortical and limbic neuronal circuitry.

The most recent permutation of this second wave of drug discovery in psychiatry concerns the demonstration that clozapine exhibited unusual properties that distinguished it from all other neuroleptics: it did not produce acute extrapyramidal side effects, it did not cause tardive dyskinesia, and it dramatically reduced negative symptoms in a significant portion of individuals with schizophrenia. Preclinical research revealed that clozapine was a complex drug with multiple neurotransmitter system interactions, including dopamine D_2, D_3, and D_4 receptors; serotonin $5\text{-}HT_2$ receptors; α_2-adrenergic receptors; histamine receptors; and cholinergic muscarinic receptors (Meltzer et al. 1989). This led to the development of the next generation of "atypical" neuroleptics that combined dopamine D_2 receptor antagonism with other actions, such as blockade of serotonin $5\text{-}HT_2$ receptors. These include risperidone, olanzapine, and sertindole, which have recently been approved for use.

This second generation of psychotropic medications exhibited substantial advances over the first generation. The serotonin-specific reuptake inhibitors and combined serotonin and norepinephrine uptake inhibitors were not compromised by the pattern of side effects associated with the classic tricyclic antidepressants because of their increased target selectivity and minimal interactions with irrelevant neurotransmitter receptors, such as the muscarinic receptor and histamine receptors, as well as with ion channels responsible for the cardiotoxic effects intrinsic to the tricyclic structure. Similarly, the new generation of neuroleptic agents exhibited much lower risk of acute extrapyramidal side effects and also possible efficacy against negative symptoms of schizophrenia. Nevertheless, the development of these drugs was largely predicated on insights into mechanisms of action of the first generation of psychotropic medications, whose discoveries were based on serendipity and not on a fundamental understanding of the pathobiology of the disorders.

Molecular Biology and Psychiatry

The conceptual approach that will drive basic biomedical research for the foreseeable future is molecular biology. Molecular approaches permit the teasing apart of the components of structure, function, and assembly of the nervous system that yield much more precise targets for drug development. Thus, biology is guiding drug discovery and not medicinal chemistry. Two converging strategies are greatly accelerating our ability to identify genes whose allelic variants confer vulnerability for brain disorders, including mental illness. Alleles connote genes with differing base sequences that affect the expression, structure, and/or function of the gene product. The two strategies are 1) *forward genetics*, when one moves from identification of a protein of interest to the isolation of the messenger RNA encoding for the protein back to its chromosomal localization and characterization of the gene; and 2) *reverse genetics*, when one identifies a gene of effect based on its close spatial association with a defined heritable marker (Hyman and Nestler 1993). Alzheimer's disease (AD) represents an example directly relevant to psychiatry in which the application of both forward genetics and reverse genetics have shed light on the molecular mechanisms responsible for the neuropathology and the cognitive decline characteristic of the disorder.

Forward genetics.   In AD, the critical pathological stigma is the senile plaque, which consists of an insoluble deposit of amyloid in the extracellular space in corticolimbic regions of the brain. The amyloid of AD is composed of aggregates of a peptide 40 to 42 amino acids in length. The peptide was purified to homogeneity from the brains of individuals afflicted with AD, and the amino acid sequence was determined. Given our knowledge of the triplicate sequence of bases that encodes for each amino acid, it was then possible to isolate the messenger RNA that contained the RNA sequence encoding for this amyloid peptide (Kosick 1992). The messenger RNA containing the sequence for amyloid in fact encoded for a much larger protein containing 699 amino acids, of which the amyloid peptide represented a small component. This protein, which is normally expressed on the surface of cells, especially neurons in the cerebral cortex and limbic system, was designated amyloid precursor protein (APP) because of the lack of a known function for the protein. With the full sequence of the messenger RNA encoding for the protein known, it was then possible to locate the gene encoding for it on the human chromosomes by its complementary binding to the gene. When the gene was localized on human chromosome 21, it was then possible to screen families with heritable forms of AD to determine if mutations in the APP gene were responsible. Accordingly, several mutations of the APP gene have been found in different families with heritable early-onset AD, albeit these mutations make a very small contribution to all cases of AD (Kosick 1992). Nevertheless, as is described below, these mutations in the APP gene provided powerful tools for determining how APP could be pathologically degraded to yield amyloid in AD.

Reverse genetics. Linkage analysis is a strategy that attempts to define loci on the human genome that are inherited with the risk for a particular disorder. With the mapping of the human genome, allelic markers distributed throughout the genome at known chromosomal locations are currently available (Weissenbach et al. 1992). A panel of these markers is scanned for their heritable association with the presence of the disorder in members of families in which the disorder occurs. If a marker at a particular chromosomal locus is transmitted from one generation to the next with a high degree of fidelity in association with the disorder, this finding strongly suggests that this locus is physically close to the gene of interest. Then the arduous task of moving from the marker locus to identifying the mutant gene is undertaken. Parenthetically, nearly a decade elapsed between the identification of the linkage association of the mutant gene for Huntington's disease on the short arm of chromosome 4 (Gusella et al. 1983) and the actual identification and sequencing of the gene itself (Huntington's Disease Collaborative Research Group 1993), although the high density of markers currently identified on the human genome has markedly accelerated this process. In the case of AD, linkage analysis indicated that one form of early-onset heritable AD was associated with a locus on chromosome 14 and another early-onset heritable form was associated with a locus on chromosome 1. The mutant gene responsible for the vulnerability to AD on chromosome 14 was first identified as a complex membrane protein of unknown function that was designated as presenilin-1. The mutant gene on chromosome 1 was subsequently demonstrated to encode for a very similar membrane protein and was designated presenilin-2 (Rogaev et al. 1995).

Modifying genes. Research on AD has also been informative with regard to genetic mechanisms that may modify disease vulnerability. Linkage mapping suggested that a locus on chromosome 19 was associated with increased vulnerability to late-onset AD. The gene ultimately identified was apolipoprotein E (Apo E), a previously characterized cholesterol-binding protein. There are three allelic variants of the Apo E gene (minor base differences common in the population) designated Apo E2, 3, and 4. The Apo E4 variant, especially in the homozygous state (two copies of Apo E4), both increased the risk for AD and decreased the age of onset (Corder et al. 1993). Allelic variants of other genes, such as anti-α-chymotrypsin, have also been implicated as affecting the risk of late-onset AD.

Transgenic mice. Molecular biological techniques now also permit the re-creation in experimental animals, primarily mice, of genetic defects identified in human disease so that the cellular mechanisms responsible for pathology can be studied in a much more rigorous fashion. With regard to AD, the mutant APP gene responsible for early-onset AD has been inserted into the mouse genome. When mice bearing and expressing this gene are bred to homozygosity (two copies of the gene), the homozygous mice develop amyloid deposits and senile plaques in the cerebral cortex and exhibit an age-related cognitive decline when compared with the control mice without the inserted mutant human APP gene (Hsiao et al. 1996). Having a mouse model with the same genetic defect and the same neuropathology as AD provides the opportunity to rigorously tease apart the cellular mechanisms that lead to the aberrant processing of APP and result in the deposition of amyloid. For example, mutations in the two presenilin genes are the most frequent causes of hereditary early-onset AD, but the relationship between these two proteins and APP remained obscure. However, the solution to this conundrum appears to be near resolution with the development of mice that are transgenic for and express mutant human presenilin-1. These mice demonstrate an overaccumulation of a form of amyloid critical to the formation of senile plaques, thereby pointing toward important interactions between the mutant presenilin and the pathologic processing of APP to yield amyloid (Duff et al. 1996).

Therapeutic implications. The reason for reviewing recent advances in the genetics and molecular biology of AD is that it represents a prototype psychiatric disorder upon which can be mapped the strategies for elucidating other major mental disorders for which family, twin, and adoption studies have demonstrated substantial risk factors for heritability. As should be expected for these psychiatric conditions, such as schizophrenia, bipolar disorder, affective disorder, and panic disorder, the genetic causes of AD are heterogeneous. Mutations in three separate genes account for the majority of early-onset forms of the disorder. Modifying genes, such as alleles Apo E4 and anti-α-chymotrypsin, affect the risk and course of the disorder (Sandbrink et al. 1996). The studies of the cellular biology of these different forms of AD strongly suggest a final common pathway, which involves the aberrant breakdown of APP that results in the pathologic accumulation of amyloid. Pharmacological strategies to treat the consequences of amyloid neurotoxicity—i.e., the degeneration of cholinergic, noradrenergic, and glutamatergic neuronal systems innervating cortex—would be temporarily palliative. The understanding of this final common pathway of pathologic amyloid deposition should provide molecular targets for drugs that would interfere with this process.

Thus, a drug that inhibits the protease that cleaves APP in a way that favors the formation of amyloid would retard the deposition of amyloid in the brain. Such a treatment strategy would be useful in slowing the progress of AD in those who are affected. But much more importantly, if this drug were administered to those at identified genetic risk before the onset of symptoms, it might actually prevent the development of AD.

Severe mental disorders. It is not difficult to speculate how the strategies applied so effectively to AD could and will be extended to other severe mental disorders such as schizophrenia and bipolar disorder. With regard to reverse genetics, promising leads on linkages to sites on the human genome have already been reported for schizophrenia and bipolar disorder. Such linkages, when extended to identified genes, will reveal critical pathways that lead to functional/neuroanatomical mechanisms responsible for the disorder. Conversely, postmortem brain studies in schizophrenia are identifying abnormal levels of neurotransmitters, receptors, or enzymes that suggest candidate genes that could be fruitful targets of genetic studies (Coyle 1996). The convergence of these two lines of inquiry, as in AD, will lead to a fundamental understanding of the causes of these disorders and the identification of molecular targets for more effective treatments.

Allelic variants in behavior. Another emerging theme at the interface between psychiatry and molecular biology is the possible genetic determinants of behavior and personality characteristics that fall under the broad rubric of temperament (Plomin et al. 1994). This line of investigation does not focus on psychiatric disease per se but may shed light on the interaction between temperamental traits and environment that could lead to psychopathology in the case of mismatch. One strategy is to exploit inbred strains of experimental animals (mice, rats, dogs) to identify gene loci that are associated with particular behavioral traits (Copeland et al. 1993; Takahashi et al. 1994). Another strategy is to exploit the wealth of information that is accumulating in neuroscience research on the role of specific neuronal systems in behavior. This is a variant on forward genetics in terms of moving from a specific protein such as a receptor to its gene to determine whether variants of the gene (alleles) are associated with specific behavioral phenotypes. A recent example of this strategy concerns the dopamine D_4 receptor.

The D_4 form of the dopamine receptor is expressed primarily in the nucleus accumbens and limbic cortex and has been linked in behavioral studies to neuronal systems involved in reward or "pleasure" (Van Tol et al. 1991). The gene encoding for the D_4 receptor has several alleles in which a

16–amino acid portion of the receptor is repeated two to nine times, resulting in a receptor with differing transduction efficiencies. Low transduction efficiency (high number of this repeat) could logically be linked to behavior that would cause increased presynaptic dopamine release in order to achieve adequate postsynaptic response. In experimental animals, stressful situations have been shown to activate dopaminergic neurons innervating the limbic cortex. In this regard, two different studies, one on an Israeli population and another on an American population, demonstrated that the less common seven-repeat form was significantly enriched in individuals exhibiting high extraversion scores on personality tests, a profile that includes risk-taking behaviors (Benjamin et al. 1996; Ebstein et al. 1996). Nevertheless, the total contribution of this association to extraversion was quite modest, representing 5% of the variance in the population. Another study has provided preliminary evidence that this allele of the D_4 dopamine receptor is enriched in individuals diagnosed with attention-deficit/hyperactivity disorder (La Hoste et al. 1996). Allelic variants of dopamine receptors have also been implicated in the increased risk for substance abuse, although this finding has been contested (Gejman et al. 1994), and allelic variants of γ-aminobutyric acid (GABA) A receptors have been shown to be associated with alcohol sensitivity in experimental animals (Korpi et al. 1993).

The clinical and societal implications of these studies in behavioral genetics are going to be a challenging topic for the twenty-first century. A misperception and misinterpretation of such findings is that genes determine behavior (genetic determinism), whereas the reality suggests that these genetically shaped behavioral characteristics interface with life experience and afford opportunities for positive and/or negative outcomes depending on developmental life experience.

Brain Imaging

Methods. A second technology that will substantially shape our understanding of the causes of mental disorders and their effective treatments in the foreseeable future is brain imaging (Rauch and Renshaw 1995). Brain imaging encompasses a number of different methods of detection: positron emission tomography (PET), single photon emission computed tomography (SPECT), and nuclear magnetic resonance (NMR) imaging. It is perhaps more useful to categorize the range of imaging technologies according to the information acquired. Through the use of radioactive ligands that bind with a high degree of specificity to brain proteins, both SPECT and PET provide the opportunity to measure biochemical markers, such as receptors, transport sites, or neurotransmitters, that occur in low concentrations in the brain. For example, [^{11}C] spiperone has been used to label dopamine D_2 receptors, [^{18}F]-dopa to label dopamine stores in dopaminergic neurons, and [^{123}I]-β-CIT to label dopamine carrier sites on dopaminergic neurons (Innis et al. 1993). The clinical advantage of SPECT over PET is that the technology for SPECT is much less expensive and that the ligands are commercially available. Nevertheless, for physical reasons, the degree of resolution with PET is somewhat better than with SPECT.

The chemical composition of the living brain can now also be visualized with an increasingly high degree of resolution by NMR spectroscopy. The limitation of this method is its sensitivity, with detection limits in the millimolar range. Nevertheless, an increasing number of brain constituents relevant to chemical neurotransmission and neuronal integrity, such as GABA, glutamate, high-energy phosphates, and *N*-acetylaspartate, can be measured with NMR spectroscopy with progressively higher spatial resolution (Rauch and Renshaw 1995). As instruments with higher power are developed, the spatial and chemical resolution will undoubtedly increase, permitting more refined studies of the living human brain. Magnetic resonance imaging is also providing an increasingly fine-grained visualization of central nervous system structures based on their water and lipid content that is providing the ability to quantify subtle structural abnormalities that have long eluded neuropathological studies in psychiatry. With the development of sophisticated and objective statistical analytic techniques, this approach is revealing regionally specific alterations in brain structure that correlate powerfully with specific symptomatic manifestations of mental disorders. For example, the quantitative measurement of the left superior temporal gyrus has shown that reductions in this structure correlate significantly with the degree of thought disorder in patients with schizophrenia (Shenton et al. 1992). These findings are rendered particularly meaningful because of the ability to correlate neuroanatomic alterations with the neuropsychological processes mediated by the structures and their connections.

Because NMR imaging does not require the use of radioactive agents, imaging can be performed repeatedly not only on adults but also on children over time. For example, a recent study has demonstrated reductions in the volume of frontal cortex in children with childhood-onset affective disorders in comparison to suitable control subjects (Steingard et al. 1996). NMR imaging also permits the performance of longitudinal and prospective studies of the developing nervous system in individuals who have or are at risk for mental disorders in a way that will provide powerful insights into the maturational anatomy and neuropathology of these conditions.

Functional imaging. Given that most psychiatric disorders likely reflect substantial changes not in brain structure but rather in the function of brain neuronal systems, the emerging area of functional brain imaging has particular salience to psychiatry. Most of the approaches rely on the inferred relationship between neuronal activity and local cerebral blood flow or oxygen consumption. In PET, this can be accomplished with ^{15}O as a reflection of oxygen consumption; in SPECT, through the use of various radiolabeled markers that are distributed with blood flow; and in NMR, through the measurement of desaturation of oxyhemoglobin. These methods are revealing regions of abnormal function that are associated with specific psychiatric disorders as well as illuminating the circuitry involved in normal cognitive functions and emotional states.

Functional brain imaging has been transformed by two developments. First, sophisticated statistical analytic methods have been brought to bear on the issue of how to resolve and identify significant alterations in blood flow and oxygen consumption under different experimental conditions both within subjects and between subjects. Coupled with refinements in image resolution, these methods have recently been able to identify activity differences in discrete structures of interest such as the amygdala and nucleus accumbens. Second, functional brain imaging has increasingly become a tool of neuropsychologists to delineate neuronal systems in human brain that are involved in cognitive functions, emotional states, learning and memory, and other physiologic processes such as sleep. This research is yielding an increasingly fine-grained understanding of human brain function and its plasticity in response to learning and experience. For example, recent studies have demonstrated that the human amygdala is uniquely activated during the apprehension of fear (Morris et al. 1996); that visual imagery activates components of the visual cortex that correspond topographically with the image (Kosslyn et al. 1995); and that mental practice of a motor activity results in expansion in the representation of these functions in the cortex (Decety et al. 1994). In addition, with clever psychophysical paradigms that exploit the visual system, functional brain imaging studies are attacking the very processes of consciousness in demonstrating that conscious awareness of visual stimuli requires their representation in the associational visual cortex and not just the primary visual cortex (Leopold and Logothetis 1996).

In the past, attempts were made to correlate abnormal function with psychiatric symptoms at a resting state. For example, several functional imaging studies in individuals with schizophrenia suggested a hypofunction of the frontal cortex, although the effect was small and variable. However, when the functional imaging was coupled with a cognitive task that required activation of the frontal cortex for its successful execution, the differences between patients with schizophrenia and control subjects without schizophrenia became dramatically apparent. Furthermore, such differences were directly linked to the symptomatic manifestations of the disorder and not to the genetic risk of the disorder, since this frontal hypofunction occurred only in the affected identical twins who were discordant for schizophrenia (Berman et al. 1992). Similarly, aberrant activation of the cingulate gyrus can be demonstrated in patients with obsessive-compulsive disorder (OCD) when they are challenged with the presence of the feared contaminated object.

By exploiting a method in which $^{15}O_2$ is repeatedly administered to develop very brief assessments of brain activity, investigators have been able to more precisely delineate systems whose activity is state dependent, using the individual as his or her own control subject. For example, recognizing that hallucinations occur intermittently in schizophrenia, Silbersweig et al. (1995) repeatedly administered $^{15}O_2$ to PET-scanned subjects with schizophrenia who had been trained to indicate when they were experiencing a hallucination. By comparing the scans that were taken while the hallucination was occurring with those taken when the subject was not experiencing a hallucination, the researchers were able to demonstrate forebrain systems that were specifically activated in association with the experience of auditory and visual hallucinations.

Treatment implications. The application of functional brain imaging techniques in psychiatry is not restricted simply to the identification of pathologic circuitry but also offers opportunities to identify processes that are altered with effective treatment of mental disorders. With the growing evidence that mental states have their representation in brain neuronal function, it is apparent that distinctions between pharmacological interventions and psychological interventions are illusory. An impressive example of this line of investigation is the study by Baxter et al. (1992) using imaging technology to correlate treatment response in OCD in which behavioral therapy was compared to pharmacotherapy with fluoxetine. Patients with OCD typically exhibit significantly elevated activity in the region of the right caudate nucleus. Patients were randomized between behavioral treatment and fluoxetine treatment, and approximately 70% in each group responded to treatment. Rescanning revealed that those who responded to treatment—regardless of whether it was behavioral or pharmacological treatment—exhibited a significant reduction in overactivity in the right caudate nucleus, whereas those who did not respond did not show change.

This study sets a clear precedent and provides a model for exploring neural mechanisms responsible for the efficacy of treatments for a host of psychiatric disorders. One might counter that this technology adds little important information, since the crucial issue is whether a treatment works or not, and not how it works. However, in fact, most treatments in psychiatry are only partially efficacious. In other words, treatments often affect certain features of the disorder without improving other aspects. For example, typical neuroleptics are efficacious in reducing positive symptoms of schizophrenia but have minimal effects on negative symptoms and cognitive impairments. Thus, imaging studies may disclose those components of functional neuronal abnormalities associated with specific disorders that respond to treatment and those that do not, thereby providing leads for alternative or complementary interventions. Furthermore, compelling evidence is being developed that psychological interventions coupled with pharmacological treatments in serious mental disorders—including schizophrenia, OCD, and affective disorders—improve long-term outcome and reduce relapse rate (Frank et al. 1992; Weissman and Markowitz 1994). Functional brain imaging will likely shed light on the complementarity of these treatments and methods for further refining the specificity and efficacy of psychological interventions.

Impact of Scientific Advances on the Practice of Psychiatry

The major effect of the expansion of managed care in psychiatry has been a rather dramatic reduction in the length of stay by patients in hospitals. The expansion of less restrictive forms of treatment, such as day hospitals, therapeutic residential care, and specialized ambulatory intensive care services, has contributed to this change. At the same time, ambulatory treatment for subacute conditions has increasingly been restricted and provided by nonpsychiatric health care workers. In many respects, these changes in care are at odds with the scientific advances that are transforming our understanding of psychiatric disorders, their pathobiology, and their treatment.

Although it is clear that more effective mechanisms for diagnosis and treatment should invariably result in a reduction in utilization of inpatient facilities, it is a misreading of trends to confuse ambulatory treatment with primary care treatment. For example, in surgery, the development of sophisticated laparoscopic technology has resulted in dramatic reductions in the morbidity associated with certain forms of surgery, so procedures that historically required several days of recuperation in the hospital can now be performed in the day hospital. If anything, more advanced forms of surgery require greater technical skills and specialized training, not a lower level of skill. By analogy, research drives refinements in diagnosis and treatment in psychiatry and delineates critical relationships between brain and life experience in psychopathology. Expertise in diagnosis and in melding the increasingly complex array of specific pharmacological and psychological interventions will require greater skills and expertise associated with psychiatric training. In support of this contention, current studies indicate that the success rate in the diagnosis and treatment of common psychiatric conditions, such as depression, is much lower when these functions are performed by primary care physicians as compared with mental health professionals. This disparity in the salience of expertise will likely become greater and not lesser.

The scientific advances that will transform the practice of psychiatry will also demand that residency training programs provide the requisite didactic and clinical experiences so that the trainees have the expertise in human genetics, clinical neuroscience, neuroimaging, and psychological interventions necessary to assume a leadership role in the diagnosis and treatment of patients (Coyle 1995). In addition, as a consequence of identification of genetic risk factors for mental disorders, it will be possible to identify presymptomatic individuals at risk within families with affected members so that preventive interventions can be instituted when appropriate. In the case of AD, the intervention might be long-term treatment with a protease inhibitor to reduce the rate of amyloid accumulation. However, such interventions will probably not be limited to pharmacological agents. For example, in the case of children born into families in which one or both of the parents have depression, psychological preventive interventions that are currently being tested might become commonplace.

Areas of concern. One concern often expressed about the "medicalization" of psychiatric practice is that it will foster a reductionistic and deterministic view of psychopathology that sunders the historical humanistic relationship between therapist and patient. However, this view results from a misreading of some of the most compelling advances in brain research, which have demonstrated the remarkable plasticity of the nervous system at all levels of organization. Furthermore, studies in which genes thought to be critical for brain function had been inactivated in "knock-out" mice on many occasions have revealed the recruitment of compensatory pathways that virtually mask the loss of function of the gene (Majzoub and Muglia 1996). As reviewed above, functional brain imaging studies in humans have repeatedly demonstrated the remarkable malleability of functional circuitry in the cerebral cortex as a consequence of experience, including psychological treatments. The psychiatrist will play a special role in the management of patients, individually as well as at a societal level, providing education about the complex and non-deterministic relationship between genetic risk, for example, and psycho-pathology.

Psychiatrists will have to take an even greater leadership role in advocating for their patients with regard to the policy implications of this new knowledge, especially in the area of genetics. These issues are already a source of debate among clinicians, ethicists, and patient advocacy groups (Lewontin and Hubbard 1996). Core issues include who owns the information and to what use it can be put. Specifically, there is considerable concern that identification of an individual as being at genetic risk can result in specific exclusion for insurance benefits or even employment. Given what appears to be at best partial penetrance of genes that may confer risk for mental disorders, there must be real concern about the ability to use these technologies in fetal diagnostic techniques as a basis for terminating pregnancy. At one level, such decisions need to take into account improved abilities to provide effective treatments and preventive interventions; at another level, they need to raise valid concerns of the positive manifestations of such risk factors, including creativity, dynamism, and leadership, that may be associated with the risk for bipolar disorder, for example.

Conclusion

In closing, the twenty-first century will see a practice of psychiatry that is deeply grounded in neuroscience and human genetics, with diagnostic and treatment decisions increasingly defined and specified by these technologies. The psychiatrist by necessity will be required to have expertise in these areas as well as a mastery of a much more complex array of pharmacological and psychological interventions that are empirically tied to diagnosis. These advances will also provide welcome opportunities for presymptomatic identification and empirically grounded preventive interventions. It is these advances that should reverse the current, expanding practice of using the least expert mental health worker to diagnose and manage individuals with mental illness. Finally, psychiatry will have to be even more vigilant in preserving its humanistic traditions and in serving as the advocate for those with mental disorders or those at risk for mental disorders to diminish stigma and to prevent discrimination.

References

Axelrod J, Whitby LB, Hertling G: Effect of psychotropic drugs on the uptake of [³H] norepinephrine by tissues. Science 133:383–384, 1961

Baxter LR Jr, Schwartz JM, Bergman KS, et al: Caudate glucose metabolic rate changes with both drug and behavior therapy for obsessive-compulsive disorder. Arch Gen Psychiatry 49:681–689, 1992

Benjamin J, Greenberg B, Murphy DL, et al: Population and familial association between D_4 dopamine receptor gene and measures of Novelty Seeking. Nat Genet 12:81–84, 1996

Berman KF, Torrey EF, Daniel DG, et al: Regional cerebral blood flow in monozygotic twins discordant and concordant for schizophrenia. Arch Gen Psychiatry 49:996–1001, 1992

Carlsson A: Antipsychotic drugs, neurotransmitters and schizophrenia. Am J Psychiatry 135:164–173, 1978

Copeland NG, Jenkins NA, Gilbert DJ, et al: A genetic linkage map of the mouse: current applications and future prospects. Science 262:57–61, 1993

Corder EH, Saunders AM, Strittmatter WJ, et al: Gene dose of apolipoprotein E type 4 allele and the risk of Alzheimer's disease in late-onset families. Science 261:921–923, 1993

Coyle JT: The neuroscience perspective and the changing role of the psychiatrist: the challenge for psychiatric educators. Academic Psychiatry 19:202–212, 1995

Coyle JT: The glutamatergic dysfunction hypothesis for schizophrenia. Harv Rev Psychiatry 3:241–253, 1996

Creese I, Burt DR, Snyder SH: Dopamine receptor binding predicts clinical and pharmacologic potencies of antischizophrenic drugs. Science 73:481–483, 1973

Decety J, Perani D, Jeannerod M, et al: Mapping motor representation with positron emission tomography. Nature 371:600–602, 1994

Duff K, Eckman C, Zehr C, et al: Increased amyloid-β42(43) in brains of mice expressing mutant presenilin 1. Nature 383:710–713, 1996

Ebstein RP, Novick O, Umansky R, et al: Dopamine D_4 receptor (D4DR) exon III polymorphism associated with human personality trait of Novelty Seeking. Nat Genet 12:78–80, 1996

Frank E, Johnson S, Kupfer DJ: Psychological treatments in prevention of relapse, in Long-Term Treatment of Depression. Edited by Montgomery SA, Rouillon F. London, Wiley, 1992, pp 197–228

Gejman PV, Ram A, Gelernter J, et al: No structural mutation in the dopamine D_2 receptor gene in alcoholism or schizophrenia. JAMA 271:204–208, 1994

Gusella JF, Wexler NS, Conneally PM, et al: A polymorphic DNA marker genetically linked to Huntington's disease. Nature 306:134–238, 1983

Hsiao K, Chapman P, Nilsen S, et al: Correlation memory deficits AB elevation and amyloid plaques in transgenic mice. Science 274:99–102, 1996

Huntington's Disease Collaborative Research Group: A novel gene containing a trinucleotide repeat that is expanded and unstable on Huntington's disease chromosomes. Cell 72:971–983, 1993

Hyman SE, Nestler EJ: The Molecular Foundations of Psychiatry. Washington, DC, American Psychiatric Press, 1993

Innis RB, Seibyl JP, Scanley BE, et al: Single-photon emission computed tomographic imaging demonstrates loss of striatal dopamine transporters in Parkinson's disease. Proc Natl Acad Sci U S A 90:11965–11969, 1993

Katz LC, Shatz CJ: Synaptic activity and the construction of cortical circuits. Science 274:1133–1138, 1996

Korpi ER, Kleingoor C, Kettenmann H, et al: Benzodiazepine-induced motor impairment linked to a point mutation in cerebellar $GABA_A$ receptor. Nature 361:356–359, 1993

Kosick KS: Alzheimer's disease: a cell biological perspective. Science 256:780–783, 1992

Kosslyn SM, Thompson WL, Kim IJ, et al: Topographical representations of mental images in primary visual cortex. Nature 378:496–498, 1995

La Hoste GJ, Swanson JM, Wigal SB, et al: Dopamine D_4 receptor gene polymorphism is associated with attention deficit hyperactivity disorder. Mol Psychiatry 1:121–124, 1996

Leopold DA, Logothetis NK: Activity changes in early visual cortex reflect monkeys' percepts during binocular rivalry. Nature 370:549–553, 1996

Lewontin RC, Hubbard R: Pitfalls of genetic testing. N Engl J Med 334:1192–1193, 1996

Majzoub JA, Muglia LJ: Knock-out mice. N Engl J Med 334:904–907, 1996

Meltzer HY, Matsubara S, Lee JC: Classification of typical and atypical antipsychotic drugs on the basis of dopamine D-1, D-2 and serotonin receptor pKi values. J Pharmacol Exp Ther 251:238–246, 1989

Morris JS, Frith CD, Perrett DI, et al: A differential neural response in the human amygdala to fearful and happy facial expressions. Nature 283:812–815, 1996

Plomin R, Owen MJ, McGaffin P: The genetic basis of complex human behaviors. Science 264:1733–1739, 1994

Rauch SL, Renshaw PF: Clinical neuroimaging in psychiatry. Harv Rev Psychiatry 2:297–312, 1995

Rogaev EI, Sherrington R, Rogaeva EA, et al: Familial Alzheimer's disease in kindreds with missense mutations on chromosome 1 related to the Alzheimer's disease type 3 gene. Nature 376:775–788, 1995

Sandbrink R, Hartman T, Masters CL, et al: Genes contributing to Alzheimer's Disease. Mol Psychiatry 1:27–40, 1996

Shenton ME, Kikinis R, Jolesz FA, et al: Abnormalities of the left temporal lobe and thought disorder in schizophrenia: a quantitative magnetic resonance imaging study. N Engl J Med 327:604–612, 1992

Silbersweig DA, Stern E, Frith C, et al: A functional neuroanatomy of hallucinations in schizophrenia. Nature 378:176–179, 1995

Singer W: Development and plasticity of cortical processing architectures. Science 270:758–762, 1995

Steingard RJ, Renshaw PF, Yurgelun-Todd D, et al: Structural abnormalities in brain magnetic images of depressed children. J Am Acad Child Adolesc Psychiatry 35:307–311, 1996

Takahashi J, Piuto L, Viaterna MH: Forward and reverse genetic approaches to behavior in the mouse. Science 264:1724–1729, 1994

Van Tol HH, Bunzow JR, Guan HC, et al: Cloning of the gene for a human dopamine D_4 receptor with high affinity for the antipsychotic clozapine. Nature 350:610–614, 1991

Weissenbach J, Gyapay G, Dib C, et al: A second generation linkage map of the human genome. Nature 359:794–799, 1992

Weissman MM, Markowitz JC: Interpersonal psychotherapy: current status. Arch Gen Psychiatry 51:599–606, 1994

CHAPTER 2

Psychoanalysis

Sidney Weissman, M.D.

W hat role will psychoanalytic concepts have in psychiatry in the coming century? Many of us assume that it will be quite different because the principal theoretical foundations for psychoanalysis were demolished by the recent advances in neuroscience that undercut the dualist thinking of psychoanalysts. Freud was a methodological dualist: access to mind is direct (i.e., by introspection); nothing mind does is easily explained by reference to bodily processes. Contemporary psychiatrists are monists: mind is mental activity; mental activity is the behavior of bodily systems, particularly the brain. Does this review justify the notion that psychiatry can only advance from its benighted past by moving toward the clear light of physiology and pharmacology? I shall be saying that this agenda is misconceived.

This chapter has two parts. The first part surveys some questions about the mind's relation to the body. The second part elaborates on the psychoanalytic concepts that will be essential to the twenty-first-century psychiatrist.

The Relation of Mind to Body

Plato and Aristotle supposed that there are three orders of soul (psyche). Vegetable soul is responsible for nutrition and reproduction. Animal soul is the power of desire, and hence movement, because animals must move to get the things they perceive or imagine and desire. Both of these aspects or kinds of soul were thought to be enmattered (i.e., as functions of body). Perception and memory, this implies, are bodily functions (i.e., activities of the brain). Compare rational soul. Thinking—the awareness of ideas—was said to be different from vegetable soul and animal soul because the latter implicate the body, and thinking does not (e.g., as thinking of circularity or mathematical equality requires an abstraction from ambient reality). Like knows like, and so the act of thinking about pure concepts was assumed to be distinct from acts of the body, as pure forms are distinct from their embodiments (Aristotle 1941; Plato 1961).

René Descartes inherited this ambivalence about soul. He agreed that bodies perceive and remember: there would be an exhaustively mechanical (i.e., physiological) explanation for these processes. He argued that some other mental activities—especially awareness, conception, and volition—do not have physiological explanations. The existence and character of mind must be independent of body, because it is inconceivable (i.e., a contradiction) that body should be aware, think (i.e., entertain ideas), or will (i.e., give or withhold assent from ideas, accordingly as they are clear and distinct—hence true—or confused) (Descartes 1985; Weissman 1996).

Notice that each of the factors Descartes emphasized when describing mind is critical for psychoanalytic theory and practice. Awareness, for example, has two orientations: one may be conscious of other things or conscious of oneself. Descartes does not emphasize this distinction, but he does imply it, as when the affirmation "I am, I exist" reports a discovery that I make about myself when I am aware of other things. There is currently no satisfactory physical explanation for consciousness of either sort: meaning that there is no theory—*theory*, not mere program—that specifies sufficient material conditions for the generation of consciousness. Brain imaging enables us to perceive the parts of the brain that are active when a subject is conscious. But this bodily activity is not an explanation for either or both kinds of awareness. For the imaging correlates with the awareness, without yet confirming a theory that explains that awareness is the effect of the processes imaged. This is not a small difference. Look at, or imagine, something that is intensely red, loud, or sweet. Where is the theory that explains the generation of both this content and our awareness of it? Hierarchically organized neural networks are likely a basis for the cross-checking and control that occur as we think. But there is, just now, no theory that explains awareness or its contents, including percepts and affective states (e.g., pain) by specifying the mechanism that generates them.

Suppose, however, that each of the three factors thought to distinguish mind from body—awareness, ideas, and will—does eventually prove to be the activity or state of the body or brain. This would be a comprehensive, ontological reduction: things of one kind are shown to be the states or activities of things of a different kind. Would this reduction entail that the yellow flowers in the vase beside me do not look yellow, or that my sore elbow doesn't feel sore? Would it entail that I am not suffused by anxiety, pleasure, or remorse? We have an answer in the consideration that specifying the sufficient conditions for a phenomenon (thereby explaining it) does not eliminate the phenomenon explained. Metabolism does not disappear (i.e., it is not eliminated) if we specify its sufficient material conditions. We would not stop being conscious, this implies, were we to know the sufficient physical conditions for being conscious. We would think, perceive, dream, and deliberate. We would be conscious of our hopes, angers, regrets. We would remember the occasions that incite one or another of these feelings, and we would know, because of having learned, how to divert ourselves from one or another affective state (e.g., from impulsive anger to attentive observation of others or ourselves).

Access to these states and activities would also be unaffected by a specification of their sufficient physical conditions. Having this access would continue to distinguish our self-perspective from that of people who observe us: physiologists would understand all the conditions for our pain, but we would know it as pain, as they would not. Nor is this access surprising if mental activities occur within a self-monitoring, closed neural loop (i.e., the circuits of the brain).

Would mind's reduction to body abolish the principal theoretical terms of psychoanalysis, including such Freudian notions as ego, id, and superego? Freud agreed that these notions are place-holders for the terms of anatomical and physiological theories that would sometime be formulated and confirmed. Never mind that this anticipated physical theory is still unavailable to us, for this other point has precedence: notions such as these three are characterized functionally, not structurally. They signify behaviors or mental activities of a kind, not the neural networks that perform them. The specification of mind's material conditions would not eliminate passion or appetite, learned social conventions, or the task of mediating between them. Indeed, knowing the sufficient physical conditions for mental activities would likely enhance our understanding of functions—including repression, impulse control, and sublimation—that Freud emphasized.

What is changed if all mental activities are only the behavior of a physical system (e.g., the brain)? Only this: we shall be able to use physical agents (e.g., drugs) to create effects that were hard or impossible to produce without them. Pharmacological agents will be ever more effective, even to the point of having the very specific effects required for treating particular patients. Psychiatry will be armed with a more powerful theory about mind's character and inception. But nothing in this implies that it should renounce the instruments currently available to us. Talk therapies are effective. Drugs that pacify do not resolve the conflicts they mask.

Can psychiatry be a science if it continues doing the things that make it disreputable in some circles? Remember that the criteria for being an empirical science are not agreed on. Karl Popper complained that Freudian claims are not scientific because they are not falsifiable: every failed prediction can be discounted by citing an unsatisfied ancillary condition (e.g., the absence of oedipal fantasies in boys raised by single mothers). Pierre Duhem and W. V. O. Quine counter that no scientific thesis is falsifiable, because every one has myriad ancillary conditions, so there is never a way of confirming that all of them are satisfied. An experiment may fail because one or many such conditions are not satisfied, not because the thesis tested is false. We can always cite or allege that one of these conditions is unsatisfied, thereby averting the conclusion that the theory is false. Adolf Grunebaum, psychoanalysis' most belligerent foe, supposes that a theory is scientific if it is empirically testable, meaning that test sentences are deducible from the higher-order sentences of a formalized (i.e., deductively organized) theory. Grunebaum faults Freudian theory because its test sentences are not confirmed. Yet, Popper (1959), Duhem (1906/1976), and Quine (1951/1976) tell us that there are many supplementary conditions that must obtain before any thesis may be tested. Grunebaum never cites the full array of ancillary conditions relevant to the theses he proposes to test. Nor does he establish that the various conditions are satisfied. It is notorious in the social sciences and psychology that experimenters are unable to control collateral conditions. Failure to prove the effects of repression in every case is therefore no evidence that repression is not a decisive variable in some or many cases. This misplaced rigor is apparent in one of Grunebaum's chapter titles, "Repressed Infantile Wishes as Instigators of All Dreams" (Grunebaum 1985), then in a discussion that easily produces the single counter-example that falsifies this generality. But psychoanalysis is not unscientific if it cannot satisfy the universality of geometry or physics.

Grunebaum's formalist rigor is misplaced. Something is missing in his conception of scientific theory: namely, the experimental character of scientific hypotheses. Such hypotheses are abductions: we infer from something thought or perceived its conditions, including causes, constituents, and laws. Seeing an apple fall, we infer the laws of motion. Hearing a patient stutter when recounting his dreams or fantasies, we infer psychic mechanisms that may explain our patient's hesitation. *Repression* is an explanatory function of this sort. The failure to confirm its operation in some or many cases does not establish that this is not a decisive factor in psychic life, or that it does not do there just what Freud says it does. There are, for example, the many specific cases in which this is a plausible explanation, one that is confirmed by predictions that assume it. Why are these confirmations less cogent than Grunebaum's disconfirming examples? Only because Grunebaum assumes that the universal application of its laws or theories is the necessary condition for status as a science. Is twenty-first-century psychiatry a science if it uses psychoanalytic concepts? Ignoring the doctrinaire formulations of the philosophers, we may reasonably believe that it is, if our theories of mental functions (e.g., id, ego, and superego) have empirical implications and if predicted phenomena do sometimes or often occur. That our theories are not the explanatory equal to theories of motion is news to no one.

Psychiatrists of the twenty-first century will work with theories more powerful than those available to Freud, because there will likely be hypotheses that describe critical mental functions (e.g., repression) against the backdrop of a physical model that enables the clinician to identify the neuronal activities that accomplish such effects. We shall not be embarrassed by always having to speak in metaphors when describing psychic functions while ignorant of the relevant physical processes. Would all this have astonished Freud? No: it is plainly foreseen in his *Project for a Scientific Psychology* (S. Freud 1895/1966). Freud sometimes despaired of ever having a physical model adequate to the functions he ascribed to mind. We can hope to be more effective because of having both the physical model and a theory or theories about mind's cognitive and affective states and behaviors.

Remember our point of departure: does having a physical model entail that mind's access to its activities is an inconsequential advantage for the purposes of therapy? It is an advantage if this access supplies opportunities for altering mind's states or behaviors. It is all the more advantageous if our physical model enables us to determine how patients are altered by clinical practice. "Tell me when it hurts," says the dentist. "I need to know." Why shouldn't psychiatrists continue to depend on more subtle intrapsychic maneuvers? Will physical models of the brain enable us to make these changes without engaging our patients (as heart surgery is not a conversation)? This is possible, though we should hesitate before intruding in this other way for a reason that is moral rather than clinical: we want patients to recover or achieve responsibility for themselves. Psychiatry is medical practice with this distinctively moral aim.

Psychoanalytic Concepts for the Twenty-First Century

Which core concepts from psychoanalysis will continue to be useful to psychiatry in the next century? Here are ten from our century that will likely be critical for understanding the thoughts, feelings, and actions of our patients.

Consciousness

Consciousness must be understood as more than simply the state of being awake. It entails the individual's capacity to be aware of and interact with both the external world and the internal world, the experience of each being shaped by the person's unique life experiences. Consciousness further includes the individual's ability to utilize all of his or her varied mental and physical capacities; of special relevance to consciousness is the capacity to use the organs of perception to gather information. By virtue of awareness of the internal world, consciousness also entails knowledge of one's unique capacities and awareness of the varied activities of the psyche that have an impact on one's behavior.

In viewing individuals' responses to similar or identical stimuli, we observe strikingly dissimilar reactions. These dissimilar reactions are in part related to the component of the psychological apparatus of which the individual is unaware—the dynamic unconscious. The dynamic unconscious exerts a significant impact on an individual's conscious functioning and must be appreciated to understand behavior.

Dynamic Unconscious

The dynamic unconscious guides behavior and thought, as noted, in ways of which the individual is not aware. Elements of the unconscious can be captured and observed, but others can only be inferred. Freud first described unconscious processes in *Studies on Hysteria* (Breuer and Freud 1883–1895/1955), in *The Psychopathology of Everyday Life* (S. Freud 1901/1960), and in *Jokes and Their Relation to the Unconscious* (S. Freud 1905/1960). His topographic model of the mind places varied drives or desires outside of the individual's awareness in the unconscious, where they exert an effect on consciousness or observed behavior. The topographic model, although 100 years old, continues to provide a vital framework to understand unconscious processes and how they are known. An example of an action determined by unconscious processes—in this case identification—would be a young man buying a suit of clothes and only later discovering that the suit is a replica of one that his father had once worn.

One cannot discuss consciousness or unconsciousness without addressing the process by which a psychic event is placed in the conscious or unconscious mind. Repression is the name given to the process that results in memories or mental activities being kept from consciousness.

Repression

Repression here refers to an action in the psychic apparatus that at times inhibits an awareness of ourselves, of certain life experiences, or of their consequences. We do not know that we repress or block from awareness or consciousness. We or others, at a later moment, are able to observe our behavior and infer the existence of something of which we are unaware—that is, that we repressed. Repression or keeping from awareness can be observed to occur in various ways, with different elements of available information being kept from consciousness.

An example can demonstrate. A woman with a clearly visible lump in her breast can repeatedly not note the existence of the lump and not visit a surgeon. She unconsciously does not allow herself to experience the existence of the lump and describes her breasts as normal. We refer to her as using denial to deal with the stress of the lump, unconsciously blocking out its existence. Another woman might observe or feel a lump and report it to others but not see a surgeon. She might say it is nothing of consequence. This woman integrates the existence of the lump into consciousness but unconsciously blocks out its importance. This woman, we say, disavows the consequences of the lump.

These examples deal with contending with a life experience. Repressive processes can also frequently account for the blocking out of painful life experiences from memory. It is important to recognize that memory also includes complex brain processes. Further, at the time of the initial painful event, the individual may not integrate or lay down memory traces of all elements of the painful event.

For these reasons, the report in psychotherapy of a lost memory must be understood by patient and therapist as a reconstruction of possible events and experiences from the past and not necessarily exactly what occurred.

Anna Freud considered repression to be one of what she called defense mechanisms. An appreciation of these processes enables us not only to understand more fully the complexity of behavior but also to understand how specific defense mechanisms can be identified with specific character types.

Defense Mechanisms

In *The Ego and the Mechanisms of Defense*, Anna Freud (A. Freud 1937/1966) defined and explored defense mechanisms at length. Defense mechanisms are unconscious processes used to maintain an individual's psychological equilibrium. The understanding of how an individual uses varied defense mechanisms will retain importance into the next century. Each individual will use a limited number of different defense mechanisms to maintain his or her equilibrium. The critical issue is that each of us develops and sustains our own specific psychological tactics (defense mechanisms), which are unconscious, to maintain our psychological equilibrium. Sometimes the use of a defense mechanism can have harmful consequences. In the example used to describe denial, although the defense mechanism may have assisted the woman in maintaining psychological equilibrium, it did so at the risk of causing serious physical harm. The major defense mechanisms used by an individual are frequently used to describe one's character.

Having described consciousness, the dynamic unconscious, repression, and defense mechanisms, it becomes clear that we cannot proceed further without a means to organize these activities of the mind. Freud developed two distinct models of the psychic apparatus. Other contributors have provided their own. Every psychiatrist, knowingly or not, has some model of their own when they see their patients.

Models of the Psychic Apparatus

Throughout his life, Freud developed new models or revised old models of the psychic apparatus or mind either to describe or to provide explanation for various psychological disorders and kinds of behavior he observed. Freud's first model was called the topographic model. It includes the concepts of consciousness, unconscious, preconscious, and the repression barrier.

These concepts, as noted, remain essential and useful descriptors of mental life. Later, in his monograph *The Ego and the Id* (S. Freud 1923/1961), Freud described his structural model of the mind. This model includes the id, ego, and superego. This model is more abstract and gives a conceptual basis to mind. Freud also includes a developmental model of how the ego and superego evolve from the id. Today, with our enhanced knowledge of development, we would not necessarily see development as Freud did, but the concepts of the ego as the agency of the mind that integrates and regulates internal bodily states in their interaction with the external would continue as a useful concept of the mind. Equally significant is the concept of the superego as the agency of the mind that governs our moral judgments and ideals. Indeed, it is difficult to describe someone meaningfully without utilizing these concepts. Freud spoke of the id being the basic energy source of the mind and serving as the repository of our drives. Newer developmental models provide more effective descriptions of drives, and the notion of the id functioning as an energy source potentially confuses psychology and brain functioning.

Other psychoanalysts have used other terms and constructs to describe the psychic apparatus. Kohut (1977) developed a psychoanalytic psychology that uses knowledge of what he calls the self, self awareness, and the essential experiences needed to develop what he terms a cohesive self to describe the psychic apparatus. His concept of self shares some of the tasks of Freud's ego but includes a number of capacities not usually included in Freud's use of the concept ego. His theory also has a number of assumptions on development that differ from those of Freud.

Freud saw one task or function of the ego as being the containment of libidinal and aggressive drives. For the contemporary psychiatrist, it remains essential to know the dimension, meaning, and force of the processes that motivate and power their patients regardless of the model of the mind that they utilize.

Drives

Drives refers to both the force and content of the sexual and aggressive urges that govern us. In considering drives it is useful to distinguish the sexual or aggressive urge from its content or object. Also, it is important to determine in our patients a baseline level of their drive-related behavior so that we may note any increases or decreases. Closely related to the concept of drives is the concept of driven behavior. That is, situations in which the individual feels propelled or compelled to act in a certain fashion. One element of psychotherapy is "teaching" the patient to be aware of his or her unique driven behavior. If, over time, we have learned that specific patterns of driven behavior signal a manic episode, then the patient can learn to effectively use medication to control this behavior by recognizing this behavior.

For example, if unusually vivid dreams are early signals of an episode, with this knowledge, an individual can increase his or her medication and abort a manic episode at the first such dream.

In observing behavior, a critical observation psychiatrists make is how individuals unknowingly take on attributes of others. We call this process identification.

Identification

The concept of identification describes how we unconsciously experience or take on a link or connection to an individual or cause of which we are not aware. The reasons for the identification can vary, but the individuals are altered in their functioning as they take on and manifest the elements of the individual or cause with which they identify. Although the process is not conscious, the individual can become aware of his or her identification. When a child pursues the same career as a parent, he or she may do so because of identification with the parent.

Two concepts elaborated on by Kohut are useful as the psychiatrist first learns about a patient and then prepares to administer treatment.

Empathy

Kohut (1959) defined empathy as vicarious introspection. By this he meant we look into ourselves to find an experience and affective state that enables us to appreciate both our patient's experience and the individual meaning of the experience. This capacity is central to understanding the complex behavior of our patients and, most importantly, to understanding the meaning of their behavior. It is seen by some as essential for performing psychotherapy. The art of therapy is the ability to communicate this understanding in a fashion that leads to healing of an impaired psychic state.

Selfobject

The concept of the selfobject was developed by Heinz Kohut to account for the way that individuals unconsciously used elements of another individual to maintain their own psychological equilibrium. Kohut believed that selfobjects are utilized throughout the life cycle to maintain equilibrium. They are first utilized by the child, who unconsciously uses the capacities of parent or caregiver initially to soothe disruptive affective states and, at times, to direct actions. One example of a selfobject relationship in adulthood may be helpful. To organize his feelings about his own competence, a researcher may unknowingly need (use as a selfobject) a senior colleague. Observers would note the importance of the relationship but would see the researcher's work as his own. An interruption of the relationship could cause the researcher to be unable to proceed in his work. The unconscious use of the senior colleague to confirm and stabilize the self and maintain its cohesion is not the same as needing the senior colleague's ideas on how to proceed. It is the unique psychological/affective support that is received, not new research ideas that are needed. In psychotherapy, the therapist must be sensitive to these unique relationships.

Finally, the twenty-first-century psychiatrist will need models to determine and classify psychological disequilibrium.

Models of Psychological Disequilibrium

The authors of DSM-IV (American Psychiatric Association 1994) have struggled to describe and define what has been known for much of the twentieth century as neurotic or character-disordered behavior. Today, we are informed from research—much of which was completed in the last quarter-century—that some of the behavior and experiences referred to as neurotic or character disordered have major genetic and biological routes. Nonetheless, we currently cannot describe all such behavior as having been caused by specific genetic coding. Even if we observe and can correlate specific brain activities to specific behavior in an individual, this knowledge does not inform us as to the unique meanings to the individuals. Symbolic communication will alter areas of the brain, but we still need a psychology to understand the meaning of the symbols. This is a role for psychoanalysis in providing models to account for a disordered psychological equilibrium with either disordered behavior or a disordered internal set of experiences or expectations. Two major models have survived the intellectual expansion of psychoanalysis in the past 100 years. One is the model of conflict between the agencies of the mind described in Freud's structural model of ego, id, and superego. For example, in this model, some types of depression are seen as being related to demands placed by the superego on the ego, with the individual feeling inadequate when he or she fails to meet the expectations of the superego.

An alternative model is proposed by Kohut, who has built his model around the self. Psychopathology is related to disorganization of what Kohut refers to as the cohesion of the self. For example, a novelist's recent book is criticized by a literary critic. The author becomes enraged and depressed. He sees or experiences his work as being of no value. The author needs, in Kohut's terms, to use the critic as a selfobject to affirm his worth. In the absence of the affirmation, he becomes enraged, depressed, and depleted. Obviously, much more is involved than is explained by either model. What is crucial is that to understand our patients and develop appropriate treatments, we must have an in-depth psychological model of the mind and the factors that lead to a disequilibrium.

Psychoanalysis alerts us to various vicissitudes of life and to the critical impact of relationships on the development of each of us. Each of our own unique life experiences further alerts us as psychiatrists to know our patients.

Perhaps the capacity to clone human life uniquely highlights the power and importance of psychoanalysis. Genetic replicas of each of us would not create copies of any of us. We are unique as individuals because of both our specific genetic structure and the idiosyncratic way our brains have developed in response to diverse stimuli. These factors in conjunction have created our specific essence. Psychoanalysis would enable us to observe the differences between us and our clones, whereas a molecular examination of our DNA would not. This illustrates the power psychoanalysis will give to twenty-first-century psychiatrists.

References

American Psychiatric Association: Diagnostic and Statistical Manual of Mental Disorders, 4th Edition. Washington, DC, American Psychiatric Association, 1994

Aristotle: De Anima, in The Basic Works of Aristotle. Edited by McKeon R. New York, Random House, 1941, pp 591–592

Breuer J, Freud S: Studies on hysteria (1883–1895), in Standard Edition of the Complete Psychological Works of Sigmund Freud, Vol 2. Translated and edited by Strachey J. London, Hogarth Press, 1955

Descartes R: Principles of Philosophy, in The Philosophical Writings of Descartes. Translated by Cottingham J, Stoothoft R, Murdoch D. Cambridge, MA, Cambridge University Press, 1985, pp 193–209

Duhem P: Physical theory and experiment (1906), in Can Theories Be Refuted? Edited by Harding S. Boston, MA, D. Reidel, 1976, pp 1–40

Freud A: The Ego and The Mechanisms of Defense (1937). London, Hogarth Press, 1966

Freud S: Project for a scientific psychology (1895), in Standard Edition of the Complete Psychological Works of Sigmund Freud, Vol 1. Translated and edited by Strachey J. London, Hogarth Press, 1966, pp 382–392

Freud S: The psychopathology of everyday life (1901), in Standard Edition of the Complete Psychological Works of Sigmund Freud, Vol 6. Translated and edited by Strachey J. London, Hogarth Press, 1960

Freud S: Jokes and their relation to the unconscious (1905), in Standard Edition of the Complete Psychological Works of Sigmund Freud, Vol 8. Translated and edited by Strachey J. London, Hogarth Press, 1960

Freud S: The ego and the id (1923), in Standard Edition of the Complete Psychological Works of Sigmund Freud, Vol 19. Translated and edited by Strachey J. London, Hogarth Press, 1961, pp 31–66

Grunebaum A: The Foundations of Psychoanalysis. Berkeley, CA, University of California Press, 1985, pp 216–239

Kohut H: Introspection, empathy, and psychoanalysis. J Am Psychoanal Assoc 7:459–483, 1959

Kohut H: The Restoration of the Self. New York, International Universities Press, 1977

Plato: Phaedo, in The Collected Dialogues of Plato. Edited by Hamilton E, Cairns H. New York, Pantheon, 1961, p 48

Popper K: The Logic of Scientific Discovery. New York, Basic Books, 1959

Quine WVO: Two dogmas of empiricism (1951), in Can Theories Be Refuted? Edited by Harding S. Boston, MA, D. Reidel, 1976, pp 41–64

Weissman D: Psychoanalysis, in Descartes R: Discourse on the Method and Meditations on First Philosophy. Edited by Weissman D. New Haven, CT, Yale University Press, 1996, pp 330–348

CHAPTER 3

Social Psychiatry

Joseph A. Flaherty, M.D.
Boris M. Astrachan, M.D.

It is a time of nearly cataclysmic change in the world of medicine and psychiatry, the kind of change that could be registered "not just on the surface of the thing, but on the thing itself" (Newman 1919). After nearly a century of enhanced post-flexnerian status and 30 years of post-Medicare prosperity, the medical profession in the United States warily views these changes as threats to its autonomy and integrity, to the time-honored sanctity of the doctor-patient relationship, to its role as the provider of "the best health care in the world," and to its previously unchallenged right to provide each patient with the most sophisticated and scientific assessment and treatment available. The very nature of these extraordinary changes also affords medical professionals an opportunity to expand beyond their traditional role in the treatment of the sick to population-based prevention and treatment, harnessing not only the basic biological sciences but also embracing their natural partners in this new endeavor: epidemiologists, public health professionals, patients, families, and communities.

During the last quarter-century, psychiatry has improved its image both within and outside the profession of medicine through rejection of the expansive and utopian promise of offering solutions to all social ills and by realigning with medicine to concentrate on nosological reliability, treatment of disease, and etiological and pathophysiological studies in neurosciences and molecular biology. Encouraged by these developments, patient, family, and consumer groups have increasingly been supportive of psychiatry, and that support has risen close to the high-water mark of the early post–World War II days. The implementation of social psychiatric theory by community psychiatrists in supporting community change to limit psychiatric disorder is largely discredited. Preventive activities have been given lower priority in academic departments of psychiatry, and the influence of social psychiatry is diminished. It is at this crossroads that social psychiatry finds itself engaged in a critical self-examination that will lead to its becoming either an endearing anachronism or a translator, developer, and bridge between the social and behavioral sciences and the world of treatment, practice, and public policy.

The basic tenet of social psychiatry is that environmental vectors play a key role in the development, recognition, and treatment of disease and in rehabilitation. The danger of returning to this position is to again be charged with expansiveness, of "riding madly in all directions" (Grinker 1964), bringing back negative reminders of the "schizophrenogenic mother" and other labels viewed as efforts to blame and alienate families and communities and "a predominance of ideology over science" (Sabshin 1990). On the other hand, the promise and potential of social psychiatry is the capacity to identify, recruit, and empower those natural, indigenous forces in communities and families to the betterment of patients. Pushing further, at a time of such social upheaval in the practice of medicine, change is occurring in social institutions, public policy, and treatment of all patients; a perspective that looks at the health care system at macro- and micro-society levels and one that recognizes the limits of the individual doctor-patient model is essential. It is this perspective that is demanded of psychiatry and requires the renaissance of social psychiatry.

Reviews of social psychiatry have attempted to chronicle the historical role its proponents have played in the development of the field and/or to outline the relationship of psychiatry to its basic social and behavioral sciences such as epidemiology, sociology, anthropology, and social and developmental psychology (Arthur 1973; Cooper 1994; Fleck 1990; Krupinski 1992; Mechanic 1995). The historical route usually begins with the efforts to provide community-based treatment in Gheel, Belgium, through foster family care and moves on to the enlightenment period and the humane treatment era with the pioneering works of Tuke (England), Pinel and Esquirol (France), and Chiaragi (Italy and Switzerland). Two modern revivals of the humane treatment era are usually discussed: the therapeutic community movement (Gruenberg 1977; Stanton and Schwartz 1954) and the community mental health movement. All these underscore the basic premise of social psychiatry: the environment has both deleterious and therapeutic effects on the lives of patients and families that, if identified and successfully used, can expand the scope of treatment beyond the traditional individual treatment and psychiatric hospital models. Too often lost in the negative backlash against the community health and mental health movements have been the extraordinary expansion of services in the community and the scientific breakthroughs that influence practice.

It is beyond the scope of this chapter to review the many contributions of the social and behavioral sciences to the field of psychiatry and the world of practice. It is possible, however, to show by example how developments in these disciplines can be successfully bridged to psychiatric treatment and public policy regarding the mentally ill. We will briefly review the relevance of sociology, epidemiology, anthropology, and ethology to psychiatry and then turn to a discussion of their potential partnership with psychiatry to address three critical social problems in the world today.

Modern sociology since Durkheim has been concerned with the development and formulation of theory to explain empirical social data. One of the most relevant paradigms related to psychiatry has been the sociological approach to the stress-illness relationship with attempts to examine causation through the use of longitudinal data to establish the independence of various stressors. Explanatory hypotheses as to why certain populations are at risk have led to a more comprehensive examination of vulnerability and protective factors, a closer inspection of the nature of stressors that lead to psychiatric illness, and consequent attempts to design psychiatric interventions to reduce the variable risk factors. The consistent finding of higher rates of mental disorder among lower social classes has moved beyond drift versus causation social theories to an examination of particular vulnerability factors with regard to education, ethnicity, and gender (Dohrenwend 1990). In considering the nature of protective factors, the construct of social support—a derivative of social network theory defined as the affective and instrumental exchanges between social network members—has proved extremely fruitful as an independent protective factor as well as one that buffers the effects of stress (Henderson 1977). Further examination of social support has yielded the finding that the presence of a close confidant may be crucial in the prevention of depression (Brown et al. 1972) and in recovery from major depression (Flaherty et al. 1983). More recent examinations have looked at other aspects of social support such as its cost (Kessler et al. 1995), gender differences in social support (Flaherty and Richman 1989), and the advantages of large support networks in both disease prevention and intervention (Leff 1976). There are many treatment and intervention derivatives of these sociological approaches that employ varying levels of mental health professionals, patients, families, and communities.

Three social (or social psychological) approaches of significance for patients with severe mental illness are social skills training, psychoeducation, and assertive community treatment. Social skills training is based on the concept that patients with severe mental illness, particularly those with schizophrenia and bipolar disorder, have neurophysiological difficulties that impede interaction with others and are reflected in problems in seeking out treatment from professionals as well as in building constructive and useful social support networks. There is an interesting link with the neurosciences in the finding that schizophrenic patients in particular have difficulty in recognizing the facial expression of emotions such as sadness, anger, and happiness. This deficit naturally leads to difficulty in maneuvering in the social sphere and to approaches to social skills training that employ affect recognition. Liberman and colleagues (1986) at the University of California, Los Angeles, developed skills training modules that are readily available. Psychoeducation (Hogarty et al. 1991) takes a practical approach toward gaining patient participation in treatment by teaching patients and family members the nature of the disorder and the scientific basis for treatment strategies.

Assertive community training (ACT) (Stein and Test 1980) was designed to provide services that would maintain clients' social adjustment, enhance the quality of their lives, and minimize the burden to families and the cost to providers. Stein and Test's original model called for the use of a single multidisciplinary treatment team that provided what the client needed, when and where the client needed it. Entry to all care was provided through the team. In the model, specialized mental health services and social services were knitted together through the use of effective case managers. Essock and Kontos (1995) reviewed literature on ACT and demonstrated how in the absence of new funding a reconfiguration of current community-based staff and staff from state hospitals can be employed effectively to develop ACT programs. Additional efforts toward using natural helpers or the helper-therapy principle has great potential for both primary and secondary prevention. Natural helping networks have been noted to be beneficial to a variety of highly at-risk individuals, including homeless people, immigrants, and psychiatric patients. Natural helpers possess important qualities that increase their efficacy such as local acceptance and skills and ideas that are consonant within a culture and social group (Gatz 1982). It is recognized that self-help groups are sometimes centered around patients and indigenous helpers; others are more family oriented and serve to reduce burden among family members; and others have effectively shown how self-help groups can be partnered with ongoing case management in a community-based treatment model. Of particular challenge to social psychiatry is identifying the most effective use of these groups while recognizing the potential limits of over-professionalizing support groups (Emerick 1989; Gottlieb 1983).

Sociology has long been concerned with issues of organization and the manner in which organization affects tasks. In 1963 major legislative acts were passed that had extraordinary impacts on practice. The Medicare and Medicaid Acts extended care to the elderly and the poor on a fee-for-service basis. In that same year the Community Mental Health Center Act was passed, continuing a program of maintaining separate services and organizational structures for the mentally ill and the physically ill, and recognizing the important role of government in mental health care as a provider. The corporatizing of health care (Starr 1982), the growth of capitated care, and the development of new organizational structures for care have again raised questions about the settings in which care ought to be provided, and—in particular for those with severe and persistent illness—the best structures and financing arrangements for providing care. The growth in privatization of public services, particularly in the health care area, has been followed with concern and studies have raised questions about the capacity to maintain quality of care in privatized services (Dickey et al. 1996).

Epidemiology, while traditionally focused on the dependent variable disease (Eaton 1994), has also examined the relative risk factors for various psychiatric disorders. From the pioneering work of early epidemiologists such as Farris and Dunham to the Midtown Manhattan Study to the Epidemiologic Catchment Area Project, studies have identified the relative risks of such traditional epidemiological predictor variables as social class, education, gender, race, and ethnicity. An expanded use of epidemiology provides data relevant to the issue of needs assessment at both the community and the national level to studies exploring aspects of help-seeking behavior and attitudes toward treatment. Epidemiology has been linked to mental health services research with the identification of specific risk factors that may be amenable to intervention. Epidemiological data helps frame studies that examine the efficacy of interventions that would reduce those risk factors. Epidemiological approaches can also provide clues into the etiology. Epidemiological findings with regard to alcoholism and depression differences by gender, race, and ethnicity have led to sociological (gender role theory), biological-genetic (bipolar illness among the Amish), and cultural (effects of rapid cross-cultural change in the development of alcoholism among Native Americans) findings that serve to focus prevention and treatment efforts. The Epidemiologic Catchment Area Project has also provided the opportunity to study the epidemiology of treatment and treatment-seeking behavior to explain the use or lack of use of mental health services in both the mental health and the general medical sector (Reiger et al. 1984). Further use of the epidemiological approach refines the capacity of different groups to identify mental illness and the benefit of such identification in terms of the epidemiology of treatment. Such efforts have also been connected to economics so that the cost/benefit ratio of identification and treatment can be examined by society.

Anthropology has offered psychiatry important explanatory models of current human behavior. The cross-cultural approach has led to the identification of such risk factors as acculturation stress and rapid cross-cultural change, to emic and etic approaches to the identification of illness (e.g., depression among Native Americans), and to the design of treatment programs that are most consonant with the cultural beliefs and values of the population to be treated. An important note is the parallel between the eradication of smallpox in the world and the discovery and utility of pharmacological treatment in psychiatric disorders. Once the vaccine for smallpox was identified and perfected it was largely assumed that the eradication of the disease would be imminent; however, the process took many years. Efforts by the World Health Organization to eliminate the disease required an extensive understanding of the cultural beliefs, practices, and attitudes toward vaccination and smallpox in each specific cultural group before acceptance of vaccination became widespread and the disease was limited. Similarly, even if the technology of both identification and biological treatment becomes apparent for schizophrenia and bipolar disorder, psychosocial and cultural understanding will be required to further define accessibility and factors responsible for the use of such services as they become available.

Ethology and animal studies have had tremendous impact on our understanding of basic developmental phenomena that may also benefit psychiatry. Through the work on attachment behavior and the subsequent animal and human studies on infant attachment, the psychology and physiology of separation and the effects of these and other childhood traumas on the susceptibility to psychiatric disorders are being elucidated. For example, using the findings derived from ethology combined with circadian rhythm data and chaotic dynamic theory, Ehlers et al. (1988) formulated the social zeitgeber hypothesis of depression that links major loss events (e.g., death of a spouse) to a change in social rhythms and subsequent circadian rhythms that can be the trigger for depression in vulnerable individuals. Likewise, modern sociobiological and evolutionary psychology approaches have equally strong potential to examine the effects of separation, population density, and aggressive behavior in humans (McGuire and Essock-Vitale 1981), despite the reductionistic thinking in popular literature that has trivialized these principles.

If social psychiatry is to be a benefit to both psychiatry and society, it should enhance our understanding and development of approaches to major social problems. We have identified three such critical social problems in the world today: substance use and abuse; violence, aggression, and trauma; and the breakdown of family bonds. In our discussion of these three social problems we will try to examine the role of social psychiatry as a bridge between the social and behavioral sciences and intervention, treatment, and prevention.

Substance Use and Abuse

Drug use and abuse are major epidemic problems in the world and United States society. Continued use of heroin, the widespread rise of crack cocaine, and the number of alcoholics who have become drug users are high both in the general population and among those suffering from mental illness. Additionally, the AIDS epidemic and the transmission of HIV through intravenous drug use has highlighted the need for drug usage treatment, prevention, and rehabilitation. Although medical efforts have identified genetic factors in disease etiology and have developed detoxification programs, social psychiatry should turn toward preventive efforts as well as social rehabilitation. The major emphasis in prevention has been geared toward early educational efforts. Kaltreider and Stpierre (1995) emphasized the use of community-based youth-serving organizations as natural settings for drug use prevention programs. Their model was adapted from a school-based drug treatment program to a boys' and girls' club serving high-risk youths. They identified key elements for success in a nonschool setting, including 1) using a team approach; 2) choosing the "right" prevention program leader; 3) creating a special prosocial bonding group for program youths; 4) involving program graduates as recruiters and positive role models; and 5) developing community support for the program. Using a family model and a child development approach, Paikoff et al. (1997) successfully developed a school-based intervention that involves parents and pre-teenage schoolchildren with strong community and school support. Their model emphasizes the examination by children and parents of conditions that foster early high-risk behavior (early sexual activity and use of drugs), such as being left in unsupervised settings, as well as teaching the type of coping skills and cognitive processes needed to resist such high-risk behavior. Donaldson et al. (1995) demonstrated the success of teaching refusal skills to combat active social pressure for alcohol and drug use in public and private high schools. In the area of adult drug treatment, relatively greater effort has been expended on immediate drug detoxification and the early (1 month) rehabilitation phase. Although these programs have been successful in the short run—using principles from psychoeducation, peer support, and 12-step models—their long-term success is not nearly as good, suggesting the need for a more comprehensive rehabilitation model that may require both booster sessions and more active community involvement. These and other data indicate that outreach services have tremendous potential and suggest the utility of a peer-driven intervention that relies on active collaboration with drug users to replace the provider-client model. Additional information suggesting that drug and alcohol treatment programs have been insufficiently sensitive to the needs of women (e.g., by not providing day care and security) provide an explanation for why women underutilize such services (Flaherty et al. 1996). One group for whom services need to be targeted are pregnant addicts, for although a number of demonstration programs have been mounted, the availability of such programs for most addicted mothers-to-be is limited.

A major arena in which drug treatment and rehabilitation efforts might be targeted is the prison system. Not only do incarcerated individuals, both men and women, have markedly higher rates of substance abuse by history, there is also striking evidence that these substance abuse patterns continue during incarceration. It would seem a minimum requirement of a just society to provide good drug rehabilitation to addicted prisoners. Intervention programs aimed at elimination of drug use and rehabilitation in the prison population have been spotty and of questionable success. Although efforts to use principles of therapeutic community in prisons are promising, successful efforts will require a more active and assertive partnership between psychiatry, the social and behavioral sciences, society, and government.

Violence, Aggression, and Trauma

There is an international epidemic of violence and aggression that has been identified both by national and international organizations such as the World Health Organization and by calls for investigations into the etiology, prevention, and treatment of violent behavior. The United States has a homicide rate of 8.9 per 100,000, the highest in the industrialized world. Although important psychological and biological inquiries into the causes of violent and aggressive behavior have been identified, there are also social vectors that provide clues and opportunities for prevention and treatment.

Overcrowding and population density have been noted in both animal and human studies to either decrease the threshold for violent acts to occur or to be the proximal cause of them. It is perhaps not accidental that increased urbanization and population density at both work and home and across social classes have been associated temporally with increases in violent acts. Related to overcrowding is a closer examination of personal space needs and the effects of reduced space on normal and impaired individuals. Previous sociological investigation into violence has focused on the "subculture of violence" by examining such variables as economic deprivation, economic inequality, and social integration in relation to violent crime and homicide rates. Using both rural and urban United States data, Kposowa et al. (1994) showed that urbanity and population density best predict violent crime. Poverty, divorce, and density figure strongly in homicide. Shihadeh and Flynn (1996) demonstrated that the spatial isolation of African Americans from whites best predicts African American homicide and robbery rates in the United States. In addition to these variables, the ready availability of handguns also has a strong association with homicides (Leenars and Lester 1997).

Several specific types of violence have had more intense study, including domestic violence, rape, and childhood sexual and physical abuse. In the area of child abuse, poverty and unemployment—particularly the recent loss of a job (McCurdy and Daro 1994)—have been strong predictors, as have being the victim of abuse and single-parent status (Garfinkel and McLanahan 1995). There is also a clear link between using corporal punishment and child abuse. Investigations have also focused on populations and communities, with the finding that neighborhoods that lack awareness of and access to social agencies, as well as those in which there is high prevalence of drug abuse, are the kinds of neighborhoods that are prone to increased levels of child abuse (Garbarino and Kostelny 1992); this inquiry had led to prevention efforts for specific communities, such as that described by Hay and Jones (1994) in Chicago's North Lawndale community. The sequelae of violence have also been studied both to identify risk factors and to identify treatment strategies. Victims and witnesses of violent acts have been noted to have higher rates of dissociative states, borderline personality disorder, suicidal behavior, poor social and interpersonal relationships, and, of course, posttraumatic stress disorder. Childhood sexual abuse victims also have higher rates of binge eating and sexual dysfunction and a greater tendency toward revictimization. In one study under conditions of urban poverty, high population density, and community disintegration, the rates of posttraumatic stress disorder as determined by structured interviews were 42% among African American mothers (Paikoff et al. 1997). An examination of the direct effects of physical trauma in urban society (Bell and Jenkins 1993) linked the effects of physical head trauma in African Americans to sleep paralysis and other disorders of attention.

While recognizing macro societal levels such as population density, poverty, and availability of handguns, other investigations have focused on identification of risk factors that may be remedied within communities, such as poor parental supervision, parental rejection, physical discipline, and parental abuse (Tolan et al. 1997). Longitudinal data on children who become criminals show that activity usually begins in elementary school with truancy and fighting, which leads to the subsequent development of juvenile delinquency in high school and increased record of arrest and violent behavior in adulthood (Haemaelaeinen and Pulkkinen 1995). These findings have suggested that one place for intervention may be at the elementary school level, and various intervention efforts to reduce aggressivity and conduct disorder have been tried at this level with the purpose of preventing adult violent and criminal behavior. These models usually incorporate programs that encourage early school success (Schweinhart and Weikart 1988) along with social skills training that promotes interpersonal problem solving; conflict resolution and support; and improving levels of success in school, family, and peer relationships (Tolan et al. 1995). Many such programs have recognized the need to bring families into the prevention plan. Parent management training programs have taught parents to interact more effectively with children around problems of aggression and acting-out behavior (Kazdin 1997).

Interventions with violent adults often begin with Hirschi's social bonding theory as the major explanation for why people refrain from crime and deviance (Gottfredson and Hirschi (1990). Lackey and Williams (1995) showed that, despite violent family histories, men who develop strong attachments to and perceive negative sanctions from significant others such as partners, friends, and relatives are more likely to be nonviolent with their female partners. Murray Strauss' power theory as well as theories of male dominance have also been used to explain society's continuing tolerance of male physical abuse of their female partners. Lenton (1995) examined the relationship of power theory to other variables in a large Canadian sample; the data indicated that a culture of male dominance is a central factor but is insufficient to explain wife abuse. Rather, a set of factors in men such as having a father who was abusive to his wife, being unemployed, being in common-law marriages, and having a low family income all create a climate in which violence is legitimized as a form of coping.

At the level of treatment and prevention of the most severe sequelae of violence, there is a developing body of literature on the types of programs that attract and are successful in treating victims of rape and domestic violence, people who have witnessed severe domestic violence or severe violence such as homicides, and individuals fleeing regions or countries affected by severe violence such as Cambodia (Mollica 1994), Central America (Locke et al. 1996), and, more recently, Bosnia (Weine and Laub 1995).

Breakdown of Family Bonds

The breakup of the nuclear family has been attributed to a variety of causes such as divorce, teenage pregnancy, dependency on public aid, and geographic mobility. Likewise, the sequelae of the breakup have been noted in the rise of single-parent families and in the loss of extended family social support and kinship and neighborhood bonds. Perhaps most importantly, families are instrumental in the transmission of caring behavior through processes such as attachment and empathy and the promotion of self-control, prosocial behavior, and positive peer relationships (Chase-Lansdale et al. 1995). Lack of family attachments has in turn been cited as a risk factor for poor school performance, truancy, childhood psychopathology, aggressivity, and depression. The need for continuing familial and other social ties is rooted in attachment theory and observations of parental bonding. The problems of single parenting have been described, as have strategies for offsetting many of these negative sequelae through the presence of an additional adult in the home. Parental capacity has been examined, and predictors of poor capacity have been identified. Intervention efforts aimed at increasing familial bonds by the identification and recruitment of family members or the establishment of peer support networks are described in a developing literature that has ramifications for both normal development and the treatment of individuals with mental illness.

In the area of child and family development it is crucial that new work and empirical data as well as theory be developed independent of the political climate and agendas. One of the clearest examples of how political and social values influence both practice and the types of research being conducted is in the area of maternal child attachment and its relationship to day care research. Ever since Bowlby's work on attachment theory, it has been commonplace to emphasize that ideal child development requires that the child be raised during his or her formative years nearly exclusively by the biological mother (McGurk et al. 1993). This idea is maintained despite the lack of data on the negative sequelae of not being raised by the biological mother (as had been traditional in upper-class European societies) as well as the anthropological evidence that demonstrates that exclusive rearing by the biological mothers occurs only for a minority of the world's children (Weisner and Gallimore 1977). It has also been assumed that failure of a single maternal child rearer leads to attachment insecurity, which has been further associated with aggressive behavior and psychopathology (Belsky 1990), although this has been shown to have a more pronounced effect in boys (Belsky and Rovine 1988). However, as Rutter (1982) argued, attachment insecurity is a concept that can include large segments of the population and as such has limited power to predict negative outcome. Maternal child rearing and attachment security have been key aspects investigated in outcome studies of children raised under conditions of day care. Studies of day care have suggested that it may have positive short- and long-term effects in terms of peer relationships (Andersson 1989) and that it may be positive for children from deprived backgrounds (Rutter 1982). The general lack of any negative findings in initial research may have been more related to the fact that many of these studies were based on high-quality, university center–based day care centers. McGurk et al. (1993) reviewed the "new wave" of day care literature that recognizes the marked complexity and heterogeneity of day care settings, the social context in which day care occurs, and the other related family and parental factors that must be taken into account. As with all major social changes, day care deserves vigorous longitudinal research that examines the type and quality of day care, the age at which the child is placed into day care, other contextual and family variables that are concurrent with the day care placement (e.g., presence and time spent with parents or other adults in the home), and the potential for a wide range of deleterious and positive outcomes in later childhood and early adult life. A similar case could be made for the need for expanded social research in the area of children of divorce and separation. The influential work by Wallerstein (1985) suggesting quite negative consequences must be considered in light of both the bias of the investigators and the populations they studied. Likewise, as geographic mobility continues, families change and rearrange, and life expectancy increases, further inquiry is needed into the successful use of grandparents (including grandfathers) and extended kin as major social forces that may be successfully harnessed in promoting well-being and decreasing the development of socially unacceptable behavior (Jendrek 1994). One specific area of investigation also in need of further exploration is the impact of the absence of fathers on child development as well as methods used to bring in positive male role models in families without fathers (Shinn 1978). We are at a unprecedented period in United States society when there is a pronounced absence of fathers among African American families living in conditions of urban poverty. In addition to the loss of fathers through homicide and incarceration, the relative loss of fathers also occurs through welfare policies that discourage the presence of fathers in the family and through substance abuse, which limits the effectiveness of any presence.

Conclusion

The central point of this chapter is to illustrate the myriad contributions, both potential and realized, of the social and behavioral sciences to psychiatric practice. We contend that the future of social psychiatry is limited only by the failure of the imagination of its practitioners. Important contributions are possible at various levels. At the most basic level is contributing to the body of knowledge of applied social and behavioral research relevant to psychiatric practice by direct collaborative work with social and behavioral scientists. This work encompasses basic investigations in such areas as child development, applied research such as the design and testing of interventions for aggressive youth, and mental health services research to examine what works best for what group of patients at what point in their illness to what outcome and at what cost. A second level is designing treatment programs that benefit from the emerging basic research. To a great extent the field of social psychiatry (including public and community psychiatry) has aimed its efforts toward disadvantaged populations served by public funding. Although this work is important, it is limited by the still predominant two-tiered system of care in American psychiatry. The emergence of managed care in both the public and private sectors and the privatization of health care in general should encourage us to examine what works for all populations. Such an approach recognizes that research directives should examine issues across a range of contextual elements and cultures. For example, if ACT works to get chronic mental patients out of state hospitals, what modifications can be made when these patients, at the earliest stages of their career, enter into the private sector? How are the indigenous forces in the community to be used with recognition of social, economic, cultural, and ethnic differences? A third level of involvement is the training of mental health professionals. Within American psychiatry, interest in social issues has declined steadily over the last 15 years. Training programs are often reduced to a short course in community and social psychiatry, which is often applied only to public-sector work. Equally important is a reaffirmation of the interdisciplinary approach to both practice and training without the boundary breakdown and role confusion between social work, psychiatry, psychology, and psychiatric nursing that occurred in the 1960s. Finally, it is also incumbent upon those in leadership positions, both national and local, to influence public policy with regard to both mental health and the treatment of people with mental illness. In this effort we need to be aware of the ways to identify social problems and the ways to reach consensus on approaches to change. Specifically, our role is not merely to be a voice of progressiveness but to take the high road of providing informed positions and recommendations based on science and data.

The dangers of overpromising and boundary diffusions are great, but the perils of passivity are even greater. We see the twenty-first century as a time of change and genuine opportunity and one in which social psychiatry must again move forward with greater confidence and stronger data to be a positive and driving force in the profession and in society.

References

Andersson B-E: Effects of public day-care: a longitudinal study. Child Dev 60:857–866, 1989

Arthur J: Social psychiatry: an overview. Am J Psychiatry 130:841–848, 1973

Bell CC, Jenkins EJ: Community violence and children on Chicago's south side. Psychiatry 56:46–54, 1993

Belsky J: Developmental risks associated with infant day care: attachment insecurity, noncompliance, and aggression? in Psychosocial Issues in Day Care. Edited by Chehrazi SS. Washington, DC, American Psychiatric Press, 1990, pp 37–68

Belsky J, Rovine MJ: Nonmaternal care in the first year of life and the security of infant-parent attachment. Child Dev 59:157–167, 1988

Brown GW, Birley JLT, Wing JK: Influence of family life on the course of schizophrenic disorders: a replication. Br J Psychiatry 121:241–258, 1972

Brown GW, Bhrolchain MN, Harris T: Social class and psychiatric disturbances among women in an urban population. Sociology 9:225–254, 1975

Chase-Lansdale PL, Wakschlag LS, Brooks-Gunn J: A psychological perspective on the development of caring in children and youth: the role of the family. J Adolesc 18:515–556, 1995

Cooper B: Sociology in the context of social psychiatry. Acta Psychiatr Scand 90 (suppl 385):39–47, 1994

Dickey B, Normand SL, Norton EC, et al: Managing the care of schizophrenia: lessons from a 4-year Massachusetts Medicaid study. Arch Gen Psychiatry 53:945–952, 1996

Dohrenwend BP: Socioeconomic status (SES) and psychiatric disorders: are the issues still compelling? Soc Psychiatry Psychiatr Epidemiol 25:41–47, 1990

Donaldson SI, Graham JW, Piccinin AM, et al: Resistance skills training and onset of alcohol use—evidence for beneficial and potentially harmful effects in public schools and in private Catholic schools. Health Psychol 14:291–300, 1995

Eaton W: Social facts and the sociological imagination: the contributions of sociology to psychiatric epidemiology. Acta Psychiatr Scand 90 (suppl 385):25–38, 1994

Ehlers CL, Wall TL, Wyss SP, et al: Social zeitgebers and biological rhythms: a unified approach to understanding the etiology of depression. Arch Gen Psychiatry 45:948–952, 1988

Emerick RE: Group demographics in the mental patient movement: group location, age, and size as structural factors. Community Ment Health J 25:277–300,1989

Essock SM, Kontos N: Implementing assertive community treatment teams. Psychiatr Serv 47:679–683, 1995

Flaherty JA, Richman JA: Gender differences in the perception and utilization of social support: theoretical perspectives and an empirical test. Social Sciences 28: 1221–1228, 1989

Flaherty JA, Gaviria M, Black E, et al: The role of social support in the functioning of patients with unipolar depression. Am J Psychiatry 140:473–476, 1983

Flaherty JA, Kim K, Adams S: The course of alcoholism in men and women, in The Principles and Practice of Addictions in Psychiatry. Edited by Miller N. Philadelphia, PA, WB Saunders, 1996, pp 155–165

Fleck S: Social psychiatry—an overview. Soc Psychiatry Psychiatr Epidemiol 25:48–55, 1990

Garbarino J, Kostelny K: Child maltreatment as a community problem. Child Abuse Negl 16:455–464, 1992

Garfinkel I, McLanahan S: The effects of child support reform on child well-being, in Escape From Poverty: What Makes a Difference for Children? Edited by Chase-Lansdale PL, Brooks-Gunn J. New York, Cambridge University Press, 1995, pp 211–238

Gatz M: Enhancement of individual and community competence: the older adult as community worker. Am J Community Psychol 10:291–303, 1982

Gottfredson MR, Hirschi T: A General Theory of Crime. Stanford, CA, Stanford University Press, 1990

Gottlieb BH: Social support as a focus for integrative research in psychology. Am Psychol 38:278–287, 1983

Grinker RR: Psychiatry rushes madly in all directions. Arch Gen Psychiatry 10:228–237, 1964

Gruenberg EM: Community care is not deinstitutionalization, in New Trends of Psychiatry in the Community. Edited by Serban G. Cambridge, MA, Ballinger, 1977, pp 257–264

Haemaelaeinen M, Pulkkinen L: Aggressive and non-prosocial behavior as precursors of criminality. Studies on Crime and Crime Prevention 4:6–21, 1995

Hay T, Jones L: Societal interventions to prevent child abuse and neglect. Child Welfare 5:379–403, 1994

Henderson S: The social network, support and neurosis. Br J Psychiatry 131:185–191, 1977

Hogarty GE, Anderson CM, Reiss DJ, et al: Family psychoeducation, social skills training, and maintenance chemotherapy in the aftercare treatment of schizophrenia, II: two-year effects of a controlled study on relapse and adjustment. Arch Gen Psychiatry 48:340–347, 1991

Jendrek MP: Grandparents who parent their grandchildren: circumstances and decisions. Gerontologist 34:206–216, 1994

Kaltreider DL, Stpierre TL: Beyond the schools—strategies for implementing successful drug prevention programs in community youth-serving organizations. J Drug Educ 25:223–237, 1995

Kazdin AE: Parent management training: evidence, outcomes, and issues. A Am Acad Child Adolesc Psychiatry 36:1349–1356, 1997

Kessler RC, Sonnega A, Bromet E, et al: Posttraumatic stress disorder in the national comorbidity survey. Arch Gen Psychiatry 52:1048–1060, 1995

Kposowa AJ, Singh GK, Breault KD: The effects of marital status and social isolation on adult male homicides in the United States: evidence from the National Longitudinal Mortality Study. Journal of Quantitative Criminology 10:277–289, 1994

Krupinski J: Social psychiatry and sociology of mental health: a view on their past and future relevance. Aust N Z J Psychiatry 26:91–97, 1992

Lackey C, Williams KR: Social bonding and the cessation of partner violence across generations. Journal of Marriage and the Family 57:295–305, 1995

Leenars AA, Lester D: The impact of gun control on suicide and homicide across the life span. Canadian Journal of Behavioural Science 29:1–6, 1997

Leff JP: Schizophrenia and sensitivity to the family environment. Schizophr Bull 2:566–574, 1976

Liberman RP, Mueser KT, Wallace CJ, et al: Training skills in the psychiatrically disabled: learning coping and competence. Schizophr Bull 12:631–647, 1986

Lenton RL: Power versus feminist theories of wife abuse. Canadian Journal of Criminology 37:305–330, 1995

Locke CJ, Southwick K, McCloskey LA, et al: The psychological and medical sequelae of war in Central American refugee mothers and children. Arch Pediatr Adolesc Med 150:822–828, 1996

McCurdy K, Daro D: Child maltreatment: a national survey of reports and fatalities. Journal of Interpersonal Violence 9:75–94, 1994

McGuire MT, Essock-Vitale SM: Psychiatric disorders in the context of evolutionary biology: a functional classification of behavior. J Nerv Ment Dis 672–686, 1981

McGurk H, Caplan M, Hennessy E, et al: Controversy, theory and social context in contemporary day care research. J Child Psychol Psychiatry 34:3–23, 1993

Mechanic D: Sociological dimensions of illness behavior. Soc Sci Med 41:1207–1216, 1995

Mollica R: Southeast Asian refugees: migration history and mental health issues, in Amidst Peril and Pain: The Mental Health and Well-Being of the World's Refugees. Edited by Marsella AJ, Bornemann T. Washington, DC, American Psychological Association, 1994, pp 83–100

Newman JH: The Idea of a University. New York, Longmans, Green, 1919

Paikoff RL, Parfenoff SH, Williams SA, et al: Parenting, parent-child relationships, and sexual possibility situations among urban African American preadolescents: preliminary findings and implications for HIV prevention. Journal of Family Psychology 11:11–22, 1997

Reiger DA, Myers JK, Kramer M, et al: The NIMH epidemiologic catchment area program: historical context, major objectives, and study population characteristics. Arch Gen Psychiatry 41:934–941, 1984

Rutter ML: Social-emotional consequences of day care for preschool children, in Day Care: Scientific and Social Policy Issues. Boston, MA, Auburn House, 1982

Sabshin M: Turning points in twentieth-century American psychiatry. Am J Psychiatry 147:1267–1274, 1990

Schweinhart J, Weikart DP: Early childhood education for at-risk four-year-olds? Yes. Am Psychol 43:665–667, 1988

Shihadeh E, Flynn N: Segregation and crime: the effect of Black social isolation on the rates of Black urban violence. Social Forces 74:1325–1352, 1996

Shinn M: Father absence and children's cognitive development. Psychol Bull 85:295–324, 1978

Stanton AH, Schwartz MD: The Mental Hospital. New York, Basic Books, 1954

Starr P: The Social Transformation of American Medicine. New York, Basic Books, 1982

Stein LI, Test MA: Alternative to mental hospital treatment, I-conceptual model, treatment program, and clinical evaluation. Arch Gen Psychiatry 37:392–397, 1980

Tolan PH, Guerra NG, Kendall PC: A developmental-ecological perspective on antisocial behavior in children and adolescents: toward a unified risk and intervention framework. J Consult Clin Psychol 63:579–584, 1995

Tolan PH, Gorman-Smith D, Huesmann LR, et al: Assessment of family relationship characteristics: a measure to explain risk for antisocial behavior and depression among urban youth. Psychological Assessment 9:212–223, 1997

Wallerstein JS: Children of divorce: emerging trends. Psychiatr Clin North Am 8:837–855, 1985

Weine S, Laub D: Narrative constructions of historical realities in testimony with Bosnian survivors of "ethnic cleansing." Psychiatry: Interpersonal and Biological Processes 58:246–260, 1995

Weisner TS, Gallimore R: My brother's keeper: child and sibling caretaking. Current Anthropology 18:169–170, 1977

CHAPTER 4

Psychiatric Diagnosis

Sidney Weissman, M.D.

I n the twenty-first century, psychiatry, in spite of major advances, faces the same dilemmas philosophers have experienced for four millennia in developing a meaningful diagnostic system. How does a diagnostic system effectively describe an individual's psychiatric disorder, inform us regarding the individual patient's treatment, and assist us in contending with the complex issues of frequency and etiology of mental disorders as they affect large populations? Additionally, do either the questions asked of patients in determining a diagnosis or the data used in our diagnostic system affect how we develop or apply therapies? At times we have adopted diagnostic systems constructed on a premise that specific theories provided information to understand mental disorders. At other times we have focused more narrowly on providing diagnostic names for disorders based on either the patient's symptoms or observed behavior. In developing this type of system, American and European psychiatrists have frequently differed as to how the diagnostic system is to evolve and be tested and still meet critical scientific rigor. The distinctions between the *International Classification of Diseases, Ninth Revision, Clinical Modification* (ICD-9-CM; World Health Organization 1978) and DSM-IV (American Psychiatric Association 1994) are examples of competing systems. A specific example of a system with an explicit theory is the notion that neurotic disorders were related to degeneration of components of the brain. Under this system, observed behaviors were attached to a specific theory (which in fact could not be supported by any empirical data). Another example of a theory being linked to a diagnosis or description of behavior—and also implicitly informing the diagnostician of the appropriate treatment—is the idea that neurotic disorders in adults were the result of unresolved aspects of the infantile neurosis. Automatically, since the concept of infantile neurosis is derived from psychoanalysis, this theory argued that for adequate treatment, a specific form of a psychoanalytic therapy was necessary. This theory also was not supported by any replicable empirical data. However, the data needed to confirm this psychological theory are of a different order than looking for brain degeneration on autopsy. Eventually, diagnostic systems derived from or implicitly supported by theories with nonvalidated foundations are unable to foster either enhanced patient care or further scientific advances in the field.

Similar restrictions can be observed in other areas that, like medicine, meld together science and art. In navigation, when data were interpreted to argue that the earth was flat and the existing model postulated that sailing too far from shore would result in falling off the end of the earth, advances in the knowledge of the world were limited. Columbus offered a new reading of the data and argued that the earth was round. Further, he proposed a way to test this theory (science) by applying his superb skills as a navigator (art). He sailed away from the shoreline and discovered the New World. Using his theory and navigational skill, he obtained new data about our world. Columbus, in contemporary scientific language, empirically confirmed with new sources of data that the earth is round and in the process added to our knowledge.

Although ascribing to data a meaning or an explanation that cannot be confirmed can stifle scientific advancement, it is also true that simply describing data alone without an underlying theory that explains the data being observed does not necessarily lead to the advancement of knowledge. For example, for many years astronomers knew that the planet Uranus did not reliably follow its orbit. Only with the use of Newton's theories involving gravity could they posit that another solar object must be exerting a gravitational pull on Uranus. Guided by theory, they correctly inferred the existence of the planet Pluto before it could be observed. This is an example where scientific advances need both effective means of observation of relevant data and effective theories to understand what is observed and lead to new discoveries. Lack of either may not lead to scientific advances. Until very recently, psychiatry has not had any underlying theories that could help explain behavior. The biological, psychological, and sociologic theories currently in existence, which have added to understanding, unfortunately have all at various times been the subject of reductionism; and, rather than adding to understanding, reductionistic advocates have slowed advances.

In psychiatry in the United States today, we have evolved and developed a means of describing (diagnosing) mental disorders on the basis of behaviors observed or symptoms reported by the patient or another significant person. This method borrows from the work of Hume: "All of our ideas derive from impressions" (observations) (Hume 1739/1985). In our attempt to make sure that the observers of the behavior (impressions) share a common ground—or, restated in contemporary "scientific" language, can develop a high degree of interrater reliability—we have not used all available data in describing our patients. We have focused on the conscious accounts by patients of their experience and actions and our direct observations (or those of other observers) of their behavior. We have not examined unconscious or inferential data about patients, nor have we examined any data about the patients' social milieu or any data based on our new understanding of genetics. These latter types of data are seen as both difficult to obtain and potentially open to varied interpretations. By neither obtaining nor utilizing these data, the current DSM-IV American diagnostic system does not attempt to inform us of the meaning to patients of either their behavior or the motivating forces governing it.

Even with the lack of this more complex psychological data, as well as genetic or environmental data regarding our patients, we are now using DSM-IV to operationally make diagnoses of psychotic and major mood disorders as well as specific disorders of brain function with great reliability. The avoidance of an assessment of motive or meaning makes it more difficult to make meaningful diagnostic statements about individuals who report painful internal states or conditions of complex repetitions of behavior in work or family situations.

The power of DSM-III (American Psychiatric Association 1980) and DSM-IV is their ability to categorize psychotic and major mood disorders. This power allows psychiatrists to clearly distinguish these patients and has assisted researchers in developing an understanding of specific brain centers and of neurotransmission and their impact on behavior. This in turn has led to the development of successive new generations of pharmacological agents. Indeed, in treating psychosis and major mood disorders, despite DSM-IV's atheoretical organization, there is a potential implication that all mental disorders have overwhelming biological causes and that psychiatrists can rely predominantly on biological interventions. This implicit view of many psychiatrists and psychiatric researchers leads to a focus on pharmacological treatments and both an absence of studying psychosocial issues in these disorders and a devaluing of psychosocial interventions for any psychiatric disorder. Indeed, the concept of the psychiatrist providing only the medication component of treatment for patients with major affective disorders or psychosis is derived from this perspective. In this model, talk is literally both cheap and of less value; and, when possibly needed by the patient, it is relegated to being provided by a nonpsychiatrist.

Clearly, for some disorders, medications are essential and are the most important element or the only element of care. Yet patients with psychosis have feelings and needs independent of their psychosis, which the psychiatrist must be aware of and potentially able to treat or respond to. I am reminded of a patient I saw while serving as an examiner for the American Board of Psychiatry and Neurology. The patient being examined was diagnosed as having chronic schizophrenia. He was taking antipsychotic medication and his psychosis was in remission. For the examination, the patient wore his only suit. Under empathic questioning by the candidate psychiatrist about his future plans, he softly spoke of how much he wanted to get married and have a family; yet he knew that his illness interfered with his relationships with women and he had to accept that this would not occur. The DSM does not allow us to factor this sense of the meaning to the patient of his illness into our diagnosis. Without this information in our diagnosis, we are limited in using DSM-IV for treatment planning. Even with psychotic patients, an impersonal diagnostic statement limits adequate description and treatment planning.

This problem in applying the DSM-IV diagnostic system to neurotic disorders is still more complex. Because many assume that DSM diagnoses imply a biological causality, there is an attempt by some to infer that all anxiety states or other neurotic disorders are disorders of brain dysfunction. Therefore, in a common scenario, upon diagnosis the proposed treatment is automatically medication—a seemingly reasonable treatment of a brain dysfunction. This is but the modern-day version of the argument that neurosis is a brain degeneration disorder.

The authors of DSM-IV, of course, do not give support to this view. However, they forget that physicians frequently look to or give a diagnostic nomenclature etiological as well as therapeutic power. This potential misuse and distortion of the role and power of DSM-IV is supported by forces external to psychiatry, which see limited interaction of patients with psychiatrists and optimal use of medications as cost-effective treatments of large populations.

Exclusive of societal pressures and potential misuse of the diagnostic nomenclature, an ideal nomenclature would contain a number of the elements already present in DSM-IV (Table 4–1). First, it would start from directly observable data. The first classification would be similar to the current DSM-IV Axis I. Indeed, DSM-IV Axis II distinctions could continue as a description of enduring patient behavioral characteristics. A new Axis III would be developed that would address issues of meaning and motive and that would include

Table 4–1. Twenty-first-century multiaxial diagnostic systems: comparison between DSM-IV and new system

DSM-IV	New twenty-first-century system
Axis I	Clinical disorders and other conditions that may be a focus of clinical attention	No change
Axis II	Personality disorders Mental retardation	No change
Axis III	General medical conditions	Assessment of motives and meanings
Axis IV	Psychosocial and environmental problems	Assessment of biological and genetic contributions to behavior
Axis V	Global assessment of functioning	General medical conditions
Axis VI	—	Psychosocial and environmental problems
Axis VII	—	Global assessment of functioning
Axis VIII	—	Therapeutic plan A. Pharmacotherapy or somatic therapy B. Psychological therapy C. Social interventions or therapy

how the patient understands his or her illness. To develop interrater reliability for this new Axis III, we might need to develop a scale similar to the one constructed for the current DSM-IV Axis V, the Global Assessment of Functioning (GAR), although such a scale would be difficult to construct using a model or language that is universal. A new Axis IV would address biological or genetic contributions to the patient's behavior, when known. The current Axis III through Axis V would become Axes V, VI, and VII. A new Axis VIII would be established that indicates proposed therapeutic interventions.

This new model parallels one used in infectious disease—for example, a patient sees a physician with a complaint of a sore throat. Examination reveals inflamed tonsils. A throat culture is taken. If it is positive for streptococcus sensitive to penicillin, the physician commences treatment with penicillin after checking that the patient is not allergic.

In psychiatry, the patient reports to the physician that he is depressed. Examination reveals classic symptoms of major depression. The patient also demonstrates a behavioral pattern consistent with obsessive-compulsive character. In the new Axis III, evaluation reveals that the patient is aware of constant demands to achieve and feels that he does not do well enough. In addition, he reports recent failure at work and his suspicion that this has contributed to illness. Relevant to the new Axis IV, the patient relates that his father became depressed at his current age and needed electroconvulsive therapy (ECT). Information on the new Axes V to VII reveals a previously well-functioning individual with no major medical illnesses who within the past week has been unable to work. Axis VIII, which relates to therapies, would argue for both a psychological treatment related to the patient's excessive self-imposed demands and a pharmacotherapeutic response related to both the severity of his disorder and the history of the same illness in his father, which was treated with ECT.

This new model would inform the therapist of the potential necessity for use or expansion of both biological and psychological treatment. A further modification of the new system could be developed to address social interaction. Failure in the twenty-first century to adopt these critical changes in our nosology would leave us with a nosology that addresses neither motive nor meaning for large groups of patients. This failure, in turn, could leave us in the long term with a potentially irrelevant diagnostic system for large clusters of patients with psychological disorders and leave open the possibility that nonphysicians will develop a system to fill the void that we create.

On the other hand, development of this new multiaxial system would require psychiatrists to generate protocols to more reliably obtain additional data from patients. Furthermore, in assessing new sources of data, psychiatrists would need to be aware of their own unique responses to a more complex data set.

For this new set of proposed axes to have a meaningful impact on the diagnostic system, a revision of the criteria used in Axis I and Axis II—which are to most clinicians the critical elements of diagnosis—would be required. The added criteria derived from the new Axes III and IV, utilizing knowledge of the motive and meaning of the patient's behavior coupled with genetic information, would enable more individualized coding of psychiatric disorders. While adding unique specificity, the new dimensions need not lose the generalizability of the DSM process. This process has facilitated the enhancement of our knowledge of mental disorders. The new specificity would add to our focused clinical power.

The diagnostic system that I have envisioned has not focused in detail on the role of society either in shaping behavior or in influencing how we interpret behavior. For example, let us suppose that a minister has informed his congregation at a Sunday service that he had a vision of God the previous day. The vision advised that he must leave the congregation to pursue missionary work. The congregation, in the absence of any change in the minister's behavior or motives, would likely support his proposed action as his responding to a higher power. The minister and his congregation share a common belief system, and no psychiatrist would be asked to intervene. A nonbeliever hearing the same story might argue that the minister and congregation share a delusion. However, in a multicultural society in which the minister's action would harm no one and his subgroup agrees, no action would be taken. What is essential to note is that in multicultural societies, differing subgroups or families have unique views that govern behavior and that can have an impact on the psychiatrist's view of what is normal, acceptable, or appropriate. Family relationships or child-rearing practices of one group can be considered abusive or bizarre by the society at large or, specifically, by the examining psychiatrist. In the expansion of many nations into multicultural societies, such as in the United States, an awareness of subgroup values is essential for the psychiatrist in determining both diagnosis and treatment.

To utilize motive and meaning in the diagnostic process, as previously noted, psychiatrists have an additional responsibility to first understand themselves and their own unique views of their own behavior (Weissman 1987). Only then can they reliably assess a given individual's behavior. Psychiatrists must always be aware of their own norms, society's norms, and the standards of subgroups. Psychiatrists who fail to maintain such an awareness will misdiagnose patients and will further confuse societal issues with individual issues.

In addition to knowing the norms of the society and of its subgroups, psychiatrists must become aware of the unique stressors faced by the various groups in their society. A middle-class psychiatrist must have some awareness of the life experiences of an impoverished unwed mother in order to develop a treatment plan for her depression. As psychiatrists become accessible to new groups, many of the questions they will be asked will not be standard treatment questions such as "what dose of medication do I take?" Some individuals will want to know how to deal with children who have school problems. Others will need to know how to deal with their elderly parents: When, for example, should one's parents sell the family home and move to a retirement home? The list of potential questions is unending. This creates an environment in which psychiatrists must develop strategies to resolve or respond to complex issues in which they may have little background. The diagnostic process, by bringing together biological, psychological, and social perspectives, will guide psychiatrists in their responses. In the social arena, it will not provide the clarity it does in diagnosing a bipolar patient, but it will allow psychiatrists to provide their patients with new insights and knowledge about themselves and their families so that the patients will be better informed to make decisions.

It might be argued that psychological or social concerns that do not necessitate the use of medications for effective treatment are not medical problems at all and would be best treated by social workers and psychologists. It is clear that there are any number of disorders that can be treated by nonpsychiatrists. However, for some complex disorders, the psychiatrist's unique perspective utilizing knowledge of the biological, psychological, and social components of behavior can be of value even if medication is not used.

Some will argue that the incorporation of information related to genetics, motives, and meaning includes an unstated theoretical basis in the diagnostic system. Few will dispute that there is a genetic predisposition to some disorders, but motives and meanings, they will contend, relate to a psychoanalytical theoretical model of the mind, and psychoanalysis is only one among many theories. Although it is true that psychoanalysis offers specific models of how to comprehend motives, it is not alone in valuing them. Indeed, it is impossible to comprehend the vast complexity of the human experience without using motives in describing an individual's behavior—ergo, in making a diagnosis. How one elects to either understand or alter motives will relate to a specific theory. Each theory, in turn, will offer its own treatment strategies. As psychiatrists, we should be able to develop means of describing these elements of the human experience as readily as we have done for the existence of hallucinations. We should not need the eloquence of Shakespeare to describe the complexity of our patients.

The proposed new multiaxial diagnostic system follows the same empirical standards as does DSM-IV. What it adds is more data to reliably advise us on varied treatment possibilities. Of course, there are theories that attempt to account for the varied mental disorders that our patients suffer. These theories, when accompanied by meaningful diagnoses, inform us about treatment alternatives. Axis VIII enables each practitioner to apply his or her unique theoretical position while using all available data to develop a treatment strategy.

In conclusion, the American Psychiatric Association's DSM-III, DSM-III-R, and DSM-IV created a diagnostic system whose descriptive labels could be agreed upon by diverse raters. Precisely because it is empirically based, it has helped distinguish unique disorders. It has served psychiatry in much the same manner that Americus Vespucius' maps of the New World served early explorers. The maps could not inform the explorers regarding the content of the New World, but they provided a sharp outline of the New World's borders and facilitated its exploration. Similarly, DSM-IV, by sharply defining the borders of psychiatric disorders, has served comparably to foster research to better understand and treat mental disorders.

With these original maps (DSM-IV), we must now develop more detailed renderings of our patients' difficulties. Knowledge of meaning and motivation as well as of biological components become critical to sharpen our diagnostic skills and enlarge our therapeutic armamentarium. The expanded multiaxial diagnostic system allows for a richness not currently available with DSM-IV. Yet it is clear that developing new axes with agreed-upon dimensions will be difficult if we are to obtain the reliability of DSM-IV, just as exploring the Americas was. However, if we fail to develop an expanded diagnostic system, we run the risk of psychiatry becoming a narrowly focused specialty. Without such a new system, it is likely that psychiatrists would eventually treat only patients with major mental disorders with medication. This would be the result of a reductionistic use of DSM-IV to focus on behaviors with presumed biological causes. These patients would then be treated with therapeutic regimens developed to meet economic concerns, not utilizing the full advances of our science. Patients with complex psychological problems would not be treated by psychiatrists and would not be seen as medical concerns. Indeed, the psychiatric profession's diagnostic schema would not likely survive as the primary diagnostic system for all mental disorders if it is perceived as not addressing numerous psychological disorders. The development of a new, expanded multiaxial system validated by new empirical studies will be expensive and time-consuming. But such a system is essential if we are to continue to expand our knowledge of mental disorders and, concurrently, to further increase the effectiveness of our therapies.

References

Hume D: A Treatise of Human Nature (1739). New York, Penguin Classics, 1985, p 54

American Psychiatric Association: Diagnostic and Statistical Manual of Mental Disorders, 3rd Edition. Washington, DC, American Psychiatric Association, 1980

American Psychiatric Association: Diagnostic and Statistical Manual of Mental Disorders, 4th Edition. Washington, DC, American Psychiatric Association, 1994

Weissman SH: The role of a personal psychoanalysis in the education of the general psychiatrist, in The Role of Psychoanalysis in Psychiatric Education: Past, Present, and Future. Edited by Weissman SH, Thurnblad RJ. Madison, CT, International Universities Press, 1987, pp 271–288

World Health Organization: The International Classification of Diseases, Ninth Revision, Clinical Modification (ICD-9-CM). Geneva, Switzerland, World Health Organization, 1978

CHAPTER 5

Normality and the Boundaries of Psychiatry

Daniel Offer, M.D.

Throughout recorded history humans have been fascinated by the insane and the pathological. Whether the insane were considered possessed by the devil or as close to God, they were often thought to be endowed with special powers that should not be tampered with. To this day some artists believe that neurotic conflicts are necessary for their work, and without them the urge to create will disappear. It is indeed a basic premise of many individuals in today's Western world that psychological conflicts are essential, emotional struggles imperative for anyone who wants to experience life to the fullest. Society is fascinated not only with mental patients. Wars and crimes, natural disasters, and, of course, the supernatural are all popular topics. So when we express scientific interest in studying what is normal, it seems to go against a well-established trend in our culture. Many people believe that "normal" means very ordinary. Normal lacks sparkle. It seems unreal, boring, and so uninteresting. Its very existence seems to be counterintuitive.

Offer and Sabshin 1991, p. 406

Offer and Sabshin (1974) differentiated the theoretical approaches to normality into the following four "functional perspectives":

The first functional perspective, "Normality as Health," includes the traditional medical-psychiatric approach, which equates normality with health and views health as an almost universal phenomenon. Many investigators have assumed behavior to be within normal limits when no manifest pathology is present.

The second functional perspective, "Normality as Utopia," which is best typified by psychoanalysis, conceives of normality as that harmonious and optimal blending of the diverse elements of the mental apparatus that culminates in optimal functioning, or "self-actualization." Such definitions emerge clearly, although most often implicitly, when psychoanalysts grapple with the complex problem of discussing their criteria for a successful treatment.

The third functional perspective, "Normality as Average," is commonly employed in normative studies of behavior. This approach is based on the mathematical principle of the bell-shaped curve and its applicability to physical, psychological, and sociological data. The "Normality as Average" perspective conceives of the middle range as normal and *both* extremes as deviant.

The fourth functional perspective, "Normality as Transactional Systems," asserts that normal behavior is the end result of interacting systems that change over time. In contrast to proponents of the other three perspectives, those who advocate this position insist that normality be viewed from a standpoint of temporal progression.

We believe that the time has come to present an up-to-date statement as to why we believe that studies of normality should be an important part of psychiatry in the twenty-first century.

The study of normality is crucial to psychiatrists because they will find that understanding normal functioning will help them in the conduct and evaluation of their work. The study of normality is an important one, as we will demonstrate below, even though it is often ignored. To understand the reason for the lack of interest in this topic among psychiatrists, we must first examine the basic premises underlying psychiatrists' understanding of mental illness.

Psychiatrists are physicians who are interested in understanding and treating mental illness. They would like to know all the factors that cause mental illness, which would allow for the primary prevention of such disorders. When such a disorder does occur, psychiatrists need to know the rate and prevalence of mental illness in a given age, gender, and ethnic group, and the availability and efficacy of treatment. Psychiatrists, irrespective of their orientation, want to help their patients back to health or normality. It is important for the psychiatrist to know the norms for the particular cultural and ethnic group the patient comes from so that the psychiatrist has a notion of what the end product of treatment should be. From a tertiary prevention point of view, when is psychiatric treatment most effective? When has psychiatric treatment achieved its goal? Who should be the judge of this? The psychiatrist? The patient? The managed care company? All may be reasonable judges, but they will produce very different outcomes. It is our contention that the differences among outcomes are due at least in part to what is defined as normal.

Historically, the specific variables that were of interest to psychiatrists varied. In the post–World War II era, there was great interest in psychoanalysis and its offspring psychodynamic psychiatry (we are including social psychiatry, for the purpose of this presentation, in psychodynamic psychiatry).

Psychological variables and conflicts were seen as causing mental illness. For example, the loss of a parent was thought to cause depression; terms such as schizophrenogenic mother were in vogue; stress was thought to cause ulcers; and psychosis was seen as having deep symbolic meaning. Although biological factors were always mentioned as being theoretically important, they were given short shrift. With the discovery of psychopharmacological agents such as chlorpromazine in 1952, the beginning of the swing toward biological psychiatry took place. This movement gained momentum in the 1970s and has been growing by leaps and bounds since then. The search has been to find genetic and biological structures that cause mental illness. As a consequence, psychological and environmental factors were seen as less important factors that only contributed to the severity of the illness. Very recently, however, there have been interesting studies on the effect that severely depressed mothers have on the development of the brain in their infant children (Dawson et al. 1997). This would be an example of how environmental factors are critical for the development of biological structures. Both fields, the psychodynamic and the biological, have strong influences on current psychiatric theories and practices.

Two Perspectives of Mental Health and Mental Illness

The psychodynamic psychiatrist sees mental health and mental illness as being on a *continuum*. No one is completely normal; it is an ideal never to be realized. And no one is completely disturbed in all areas of personality and functioning. The therapeutic movements within the continuum are from being relatively mentally ill to being relatively mentally healthy.

The concept of mental illness held by the psychodynamic psychiatrist is that "to be human is to be neurotic." Some individuals have severe mental disorders (e.g., schizophrenia), but everyone has personality problems and psychological symptoms. Mental problems are universal, and it is mainly chance that leads a particular individual to see a therapist. The coincidence is influenced by factors such as availability of therapists, insurance policies, and cultural and ethnic attitudes of people toward psychiatry. Whether a person sees a psychotherapist does not, however, depend on that person being mentally healthy or mentally ill. It depends on the individual's wishes. The therapist asks a patient what his or her wishes are. The patient may say, "I want to be happy," and sets this as a goal. A second patient's goal is to rid himself of voices. Both goals are reasonable to the respective patients. However, psychotherapy is really never over for the first patient, as happiness is very elusive. Thus, psychodynamic psychiatrists have a theory of mental illness that is *relative:* all individuals suffer from psychiatric disorders or emotional problems— some more, some less.

The biological psychiatrist has a *categorical* approach to mental health and mental illness. The patient either has an illness or not. The concept of illness held by the biological psychiatrist is the traditional one that medicine has taken toward physical illness. Only if one has a specific cluster of signs and symptoms in addition to specific laboratory findings does one have the clinical entity known, for example, as diabetes. The whole approach is illness oriented. The physician's role is to manage the illness and, if possible, to cure the patient and bring him or her back to health or normality. The biological psychiatrist loses interest in his psychiatric patients when they no longer suffer from a specific mental illness. Most persons are free of mental illness, and only a fraction have diagnosable psychiatric disorders, say 20% of the total in any age, gender, or ethnic group. Among the 80% who are free of symptoms at any point in time, a certain percentage (i.e., 20%) are also at risk for mental illness; this group has recently been of great interest to biological psychiatrists. The other 60%, the majority, are of no particular interest to biological psychiatrists.

For biological psychiatrists the theory of mental illness is one of *absolutes:* either one has the disorder or one does not. Thus, the biological psychiatrist is interested only in the small group of individuals who suffer from severe mental illness (e.g., schizophrenia, bipolar disorders). This group does not include the personality disorders or the mild depressions and phobias. The biological psychiatrist believes that the latter groups can be cared for by professionals other than physicians, such as social workers and psychologists. The biological psychiatrist is also not interested in caring for individuals who have no overt behavioral or emotional problems.

It is our contention that one must have a concept of what is normal or mentally healthy (we are using the terms *mental health* and *normality* interchangeably) when studying mental illness because it is the "other side of the coin." But psychodynamic psychiatrists, in general, have not been interested in normality. They assume, we believe, that normality is the lack of mental illness. But underlying this assumption is the notion that normality really does not exist at all. Normality is a utopian ideal. All humans are really potential patients to be treated. For the psychodynamic psychiatrist, normality means not just freedom from symptoms, but moving the patient on the continuum as close as possible to optimal functioning.

For the biological psychiatrist normality means freedom from symptoms. For the psychodynamic psychiatrist it is a categorical issue: the move from illness to health is discrete. To highlight the difference between the two generic psychiatrists let us use a simple example. Let us say the psychodynamic psychiatrist is like a personal trainer. He wants to help the individual be in the best possible physical condition. The trainer knows full well that no one can be in perfect condition. On the other hand, the biological psychiatrist, when in the role of personal trainer, is interested in teaching the individual the principles of physical conditioning and leaves the individual with the tools to accomplish this on his or her own.

For the managed care company, normality is an ever-expanding universe, as psychopathology continues to shrink. The catch phrase for the 1990s is "disease management." Treatment of four sessions "should be sufficient time for the client and the provider to form a working alliance and to initiate the treatment plan. The working alliance should include a mutual agreement between the client and the provider about specific symptoms and behaviors targeted for change" (letter from a managed care company, April 2, 1996). In other words, normality is extremely diverse and only the most extreme forms of disorders should be treated. This approach to psychiatric care differs markedly from the other approaches described above and results, at least in part, from a different perspective of normality.

General Considerations

Psychiatrists are trained to recognize psychopathology and disorder. They are good at it. But how good are they at recognizing the normal? From a social psychological point of view, is it possible that psychiatrists are trained to see psychopathology and so they develop a cognitive model of psychopathology everywhere that does not allow them to see other aspects of their patients' psychological state? This tendency of the psychiatrist to overgeneralize has been called "illusionary correlation" (Fiske and Taylor 1984). As we stated in another context (Stoller et al. 1996), "psychiatrists may view psychopathology as an all or nothing event." Once they observe a correlation between psychiatric disturbance and some aspect of behavior, psychiatrists may extend that correlation to *all* of the other aspects of a person's behavior. This will generally lead psychiatrists to believe that their patients have problems in all areas, a belief that is most often incorrect.

Normality usually means freedom from mental illness. The problems, or symptoms, that bring individuals to the psychiatrist's consulting room vary. Severe symptoms almost always bring the patient—or, in the case of children and adolescents, the family—to the psychiatrist. In some segments of society, patients seek therapy because they cannot form a meaningful relationship or because they feel unfulfilled. These are the ones who suffer from personality disorders. Attitudes toward psychiatry are not consistent, even within the American culture. They are based on differences in subculture, ethnic group, gender, age, and class. From a practical point of view, they also vary with the kind of insurance one has.

A concept that has been often used to illustrate the bottomless pit of mental health services is that of the "worried well." These are individuals who are considered by many to be well-functioning—that is, normal—individuals who cannot be considered to be medically or psychiatrically ill. (See, for example, "Treating Mental Illness Fairly," by Richard Estrada, which appeared in *The Chicago Tribune* on June 4, 1996.) There are no studies on this particular group, although the term has been used for some time. For example, the term *worried well* was used by the community mental health movement in the 1960s (H. Visotsky, personal communication, 1996). According to Visotsky it referred to the notion that the mental health workers in the community mental health centers were interested in working with the worried well, who did not really need treatment. The seriously mentally ill patients were sent to state hospitals.

We have used the term *worried well* in the context of discussing mental health services in underdeveloped countries. We stated, "at the present time there is little likelihood that psychiatrists in China, India, and other underdeveloped nations will deal with the 'worried well'; their emphasis has to involve adequate systems of treatment for those with gross mental symptomatology" (Offer and Sabshin 1984, p. 429). We obviously used the term *worried well* to represent individuals with emotional problems but not with severe mental illness.

To illustrate the dilemma that puts an undue burden on psychiatry, let us give two recent and very real examples from practice. First is the worried well individual who is stuck in an unhappy marriage. The person is a successful practicing attorney. He has no Axis I diagnosis according to DSM-IV (American Psychiatric Association 1994). He has an obsessive-compulsive personality disorder (DSM-IV 301.4) and partner relational problems (DSM-IV V61.1). He is asking for mental health services for 20 sessions to help him deal with this problem and extricate himself from it. Total cost of the mental health services is $2,800 (20 sessions at $140 per session), of which the insurance company would pay $1,980; there is a preferred provider organization (PPO) reduction of $560, and the patient would pay $260 out of pocket. The patient is denied the service because it is not "medically necessary."

Second is a physically healthy individual who for the past 8 years has been suffering from paroxysmal supraventricular tachycardia (PSVT), a benign nonprogressive medical condition that affects 5% of the population. The patient gets attacks once a month, at which time his pulse goes up to 140 per minute and he has to lie down for 2 to 3 hours until the tachycardia goes away. In the past 8 years the patient had to cancel going to the opera once and twice had to cancel his afternoon appointments. A catheter ablation procedure was recommended, since it can cure this condition 50%–95% of the time (Evanston Hospital 1995). The procedure was performed on May 21, 1996, and it cost $24,119, of which the insurance company paid $18,378; there was a PPO reduction of $1,622, and the patient paid $4,119 out of pocket. The procedure improved the quality of life of this individual. Because the procedure was a surgical one, it was approved without problem.

These two examples demonstrate the bias against mental health care in our society. It seems reasonable to believe that an unhappy marriage would result in stress, which would cause a reduction in the protective nature of the immune system of the individual and make him or her more vulnerable to illness. There are definite costs associated with unhappy marriages. Like the cardiac condition, it is treatable, although the treatment of both conditions is not always successful.

We searched the *Encyclopedia Britannica* and the *Oxford English Dictionary* for the term *worried well* and did not find any reference to it. The only references that were found were in the medical literature. We found six references to physically healthy individuals who worried about contracting AIDS. They were described by the authors as "worried well" individuals.

In talking informally with colleagues we have found that there are wide discrepancies in what psychiatrists believe the concept *worried well* means. Some believe that it is clearly a mild psychiatric disorder (for example, DSM-IV 300.40). More commonly it is thought to refer to individuals who consult family physicians for psychosomatic problems or those who are obsessively concerned about their health (see, for example, Meador 1994). Others think that it includes individuals who are genuinely unhappy and would like to "be happier." It is possible that these individuals equate normality with happiness—a daunting prospect! Others, us included, think that maybe we should look at the worried well as individuals at risk, like those who have a preclinical disorder. We believe that future research on nonclinical populations will be needed to demonstrate which is which.

Worrying as a psychological state has been studied by a number of psychologists. Their studies clearly demonstrate that worrying is often closely linked to psychiatric disorders (e.g., obsessive-compulsive disorder, panic disorders). However, these investigations do not include any studies on the worried well (see, for example, Davey and Tallis 1994).

The current sophisticated neuroscience research on markers for psychiatric disorders has demonstrated advances in areas such as schizophrenia and bipolar disorders. Recently, even in areas such as personality disorders, there have been promising findings concerning genetic makeup. There has not been, to our knowledge, any study concerning markers for coping or a gene for novelty seeking. It would be reasonable to assume that genetic loading would exist for normality and health, as well as for psychiatric disorders, although future research will have to discover it.

Psychiatrists, in general, have not focused enough on the normal aspects of their patients' behavior. It is our belief that psychiatrists have to pay careful attention to a person's coping skills. As Sabshin pointed out, "We do need to be able to understand better how and why many individuals cope with specific biological, psychological and social stresses. Adaptation will be studied in its own right, not simply by studying low scores in a scale of maladaptation. A totally new language of coping should emerge by the middle of the twenty-first century. There are many implications of this development including understanding of the boundaries between health and disorder and developing techniques to reinforce coping patterns" (Sabshin 1995, p. 5).

Returning to our original premise, that the study of the normal is important for psychiatrists, here are three of the benefits that come to psychiatrists from studying normal behavior and development:

1. It will allow psychiatrists to better understand the totality of behaviors on the continuum from extreme psychopathology to superior functioning. A result of this understanding will be the tempering of the golden ideal. It will be to demonstrate to the public in general, and the psychiatric profession in particular, that normal people do exist. The studies will show in detail how the vast nonpatient population approaches problems and solves them successfully.

2. It will help psychiatrists to better understand the factors that help some patients stay symptom free while others, with the identical cluster of symptoms, are unable to change. It is also of tremendous interest to any clinician to know what causes recurrence and what helps keep patients in

remission (see, for example, Moos 1995). Is it not possible that coping ability and strength are just as important as psychopathology or disorder? We need to find out more about the totality of human behavior before we can answer these important questions.

3. A better understanding of the normal will help psychiatrists establish a realistic end point of psychiatric treatment. Different end points will have to be established for the mostly diverse population. New ways will have to be found to reinforce coping skills among psychiatric patients.

An example of a recent study of normal individuals using different psychiatric and psychological methodology is "Normal Adolescent Males: A 25-Year Follow-Up Study" (Offer et al., in press). The investigation is a 25-year follow-up study of normal adolescent males who were originally studied between 1962 and 1971 to identify patterns of normal adolescent development from early adolescence to adulthood.

There are four objectives of the study. The first is to determine predictors of mental and physical health in middle age based on developmental patterns occurring during adolescence and young adulthood. The second is to study the patterns of relationships that men form with the significant people in their lives, including colleagues, parents, children, spouses, and friends. The third objective is to identify the coping strategies of these subjects. The fourth objective is to study subjects' memory of specific events that happened during their adolescence.

The investigators have located all of the original 73 subjects, whose average age is 48. Two have died, both of cancer. The study subjects were originally from two Chicago-area communities. Sixty percent now live throughout the United States and 40% are in the Chicago area. Ninety-three percent (all but three) of the subjects have agreed to participate.

Individual detailed interviews and standardized assessments are conducted with each subject. Interviews focus on major life events since their last interview at age 22. Major changes and influences in their lives are included, as well as assessments of work, family, and physical and mental health. Several sets of questions from the original interviews are repeated in order to examine continuities and discontinuities in adaptation from adolescence to middle age.

Our previous research resulted in the determination of three routes of development from adolescence to young adulthood. They are 1) continuous growth, 2) surgent growth, and 3) tumultuous growth. We now turn our attention to the sample in middle age to examine what has happened, developmentally, to these subjects.

We are near the end of the data collection phase. We are most impressed with the coping abilities of these subjects, despite the many traumas and stresses that they encountered. There is a relatively minimal amount of symptomatology (as measured by the symptom checklist). The subjects are reliable and most cooperative in the research process, especially considering the fact that the data collection phase, or interview, takes 4 hours.

This study, and other studies like it, will help psychiatrists bridge the knowledge gap that currently exists. As we stated above, the three benefits that come to psychiatrists from learning more about studies like ours will enhance their understanding of their patients as well.

References

American Psychiatric Association: Diagnostic and Statistical Manual of Mental Disorders, 4th Edition. Washington DC, American Psychiatric Association, 1994

Davey G, Tallis F (eds): Worrying: Perspectives on Theory, Assessment and Treatment. New York, Wiley, 1994

Dawson G, Frey K, Hessl D, et al: Infants of depressed mothers exhibit atypical frontal brain activity: a replication and extension of previous findings. J Child Psychol Psychiatry 38:179–186, 1997

Estrada R: Treating mental illness fairly (editorial). Chicago Tribune, June 4, 1996

Evanston Hospital: Cardiac Electrophysiology. Evanston, IL, Evanston Hospital, June 1995

Fiske S, Taylor S: Social Cognition. Lexington, MA, Addison-Wesley, 1984

Meador CK: The last well person. N Engl J Med 330:440–441, 1994

Moos R: Development and application of new measures of life stressors, social resources, and coping responses. European Journal of Psychological Assessment 11:1–13, 1995

Offer D, Sabshin M: Normality: Theoretical and Clinical Concepts of Mental Health. New York, Basic Books, 1974

Offer D, Sabshin M (eds): Normality and the Life Cycle. New York, Basic Books, 1984

Offer D, Sabshin M (eds): The Diversity of Normal Behavior. New York, Basic Books, 1991

Offer D, Kaiz M, Howard KI, et al: Emotional variables in adolescence—their stability and contribution to the mental health of adult men: implications for early intervention strategies. Journal of Youth and Adolescence (in press)

Sabshin M: Psychiatry in the 21st century: new beginnings. Paper presented at the Regional Symposium of the World Psychiatric Association in Prague, Czech Republic, September 1995

Stoller CL, Offer D, Howard KI, et al: Psychiatrists' concepts of adolescent self-image. Journal of Youth and Adolescence 25:273–283, 1996

CHAPTER 6

The Evolution of Psychiatric Subspecialties

Lois T. Flaherty, M.D.

Background and History

Specialization and subspecialization have been part of the development of medicine throughout its history. The understanding of illnesses and their treatment naturally lent itself to categorization; early treatises dealt with diseases according to the part of the body or organ system affected or the type of patient. Growth in the number of practitioners of a subspecialty occurs in response to new technologies, expansion of the knowledge base, and market forces. The latter include consumer demand, social trends, and legal mandates or entitlements.

Subspecialization in Psychiatry Compared With Other Medical Specialties

The trend toward subspecialization has been much less pronounced in psychiatry than in other specialties. It is possible that the preeminence of psychoanalysis in the United States and in academic departments was responsible for this. Psychoanalytic theory, whether classical or otherwise, supports a unified view of human existence and psychiatric disorders. This view is a developmental one, in which the unfolding of personality and psychopathology can be understood as part of a universal process that affects all human beings throughout the life cycle. Diversity may be seen as variations on a theme; rather than to classify and compartmentalize, the goal is to understand the uniqueness of the individual in the context of underlying truths.

In contrast, the emphasis on biological and phenomenological psychiatry in our current era has fostered a segmented approach, which lends itself to research. The development of subspecialty clinics is one example of this. Such clinics allow for intensive investigations into the phenomenology and responsiveness to interventions of a single disorder. They also serve a purpose in marketing particular areas of expertise to the public.

Yager and colleagues predicted that psychiatry would inevitably "evolve into a discipline with multiple subspecialties" (Yager et al. 1987, p. 136) and that psychiatrists, while firmly grounded in general psychiatry, would increasingly focus on highly circumscribed tertiary spheres of care, built on a strong biopsychosocial knowledge base. They identified natural areas of subspecialization as by population groups, disorders, techniques, and domains. They argued in favor of a cadre of subspecialists who could teach residents, but they pointed out that more subspecialization did not necessarily mean more certificates would or should be granted.

Others have argued that increasing subspecialization will bring about undesirable fragmentation in the field, just as has been decried in internal medicine and pediatrics (Romano 1994).

Regulatory Organizations

In the United States, control over medical education and credentialing is exerted by several interlocking voluntary organizations. This is a unique situation that does not prevail anywhere else in the world. These organizations have power, in part because their members agree to abide by their rules, and also because governmental agencies that control licensing and reimbursement accept their standards and regulation. Partly because of concern about antitrust laws and partly because of their independent spirit, these organizations have not attempted to control the amount and distribution of medical workers, and this accounts for some of the proliferation of subspecialty training and subspecialists in the United States.

In medicine nearly all of credentialing for specialties and subspecialties is done by the 24-member American Board of Medical Specialties (ABMS). The ABMS was formed in 1933, and the formation of the American Board of Psychiatry and Neurology (ABPN) occurred in 1934. Oversight of residency training programs is done by the Accreditation Council for Graduate Medical Education, with its Residency Review Committees corresponding to the areas of specialization recognized by the ABMS. Although in theory subspecialty training programs could be accredited without a corresponding credentialing process for their graduates, in practice this has not occurred.

Child Psychiatry—The First ABPN Subspecialty

It was more than 20 years after the formation of the ABPN before the first subspecialty examination—in child psychiatry—was given in 1959. Certification in this field was first proposed to the ABPN in 1949 (Beiser 1991). Because of its strong ties to pediatrics (in the 1950s, the majority of child psychiatrists had begun their careers as pediatricians), there was much debate over whether child psychiatry more appropriately belonged to pediatrics or to psychiatry.

The triple-board program, a 5-year Pediatrics–Psychiatry–Child and Adolescent Psychiatry training track leading to eligibility for certification in pediatrics, general psychiatry, and child and adolescent psychiatry, is another step in the evolution of subspecialization in child and adolescent psychiatry. In 1993, after an experimental period of several years, the ABPN agreed to continue this training and to work out training guidelines with the American Board of Pediatrics.

Development of Other Psychiatric Subspecialties

Following the recognition of child psychiatry in 1955, there was a long period during which no new subspecialties were recognized by the ABPN, although new fields were developing. Subspecialty societies were formed, journals were launched, and knowledge advanced rapidly in many areas. In the 1980s groups began to press for certification in their fields, and some actually developed their own certifying examinations.

Introduction of "Added Qualifications" by the ABMS

Concerned about increasing fragmentation—a negative effect of subspecialization on core specialties—the ABMS developed a category of "added qualifications" or "added competence" in 1985. The certificate of added qualification (CAQ) was in contradistinction to a certificate of special qualification (CSQ). The purpose of this classification was to preserve the integrity of the core specialty, as the initial certification as well as recertification had to be in the core. In contrast, the notion of special qualifications implies more of a "standalone" quality for a subspecialty. Diplomates who hold CSQs may be recertified in the subspecialty without renewing their certification in the core specialty. Within psychiatry, only certificates in child and adolescent psychiatry are CSQs; all of the new areas of specialization approved by the ABPN have involved added qualifications rather than subspecialization.

Areas of special competence considered by the ABPN. In a 1986 meeting in Aspen, Colorado, the ABPN held what were essentially hearings that gave the various subspecialties an opportunity to argue in favor of certification. Some of these, such as administrative psychiatry and forensic psychiatry, had already developed their own board examinations, and others were considering doing so. Psychoanalysis had long had its own process of certifying graduates of accredited institutions. Consultation-liaison, addictions, and geriatric and adolescent psychiatry were also represented. Out of this initiative, the ABPN began a process that involved responding to requests from the field and developing a formal application process for consideration of new subspecialties.

Guidelines developed by the American Psychiatric Association. As the leading representative of the field of psychiatry, the American Psychiatric Association (APA) assumed a crucial role in organizing the clamor for subspecialty recognition. To deal with the demands from various constituent groups for recognition as subspecialties, the APA developed a Commission on Subspecialization to review such requests, which, following approval by the commission, would be voted on by the APA Assembly and Board of Trustees. In this way, the APA could represent the views from the "field" in communicating with the ABPN regarding new subspecialty applications. This component of the APA developed criteria to be used to determine whether or not a field qualified for recognition as a subspecialty. These include focus on a discrete patient group by virtue of age or major diagnostic category, the existence of a scientific body of knowledge and research, a requirement for special knowledge and skills, a conceptual basis, and need (American Psychiatric Association 1990). The APA has been particularly concerned about the need to establish standards for fellowship programs and has advocated accrediting such programs even where no certification exists.

Other subspecialties recognized by the ABPN. Geriatric psychiatry was the first subspecialty to be granted a CAQ, receiving this status from the ABPN in 1989. Next to be recognized were clinical neurophysiology (recognized in 1990), addiction psychiatry (1991), and forensic psychiatry (1992). Clinical neurophysiology is shared with neurology—that is, either psychiatrists or neurologists may qualify to take the examination. Thus, after a long hiatus, four CAQs were approved within a span of 4 years.

Existing and Emerging Subspecialties

Although other subspecialties exist and are pressing for recognition, forces outside the field of psychiatry that are antithetical to increasing subspecialization make it uncertain whether any of them will be recognized in the near future. A brief history of the major subspecialties follows.

Geriatric Psychiatry

Geriatric psychiatry is a good example of how a confluence of forces outside psychiatry led to the development of a subspecialty. Foremost is the impact of demographics; the increased numbers of aging persons means that there will be more of them with psychiatric disorders. The expansion of the knowledge base is exemplified by the finding that many illnesses presumed to be dementia are actually depression with associated cognitive impairment. In addition, the advent of Medicare with its provisions for mental health coverage, albeit limited, meant that psychiatric services to the elderly became reimbursable. Finally, the improved overall health status of the elderly resulted in their increasing concerns about quality-of-life issues. All of these factors combined to increase the demand for geriatric subspecialists. That there is a significant demand for certification in this field is demonstrated by the fact that 1,647 certificates were issued during the 5-year period from 1991 through 1995. This compares with 1,357 certificates awarded in child and adolescent psychiatry during the same period.

Clinical Neurophysiology

Involving electroencephalography and evoked potentials, clinical neurophysiology is mainly of interest to neurologists. For this subspecialty a certificate in more than one specialty can serve as a prerequisite: both neurologists and psychiatrists are eligible to take the examination, although to date few psychiatrists have elected to do so.

Forensic Psychiatry

Although it is the most recent subspecialty to be recognized, forensic psychiatry may have the longest history, with roots in the nineteenth century in the United States (Quen 1994). Its parent organization, the American Academy of

Psychiatry and the Law, along with the psychiatry section of the American Academy of Forensic Sciences, sponsored the establishment of the American Board of Forensic Psychiatry. That organization began administering examinations in 1979 and issued more than 200 certificates between then and 1992, when the ABPN began to offer a CAQ in forensic psychiatry.

Administrative Psychiatry

Certificates in administrative psychiatry were offered by the ABPN in the 1950s but were subsequently discontinued; this function was later assumed by the Committee on Administrative Psychiatry of the APA, which developed a curriculum and its own examination. This examination, with both a written and an oral component, is given on a yearly basis. Preparation consists mainly of self-study, but applicants must demonstrate experience and/or formal training in psychiatric administration. The number certified each year is small, averaging under 10, but demand has been steady and growing.

Adolescent Psychiatry

Developments in adolescent psychiatry can be contrasted with those in geriatric psychiatry. Despite evidence that the majority of adolescents in need of mental health services do not receive them, and recurrent alarms about delinquency, risk-taking behavior, teen pregnancy, and suicide, services for adolescents continue to be underdeveloped, and this field has not achieved formal recognition from the ABMS as a subspecialty. A British psychiatrist, Parry-Jones (1995), argued that the fusion of adolescent psychiatry with child psychiatry has retarded the development of the former in terms of research and training in the United Kingdom, and the arguments he presents are applicable to the United States as well. An application to the ABPN in 1986 by the American Society for Adolescent Psychiatry (ASAP) for certification in adolescent psychiatry was denied on the grounds that existing certification in child psychiatry was sufficient for the needs of the field. To underscore this decision, the Committee on Certification in Child Psychiatry and the American Academy of Child Psychiatry added adolescent to their names shortly afterward. The response of the ASAP was to encourage the development of an independent certification process and accreditation standards, with the formation of the American Board of Adolescent Psychiatry and Council on Accreditation of Fellowships. More than 300 psychiatrists have been awarded certificates through this mechanism.

Psychoanalysis

The American Psychoanalytic Association has certified graduates of its accredited training institutions through a detailed process involving written case studies and oral examinations; such certification in fact predates the ABPN certification in psychiatry. Beginning in 1939 and extending more or less continuously until 1975, discussions have taken place on establishing an ABPN certificate in psychoanalysis (Hollender 1991). Among psychoanalysts there was, on the one hand, a wish to have psychoanalysis firmly associated with psychiatry as a medical discipline, but on the other hand a reluctance to have it become a subsidiary of general psychiatry. In response to pressures from nonphysicians to become certified psychoanalysts in the 1980s, the American Psychoanalytic Association again pursued ABPN certification but did not go beyond presentations at the 1986 meeting in Aspen, Colorado.

Consultation-Liaison Psychiatry

Consultation-liaison psychiatry is currently seeking recognition by the ABPN (Ford et al. 1994). It has a very active constituency and the support of several national organizations; like administrative psychiatry it is an example of a domain-oriented subspecialty. Its proponents have cogently argued that the skills of consultation are particularly necessary as psychiatrists increasingly serve as tertiary care providers and that certification is necessary to preserve consultation-liaison divisions in academic departments and establish and maintain training standards.

Other Subspecialties

Sleep medicine has sought formal credentialing and has been denied. Other areas of subspecialization include infant psychiatry, community psychiatry, and various treatment modalities; none of these have plans to seek formal credentialing at present.

Trends Toward Informal Subspecialization

Much of subspecialization occurs informally. Individual psychiatrists gravitate toward areas of particular interest and—through patient care, research experience, attendance at conferences and courses, and self-study—become expert in these areas. Data from the 1988–1989 APA survey of approximately 20,000 member and nonmember psychiatrists document a trend toward subspecialization. Of respondents to the workforce survey expressing interest in a subspecialty, more than 30% indicated adolescent psychiatry, alcohol abuse, consultation-liaison, or geriatric psychiatry. Other areas include administration, community psychiatry, forensic psychiatry, and research. Respondents frequently indicated multiple subspecialty interests (Dorwart et al. 1992).

Subspecialty organizations. Subspecialists naturally tend to form organizations to share information; these organizations establish journals, sponsor scientific meetings, and recruit new members. All of these activities serve to strengthen their members' identities as subspecialists and provide a way for members to unite and seek formal recognition. Many of the APA components are actually groups of subspecialists who focus on issues relevant to them. Examples of these include the Councils on Aging; Addictions; Psychiatry and the Law; Children, Adolescents and Their Families; and the Committee on Administration. Responses to the APA workforce survey indicated that organizational membership was a common expression of subspecialty interests (Dorwart et al. 1992).

Fluid Boundaries Between Subspecialties

One can argue that formal subspecialization is counterproductive to new areas of research. Most of the research in psychiatry has been done by general psychiatrists. These investigators' lack of a developmental perspective, for example, has hindered the understanding of ways in which major psychiatric disorders such as schizophrenia manifest themselves in children and adolescents. Within research, education, and clinical practice, one can argue strongly against rigid boundaries that would exclude psychiatrists from pursuing greater knowledge of specialized areas of interest outside of formal subspecialty training.

It is important to remember that the boundaries between subspecialties and specialties are not firm and are in fact quite fluid. Within pediatrics, new subspecialties have developed that overlap with psychiatry; the recently approved neurodevelopmental pediatrics is an example. The availability of a training pathway through either internal medicine or pediatrics to adolescent medicine is an example of a subspecialty that has roots in both parent specialties.

The Impact of Subspecialization

Impact on Academic Departments

As new subspecialties develop within departments of psychiatry, departments are challenged with deciding how many resources to commit to the training of specialists versus the training of general psychiatrists. Their incentives are to focus on training of subspecialists, and generalists—like the undergraduates in universities—do not always have first claim on the faculty's time and energy. The result is that the teaching of the nonspecialist becomes diluted. At the same time, from the point of view of the trainees, specialties are increasingly seen as the exclusive province of the specialists, and generalists do not consider these areas as being within their ken. This view is fostered by the inevitability that, as the knowledge base expands, it becomes more difficult for the generalist to keep up with expertise in all of the specialty areas. Thus one can argue that the development of subspecialties erodes the core specialty.

Research. Subspecialization is essential to academic research, which involves the ability to focus intensively on a limited area. The ABMS requires that any new specialty be grounded in research. However, an unfortunate consequence of formal recognition of subspecialties can be the draining of academic resources to establish subspecialty divisions with their own faculty and training programs, diverting faculty resources that might have been devoted to research to administrative and teaching tasks. This problem has been wrestled with in many medical specialties; many have formal research requirements as part of subspecialty training. This is not the case with the psychiatric subspecialties, which simply require that residents have opportunities to do research, although the establishment of a requirement for research has been strongly considered.

Economic and Political Issues Raised by Subspecialization

Impact on Medical Economics

The advent of efforts to cut medical costs has been accompanied by the mantra that there are too many specialists and it is specialists who are driving up the costs of medical care. In a fee-for-service environment, increased numbers of physicians increase medical costs as they vie to perform ever more procedures that will generate income. Doctors have been motivated to subspecialize in fields that have procedures because of the competitive advantage in being able to perform costly procedures. In effect, increasing supply has increased demand; it has also been true that where there are too many doctors seeing too few patients, fees rise as doctors attempt to maintain their incomes at the same level despite reduced volume of work (Petersdorf 1984).

The actual impact is difficult to measure, however, as many subspecialists in fields such as internal medicine and pediatrics actually practice as primary care physicians, and even psychiatrists provide some primary care for their patients. In psychiatry, a cognitively based specialty, subspecializing does not raise incomes, as illustrated by the fact that child and adolescent psychiatrists' fees and incomes are not appreciably different from those of general psychiatrists.

In a managed care environment where there are too many specialists, managed care companies are able to drive costs down by contracting with the lowest bidder. Subspecialists have an advantage in getting on "provider panels" as managed care companies seek to have a full range of expertise that they can advertise to employers and the public.

Impact on costs of graduate medical education. Graduate medical education costs money. In the United States a significant share of the costs of residency training has been borne by public tax dollars, in the form of payments from Medicare and Medicaid funds to teaching hospitals. Various carrot-and-stick approaches have been implemented to influence graduate medical education in the direction of training fewer subspecialists. Funding for residency training is currently capped at 5 years of training or up to the point of eligibility for the first board certificate, whichever comes first. This excludes much subspecialty training (but not the psychiatric subspecialties, all of which are designed as 1-year fellowships in postgraduate year 5, or child and adolescent psychiatry, which may be taken during postgraduate years 4 and 5). Excepted from this rule are geriatrics and preventive medicine, deemed shortage specialties. The Clinton health care proposal of 1993 included a plan to cap the total number of residency slots, and Congress proposed changing the Medicare law so that funding of residents would be fixed at the number of slots in existence on 1 August 1995. These measures did not pass but are likely to reappear.

Apart from any government mandates, the movement of Medicare and Medicaid enrollees into managed care organizations will reduce public funding for graduate medical education, as managed care organizations are not mandated to make payments to academic medical centers on behalf of these patients.

One very likely effect of reduced funding for graduate medical education will be a reduction in subspecialty training, as departments decide that they can no longer afford the faculty or residents involved in such programs. We are already seeing declines in the number of medical school faculty in all fields except family practice and emergency medicine (Barzansky 1996). Whether the changes in the health care system that limit access to physicians and favor primary care specialties will in and of themselves provide a correction factor to the excess—or whether governmental controls will be implemented—remains to be seen.

Impact on the Field of Psychiatry

For the field of psychiatry itself, one of the most pressing questions about the effect of increasing subspecialization is about its impact on the generalist. What will be left for the general psychiatrist to do if every age group and technique is the province of some specialty? As child and adolescent psychiatry is clearly the most well developed of all the subspecialties at this point, one may ask whether its diminished role within general psychiatry has come about as the result of the growth in its subspecialty status. Although clearly some of this growth (and increasing separateness) involves a real and dramatic expansion of its knowledge base, part of it is also due to the political power of its practitioners, whose primary organization, the American Academy of Child and Adolescent Psychiatry, has been extraordinarily active in public relations, political lobbying, and advocacy for children as well as the field. This organization has issued position statements advocating that care of children and adolescents be delivered only by child and adolescent psychiatrists.

The advent of managed care has greatly changed the landscape of medical practice in all of the specialties. By relying on primary care physicians to serve as gatekeepers and eliminating direct access to specialists, the demand for specialists has been reduced and that for primary care physicians has increased. In these settings, referrals are likely to be made only for treatment failures or more complicated cases. Psychiatrists who have expertise in handling particular kinds of problems will more easily receive referrals of these cases.

Other trends are likely to increase demands for psychiatric subspecialists who deal with special populations. We have already seen that Medicare has had a dramatic effect on health care for the elderly and has increased the demand for geriatric psychiatrists. Despite its many shortcomings, managed care has increased access to basic medical care for children and adolescents, who now have well-child visits covered. States are implementing improved insurance coverage for children and adolescents in response to federal initiatives to reduce the numbers of uninsured in this age group. Improved access to basic health care for special populations increases the likelihood of referrals to psychiatric subspecialists serving these groups.

Current Challenges—
Summary and Recommendations

Subspecialization has accompanied the growth in the knowledge base and technical advances in psychiatry, albeit at a slower rate than in other medical specialties. Educators and policymakers disagree on whether this trend is desirable for the field and for patients. Certainly patients can benefit from the availability of experts with specialized knowledge and skill to treat their particular disorders; institutions can benefit from psychiatrists with administrative or legal expertise; and special populations, such as children, benefit from doctors who know how to communicate with them and help them. But subspecialization can bring fragmentation, territorial feuds, and diffusion of scarce academic resources. To the extent that subspecialization is linked to expansion of the knowledge base and technology, it is a sign of health for the profession; to the extent that it reflects simply professional pride and desire to carve out exclusive turf, it is destructive.

If the future role of the psychiatrist is to be a provider of tertiary care and to be a consultant to primary care physicians and nonphysicians, then specialized expertise in the more complicated problems faced by these other clinicians will be an important asset. In addition to special expertise, skill in consultation with primary care physicians and other professionals will become increasingly important. At the same time, flexibility will be important; rapid changes in the health care system are likely to continue, and we are in an era of "shifting sands" with regard to graduate medical education (Dunn and Miller 1996). Continued emphasis on preservation of the biopsychosocial model; the retention of the core of general psychiatry as a specialty that deals with the whole person throughout the life span; and a thoughtful, reasoned approach to the formal recognition of subspecialties will ensure that psychiatry will meet the challenges of evolving health care systems.

References

American Psychiatric Association: APA Criteria for Becoming a Subspecialty. Washington, DC, American Psychiatric Association, 1990

Barzansky B, Jonas HS, Etzel SI: Educational programs in U.S. medical schools 1995–96. JAMA 276:714–719, 1996

Beiser HR: Certification in child and adolescent psychiatry, in The American Board of Psychiatry and Neurology: The First Fifty Years. Edited by Hollender MH. Deerfield, IL, American Board of Psychiatry and Neurology, 1991, pp 81–88

Dorwart RA, Chartock LR, Dial TD, et al: A national study of psychiatrists' professional activities. Am J Psychiatry 149:1499–1505, 1992

Dunn MR, Miller RS: The shifting sands of graduate medical education. JAMA 276:710–713, 1996

Ford CV, Fawzy FI, Frankel BL, et al: Fellowship training in consultation-liaison psychiatry. Psychosomatics 35:118–124, 1994

Hollender MH: Certification for psychoanalysis, in The American Board of Psychiatry and Neurology: The First Fifty Years. Edited by Hollender MH. Deerfield, IL, American Board of Psychiatry and Neurology, 1991, pp 69–76

Parry-Jones WLL: The future of adolescent psychiatry. Br J Psychiatry 166:299–305, 1995

Petersdorf RG: The physician's education—generalist versus specialist, in Medical Education for the 21st Century, A Sesquicentennial Conference of Ohio State University. Edited by Warren JV, Trebiatowski GI. Columbus, OH, Ohio State University, 1984, pp 81–98

Quen JM: Law and psychiatry in America over the past 150 years. Hospital and Community Psychiatry 45:1005–1010, 1994

Romano J: Evolution of psychiatric education in the United States, 1849–1993, in American Psychiatric Press Review of Psychiatry, Vol 13. Edited by Oldham JM, Riba M. Washington, DC, American Psychiatric Press, 1994, pp 9–25

Yager J, Langsley D, Peele R, et al: The future psychiatrist as subspecialist: there is no alternative, in Training for Psychiatrists for the '90s: Issues and Recommendations. Edited by Nadelson CC, Robinowitz CB. Washington, DC, American Psychiatric Press, 1987, pp 129–137

The Discipline of Psychiatry, Part II

The Impact of Research Findings on the Shape of Psychiatry

INTRODUCTION

The next two chapters take us to the frontier of neuroscience research. Here are presented with the basic tools to proceed with future exploration.

In Chapter 7, Looking to the Future: The Role of Genetics and Molecular Biology in Research on Mental Illness, by Steven Hyman, the pathway laid down by Coyle is elaborated on in the field of genetics and molecular biology. Hyman presents the core language and scientific principles to understand how genes (DNA) regulate the biological processes of the body. He notes that the brain is a uniquely complex organ with over 100 neurotransmitters and hundreds or thousands of cell types. Hyman presents a model of how we can understand gene involvement in the expression of behavior and how the role of "environment" varies with an individual's age. He concludes the chapter with a review of how molecular biology informs our understanding of the action of psychopharmacological agents and a specific discussion of why and how the therapeutic action of certain drugs is not experienced for an extended period of time.

In Chapter 8, Functional Brain Imaging: Future Prospects for Clinical Practice, Joseph Callicott and Daniel Weinberger pursue another path demarcated by Coyle and address the complex area of brain imaging in much the same manner that Hyman reviewed questions in molecular biology. They review a number of the methods used in imaging and the respective uses of specific imaging techniques. They note: " . . . it is clear that . . . functional tests are capable of differentiating ill from healthy populations. . . . For additional reasons, we are not ready to place a subject in the machine and generate a diagnosis." Although they note current limitations on immediate use of these approaches, they observe that ultimately these neurofunctional tests, although not diagnostic, may have the ability to suggest early signs of illness or perhaps even identify early risk factors that could be helpful in management. They further report potential uses of functional neuroimaging to follow and correlate in a given patient the potential response to treatment. In sum, this chapter provides the reader with the current outer limits of functional neuro-imaging and a map of its future course and potential power.

CHAPTER 7

Looking to the Future

The Role of Genetics and Molecular Biology in Research on Mental Illness

Steven E. Hyman, M.D.

The recent revolution in genetics and molecular biology has provided significant new opportunities for psychiatric research. This brief chapter can only focus on some of the most exciting of these and obviously does not address other significant areas of psychiatric research, including integrative neuroscience, basic behavioral research, and clinical research—areas that are addressed in other chapters.

Scientific and technological developments in genetics and molecular biology have been rapid and profound during the last 15 years; as a result, the use of molecular tools should drive a great deal of progress in research on mental disorders and their treatments as we approach the new millennium. At the same time, however, it is critical to recognize that molecular approaches cannot achieve the core goals of psychiatric research by themselves. Understanding mental disorders, discovering more effective treatments, and possessing—eventually—effective approaches to prevention demand that what we learn

Portions of this chapter are updated from Hyman 1996 and Schulman and Hyman 1999, with permission.

from molecular biology and genetics be put in the context of what we are also learning at higher levels of integration; for example, from neuroscience and behavioral science. As is described in this chapter, for example, the pathophysiology of mental disorders depends on the complex interaction of genetic ("bottom-up") factors and environmental ("top-down") factors affecting the development and subsequent function of the brain, and hence our mental lives and behavior. The eventual discovery of genes that confer vulnerability to (or that protect against) mental disorders will not supersede research on environmental factors; indeed, studies of the inheritance of mental disorders, most notably studies of monozygotic twins (i.e., twins with identical genomes), have demonstrated that genes confer vulnerability but not the certainty of mental disorder. Genes collaborate with environmental "second hits" to produce *illness per se*, as well as the individual's particular pattern of illness. Thus the identification of disease vulnerability genes will provide important clues not only to neuroscientists trying to understand pathophysiology, but also to behavioral scientists and others trying to identify environmental factors that lead to illness or resilience.

Deoxyribonucleic Acid

Deoxyribonucleic acid (DNA) is the macromolecule that encodes the genetic blueprint for all living organisms from bacteria to humans. (In certain viruses, ribonucleic acid [RNA] substitutes for DNA, but is actually reverse-transcribed into DNA during the viral life cycle.) As is well known, DNA is an extended double helix, each strand of which is a linear polymer constructed of varying sequences of four building blocks called nucleotides. The four nucleotides that make up DNA are the purines adenine (A) and guanine (G) and the pyrimidines cytosine (C) and thymine (T). In RNA thymine is replaced by another pyrimidine, uracil (U). In the DNA double helix, there is a backbone formed of deoxyribose-phosphate, with the nucleotide bases oriented toward the inside. The bases from opposing strands pair with each other to form a ladder-like structure. In DNA a purine is always found directly opposite a smaller pyrimidine, with the rule being that A always pairs with (or is complementary to) T, and G with C. Any other arrangement of bases destabilizes the double helix. Within living cells such mismatches are corrected by DNA repair enzymes.

Complementary base pairing provides the fundamental mechanism for information transfer—that is, for DNA replication—and also for the first step in gene expression, the transcription of DNA into RNA. It is also exploited in molecular cloning techniques and in techniques that permit the detection of particular DNAs and RNAs in tissue samples: under appropriate laboratory conditions, a selected single-stranded DNA or RNA "probe" will hybridize (bind) only to its correct complement (reviewed in Hyman and Nestler 1993). In DNA replication, which is required for cell division, the double helix unwinds and each existing strand of DNA serves as a template for the synthesis of a new complementary strand of DNA. This process is described as semi-conservative, since each new double helix contains one old strand and one newly synthesized strand. In RNA synthesis (transcription), the DNA unwinds in a local region of the chromosome and only one of the two DNA strands is used as a template for the synthesis of a single-stranded RNA, which then dissociates from the DNA, permitting the original double helix to re-anneal.

Information Flow From DNA to RNA to Protein

Because DNA is a linear polymer, it is an ideal template for the synthesis of other macromolecules: enzymes processing down unwound or otherwise single-stranded DNA can add a succession of nucleotides complementary to those in the template strand. However, its chemical simplicity and relatively rigid helical structure limit its functions in the cell to information storage and transfer. The information contained within DNA must therefore be expressed through other molecules: RNA and proteins (reviewed in Hyman and Nestler 1993). RNA, like DNA, is a linear polymer of four nucleotides, but unlike DNA it is a nonrigid single strand, free to fold into a variety of conformations, giving it far greater functional versatility than DNA.

Within the cell nucleus, DNA is organized into discrete chromosomes that are composed of extremely long molecules of DNA wrapped in structural proteins, such as histones, and regulatory proteins. Each chromosome contains multiple segments of DNA called genes and far greater numbers of sequences of unknown function between genes. A gene is a region of DNA that is transcribed to form a discrete RNA. Some RNAs subserve cellular functions directly (e.g., ribosomal or transfer RNAs). Other RNAs—i.e., messenger RNAs (mRNAs)—are intermediates for the synthesis of proteins. Following transcription, mRNAs are processed and exit the nucleus, where they are translated into proteins on organelles called ribosomes.

In the human genome only about 1% of the chromosomal DNA is required to contain the approximately 100,000 genes that produce structural RNAs or protein-coding mRNAs. The remaining DNA is found not only between genes but within them. Whereas in bacteria, proteins are encoded by a single uninterrupted stretch of DNA, in higher organisms most protein-coding genes have the sequences of their mRNAs interrupted by intervening DNA sequences. Only the sequences that encode the mature mRNA enter the cytoplasm, where they can be involved in the synthesis of proteins. The sequences within a gene that code for a segment of mRNA that will be exported from the nucleus within an mRNA are called exons; the intervening sequences are called introns. When a protein-coding gene is first transcribed, a long RNA, the primary transcript, is produced that is collinear with the DNA and therefore contains both exons and introns (Figure 7–1). RNA that contains both introns and exons is called heteronuclear RNA (hnRNA). Before this RNA exits the nucleus, the introns are removed and the exons are spliced together to form a mature mRNA. Once splicing is completed, the mRNA leaves the nucleus and binds to a ribosome in the cytoplasm, where it can direct the synthesis of a protein.

The rules governing the translation of mRNA into protein are called the genetic code. The sequence of nucleotides in the mRNA are "read" on ribosomes in serial order in groups of three. Each triplet of nucleotides, called a codon, specifies a single one of the 20 amino acid building blocks of protein. The codons within a messenger RNA do not interact directly with the amino acids they specify; the translation of mRNA into protein depends on the presence of adapter RNA molecules, called transfer RNAs (tRNAs), that recognize the three bases within a codon and carry a corresponding amino acid. There is a specific tRNA species for each codon triplet that specifies an amino acid. Ribosomes, which are themselves composed of both proteins and specific ribosomal RNAs, provide the structure on which tRNAs can interact with the codons of an mRNA in sequential order. The ribosome finds a specific start site on the mRNA and then moves progressively along the mRNA molecule translating the nucleotide sequence one codon at a time, using tRNAs to add amino acids to the growing end of the polypeptide chain. When the ribosome reaches the end of the message, both the mRNA and the newly synthesized protein are released from the ribosome, which then dissociates into individual subunits. Following (and often coincident with) translation, proteins often receive additional chemical modifications, undergo appropriate folding, and are targeted to their appropriate location within the cell—for example, neurotransmitter receptors to the cell membrane, hormones to secretory vesicles, and many metabolic enzymes to the cell cytoplasm or to mitochondria.

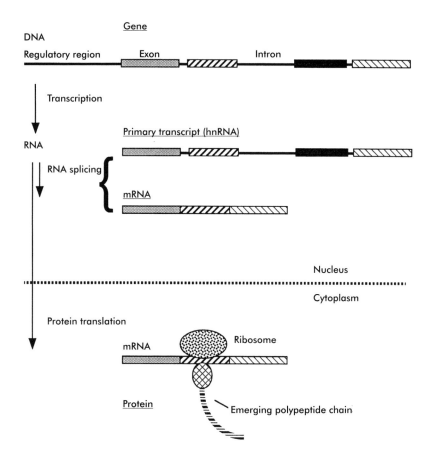

Figure 7–1. A schematic representation of steps in the expression of genes from the DNA to the protein. The nucleus is at the top and the cytoplasm at the bottom. DNA regulatory regions and introns are shown as *black bars*. Exons are shown as *stippled, black,* or *cross-hatched rectangles.* In the diagram, the region to the left (upstream) of the first exon is shown as the regulatory region of the gene, but *cis*-regulatory elements (see text) are occasionally found within introns or even downstream of the last exon of a gene. The primary transcript contains both exons and introns; the introns are spliced out to produce a mature mRNA, which is exported to the cytoplasm for translation. hnRNA = heteronuclear RNA.

Molecular Cloning

The fruits of molecular biology are not only relevant to understanding the inheritance of vulnerability to mental disorders. Although the limited scope of this chapter precludes an extended discussion of many important aspects of molecular neurobiology, the power of molecular approaches can be illustrated by recent progress in identifying neurotransmitter receptors.

Before the molecular revolution, the existence of a new receptor type was hypothesized either because a drug had an unexpected physiological effect or because it had novel binding properties in a given tissue. Such traditional pharmacological approaches are powerful but are entirely dependent on the availability of drugs that reliably distinguish among different receptors. Many receptors could not be identified because they were found only in tissues where they were mixed with other receptors that masked their contributions to physiology or binding, or, more commonly, because of the lack of selective drugs altogether.

In the case of several receptors, such as the β-adrenergic receptor, traditional pharmacological and biochemical methods permitted identification and protein purification followed by determination of part of the amino acid sequence of the receptor. Using the rules of the genetic code, artificial DNA probes were synthesized that could encode the amino acid chain that had been identified. These probes, tagged by radioactivity, were then used to fish through "libraries" containing DNA complementary to all of the expressed genes (i.e., all of the mRNAs) within a cell type or tissue known to express the receptor. The complementary DNA (cDNA) encoding the receptor could be isolated because it hybridized to the radioactive probe, and its DNA sequence could then be determined. The receptor protein itself could be expressed in cells of the investigator's choosing by "transfecting" the receptor encoding cDNA into those cells. The cDNA encoding the receptor could also be mutated, and the mutated receptor could be expressed in cells to investigate in systematic fashion the function of different parts of the receptor protein.

In addition, molecular tools have been used to clone the cDNAs of receptors that had not been purified biochemically and, in some cases, that had not even been suspected to exist. Thus, for example, traditional pharmacological approaches identified two types of dopamine receptors, D_1 and D_2; but, based on the existing agonist and antagonist drugs, the D_5 receptor could not be distinguished from the D_1 receptor and the D_3 and D_4 receptors could not be distinguished with certainty from the D_2 receptor. The discovery of novel dopamine receptors has been critical, however, to understanding the pharmacology of antipsychotic drugs. The apparently selective activity of clozapine in limbic brain regions rather than in the caudate nucleus and putamen, where typical antipsychotic drugs produced extrapyramidal side effects, partly reflects its relatively greater affinity for the D_4 receptor than for the D_2 receptor compared with other antipsychotic drugs. The differences between clozapine and other drugs were not so great, however, as to permit the identification of the D_4 receptor by traditional pharmacological means. Rather, it was only after cloning the gene encoding the D_4 receptor and expressing it in cells that lacked background expression of any dopamine receptors that the critical details could be worked out.

It was possible to discover the D_3, D_4, and D_5 receptors because molecular approaches permit the cloning of genes encoding novel receptors based on the similarity of their DNA sequences to previously cloned receptor-encoding genes—regions preserved by evolution—in the absence of any prior knowledge of the pharmacology of the receptor. These approaches utilize principles of complementary base pairing, but at reduced "stringency"; that is, conditions in which probes will hybridize with sequences that are approximately complementary, but not necessarily exact complements. The combination of traditional pharmacology with molecular biology has vastly expanded our knowledge of neurotransmitter receptors, neuropeptides, neurotrophic factors, intracellular regulatory proteins, and many other key molecules involved in the function of the nervous system. The identification of molecules involved in the development and differentiated functioning of the nervous system is an important area that, as it progresses, will provide tools for the investigation of mental disorders and their treatment. Important goals of psychiatric research are to clone the genes involved in the development of the brain and in brain function relevant to emotional and cognitive functioning. Many such genes may encode proteins that are potential targets for therapeutic agents.

Genes and Mental Illness

We must study genes not only because this is a very efficient way of discovering the molecules that govern the development and functioning of the brain; we must also study genes because particular versions (alleles) of certain genes in the human genome appear to play critical roles in the pathogenesis of mental disorders. There is a long tradition of studying the familial transmission of mental disorders. Studies of adoptees and twins have made it clear that in many cases the familial nature of mental disorders is explained by genes. But the same types of studies have made it equally clear that genes interact with environmental factors both in normal psychological development and in the pathogenesis of major mental disorders, including schizophrenia, bipolar disorder, major depression, panic disorder, and obsessive-compulsive disorder. While underscoring a role for genes, current methods for understanding the mode by which vulnerability to mental disorders is inherited have demonstrated that the genetics of mental illness is extremely complex.

Based on the work of the pioneering geneticist Gregor Mendel, who analyzed the inheritance of relatively simple traits in pea plants, traits are described as "mendelian" when they are inherited as a single major genetic locus—a locus being any chromosomal location of interest, ranging from a single base pair of DNA to a gene cluster. Many of the loci of interest in genetic studies are single functional genes (as they were in Mendel's studies), deleted chromosomal regions, or locations of abnormal chromosomal expansion, as occurs in Huntington's disease. Simple mendelian disorders may be either recessive (requiring two abnormal alleles) or dominant (requiring only a single abnormal allele). Cystic fibrosis is a mendelian recessive disorder. An individual who inherits two defective alleles of the relevant gene, which encodes a critical transmembrane channel, will develop this ultimately lethal disorder. Huntington's disease is a mendelian dominant disorder. An individual who inherits a single appropriately mutated copy of the Huntington's disease gene will, if he or she lives long enough, invariably acquire the disorder. The precise mechanism by which the Huntington's mutation (Huntington's Disease Collaborative Research Group 1993) produces disease is not yet certain, but, like most dominant disease genes, it is thought to produce a novel pathogenic protein (a so-called gain-of-function mutation) that has devastating consequences for a subset of neurons in the brain, especially—but not exclusively—neurons in the caudate nucleus.

In contrast to cystic fibrosis or Huntington's disease, none of the major mental disorders results from such a seemingly direct unfolding of genetic information. Studies of monozygotic twins, for example, reveal that if one twin has schizophrenia, the other twin has a 30%–50% risk of developing schizophrenia. This is far above the 1% risk found in the general population but also clearly less than 100%. The concordance rates differ among mental disorders but, with the possible exception of Tourette's syndrome, they are all less than 100%. Thus, the genetics of mental disorders reflects incomplete penetrance; that is, additional developmental or environmental factors must interact with genes to produce disease.

In addition, all mental disorders exhibit variable expressivity. Even if both members of an identical twin pair develop a mental disorder, the pattern of disease may differ substantially. Among family members who are not monozygotic twins, differences in the pattern of disease may reflect the interaction of vulnerability genes with additional unshared genes, but studies of monozygotic twins remind us that in addition to gene–gene interactions, we must also think in terms of gene–environment interactions to understand each individual's pattern of illness.

Although the interactions of genes with developmental or environmental second hits introduce an important level of complexity into the inheritance of mental disorders, there are others. Based on current genetic methods (reviewed in Lander and Schork 1994) it appears likely that, in addition to reduced penetrance and variable expressivity, there are additional layers of complexity to the inheritance of vulnerability. In any given individual, vulnerability likely reflects the collaboration of multiple genes, each of which makes a partial contribution to heritability. Moreover, within the population there are likely multiple genetic pathways to vulnerability; indeed, there may be no single obligate mutation shared by all individuals with a given disorder. The rate at which the field will succeed in discovering vulnerability genes will be greater if there are a subset of genes that contribute substantially to heritability and are therefore more readily detectable by current genetic methods. If, in contrast, vulnerability to any given disorder is due to a very large number of genes each making a very small contribution, progress will be very slow indeed (Lander and Schork 1994; Risch and Merikangas 1996).

Despite the difficulties, the effort to identify disease vulnerability genes is critical. Researchers have searched, without significant success, for the past 30 years for biological markers that might correlate with particular mental disorders. This failure almost certainly reflects the inadequate tools that were available for investigating brain function in a living human being. Unlike peripheral organs, the brain is characterized by hundreds if not thousands of distinct cell types, with an exquisitely specific architecture subserving the functioning of diverse circuits. Cell–cell communication involves more than 100 different neurotransmitters and peptides interacting with a far greater number of receptors. The more we learn about the brain, the less likely it appears that some simple peripheral chemical measure, such as a hormone level or receptor binding on a peripheral blood element, would give us information about vulnerability to mental disorders, disease states, or disease subtypes. The identification of disease vulnerability genes would provide much needed "independent variables" for biological and environmental studies of individuals at risk of developing specific mental disorders. In addition, vulnerability genes would provide tools for the investigation of the brain. We could ask in what cells these genes were expressed, and under what circumstances. We could ask how the gene or genes in question alter development or mature cellular function. The resulting information might not provide straightforward clues to pathophysiology—a lesson underscored by the continuing mysteries of the Huntington's disease gene and the protein it encodes (Sharp and Ross 1996)—but it would certainly provide a start.

Gene–Environment Interactions

As described above, one of the important results of finding disease vulnerability genes would be the possibility of studying populations known to be at risk in order to uncover environmental second hits that collaborate with genes to produce illness. In addition to contributing to our understanding of pathophysiology, it is to be hoped that environmental second hits, whether perinatal insults, viral or bacterial infections, drug exposures, or intense forms of human experience, may prove amenable to preventive interventions.

How might environmental factors interact with genes to produce illness? The possibilities are many, but they can conceptually be divided into three broad types of interactions. The first type of interaction reflects that fact that expression of genes within cells is regulated by extracellular signals. Every cell in an individual's body shares a common genome comprising approximately 100,000 genes. The identity of cells depends on the developmental processes by which a subset of genes in a given cell are activated and the remainder inactivated to produce the characteristic set of proteins that determines the structure and function of that cell. Thus, red cell precursors in our bone marrow express globin genes (among others) at high levels, whereas cells in our embryonic midbrain do not express the globin genes—even though the genes are contained within their nuclei—but instead express genes required for the synthesis of the neurotransmitter dopamine. Chemical messengers from the cell itself (autocrine signals), from neighboring cells (paracrine signals), and from the maternal environment (e.g., hormonal signals and diverse chemicals) play key roles in these processes.

These developmental processes are not the end of gene–environment interactions, however. A critical insight into the plasticity of the brain is based on the recognition that once genes are rendered active by developmental processes (i.e., are in a potentially expressible form) in a cell, the rate at which those genes are expressed—that is, the rate at which the DNA is read out to produce mRNA and thence protein—remains subject to regulation by environmental signals throughout life. To a great extent, such regulation underlies the remarkable abilities of our brains to learn and adapt throughout life; we will return to the mechanisms of such gene–environment interactions later in the chapter.

The second type of gene–environment interaction that we must consider is really a special case of the first. Genes interact with environmental regulators to build the brain (and other organ systems, such as the immune system) during development. Unlike alterations in the rate of gene expression that occur in mature organisms, environmental inputs, including pathogenic perturbations early in life, may alter the developmental trajectory of the brain in ways that are irreversible, because they occur during a transitory developmental window or because other processes are dependent on the process that is perturbed. Put another way, environmental factors might exert important and perhaps permanent influences on brain function if they occur (or fail to occur) at times when relevant systems are undergoing development. For example, it has been shown in animal models that there are critical periods in the development of primary visual and somatosensory cortices that occur in early postnatal life. During such periods synapses that are actively used are stabilized and inactive synapses are selected against. After the end of those critical periods, the resulting patterns of synaptic connections are relatively resistant to further change, barring catastrophic damage to the nervous system. Although at present there is no direct evidence for critical periods of heightened plasticity in brain regions involved in emotional or cognitive development, such periods of enhanced plasticity might exist and would represent periods of increased vulnerability to noxious environmental factors.

The third type of gene–environment interaction is that in which genes yield phenotypes that produce disease when the organism interacts with adventitious environmental factors later in life. This type of interaction is illustrated by certain autoimmune disorders. Based on genes and developmental factors, an individual's cells may display a particular antigen that is similar to a bacterial or viral protein. Should the individual encounter that protein later in life and mount an immune response, the organs displaying that antigen may then become innocent bystanders in an inappropriate immune response. Thus certain streptococcal infections may lead to acute rheumatic fever with an inappropriate immune response directed against the heart (carditis) and the brain. There is increasing evidence that the striatum is a key structure affected by acute rheumatic fever, resulting in Sydenham's chorea, which is often accompanied by obsessive-compulsive disorder (OCD). Although this mechanism does not account for all instances of OCD, it is an important reminder of how broadly we must cast our net in the search for second hits that produce mental disorders (Swedo et al. 1997). Other phenotypes emerging from developmental processes may be more complex; for example, one might hypothesize phenotypes affecting the sensitivity of specific neural circuits. Such phenotypes might render an individual more or less vulnerable to post-traumatic stress disorder, for example, should a powerful psychological trauma be encountered later in life.

Based on these considerations, it should be apparent that the influence of environmental factors on gene expression may explain how even identical twins may exhibit significant phenotypic differences (e.g., discordance for schizophrenia). If this complexity were not enough, it has also been recognized that in normal psychological development, and perhaps the development of some types of mental disorder (e.g., the addictive disorders) in which interpersonal and contextual factors appear to play a substantial role, gene–environment interactions become a reverberating hall of mirrors that cannot be easily dissected. For example, genes and early developmental regulators collaborate to produce a child's temperament. A child with a certain temperament (e.g., a ready smile and an even disposition) will elicit a different set of reactions from many parents or siblings than a child with a different temperament (e.g., an irritable, often inconsolable baby). In this sense the "genome" will influence the effective developmental environment, which may in turn influence the further readout of the genome. Similarly, depending on factors such as fearfulness, curiosity, and even more particular "tastes," a child may find certain experiences salient and others not, so that even in the same room, two different children may experience a profoundly different environment. Because of the likelihood that many genes contribute to different aspects of temperament and personality, and because of the complexities introduced by the gene–environment covariation described above, this is an area of great difficulty in which progress will require immense effort and sophistication. It is also an area of great importance to human self-understanding and well-being.

Animal models of altered gene expression. To understand the contribution of genes to a wide variety of phenotypes, including behavioral phenotypes, and to go beyond correlations to the study of mechanisms underlying the gene–environment interactions that contribute to behavior, it is critical to have animal models. Although modern approaches to human genetics can identify alleles that confer vulnerability to a disorder or protect against it, it is not feasible to perform studies of the underlying molecular mechanisms in humans. Rats have arguably been the most important organism for the study of brain structure and function, although many human behaviors are best studied in nonhuman primates because of their evolutionary relatedness to us.

However, the organism that appears to be the most promising mammalian model for genetic studies is the mouse. A large variety of well-characterized inbred mouse strains exist, and mice are smaller than rats and therefore more practical to breed in large numbers. There is also a substantial base of information on mouse genetics, but perhaps most important is our increasing ability to manipulate the mouse genome at will.

By the early 1980s, it was routinely possible to produce transgenic mice—that is, mice expressing any cloned gene of interest—by microinjecting DNA into mouse embryos at the single-cell stage and then reintroducing the embryo into the oviducts of a prepared female. The addition of a "transgene" to the mouse genome permitted the study of "gain-of-function" mutations. Examples include the overproduction of certain gene products, the targeting of proteins of interest such as oncogenes or toxins to certain cell types, or the expression of "reporter" or marker genes under the control of identified DNA sequences to investigate developmental or other physiological processes in gene regulation. This conventional approach to the production of transgenic mice suffered from an inability to control the integration site of the transgene within the mouse genome, with the result that there was poor control over levels of transgene expression, including the possibility of expression in inappropriate cell types or lack of expression in expected cell types.

More recently it has been possible to disrupt any existing gene within the mouse genome, leading to the possibility of studying "loss-of-function" mutations. The production of such "knock-out" mice was dependent on the ability to grow pluripotential embryonic stem (ES) cells in culture, to introduce genes into them in a manner that would permit the selection of cells in which homologous recombination events had occurred (i.e., events in which the mutated gene replaced its precise homologue), and the injection of the manipulated ES cells into mouse embryos. Because they were pluripotent, the manipulated ES cells could contribute to the formation of all tissues in the resulting mice, including the germ line; when ES cells contribute to germ cells, it is possible to propagate lines of mice in which the gene of interest is knocked out.

This same technology makes it possible to replace mouse genes not only with nonfunctional genes (knock-outs), but also with subtle mutations or with unrelated genes that will now be targeted for expression to the cells in which the replaced gene would have been expressed ("knock-ins"). There is still no fully reliable method of activating homologous recombination in mature mice—with few exceptions the knock-out or knock-in mutation is expressed from the very beginnings of development—but such methods are on the horizon.

A large number of transgenic and gene knock-out mice have been reported that exhibit interesting behavioral phenotypes. Until the problem of temporal control of the recombination event is solved, it is most often impossible to know whether the resulting phenotype is due to the introduced mutation or to the developmental compensations that the lack of a critical gene product might engender. Moreover, some gene knock-outs cannot be studied in adult mice at all because they produce embryonic lethality. Despite these caveats, many mouse strains with significant behavioral phenotypes have been produced. For example, a mouse strain in which the gene encoding a key transcriptional regulatory protein, fosB, has been knocked out (Brown et al. 1996) resulted in a striking and unexpected phenotype in which mothers do not learn how to nurture their young. A strain lacking the dopamine reuptake transporter (Giros et al. 1996) resulted in spontaneous hyperlocomotion and lack of a locomotor response to cocaine or amphetamine. A strain in which the gene encoding the endogenous opioid enkephalin peptides is knocked out (Konig et al. 1996) yielded mice with altered central analgesic responses and increased anxiety as measured by several standard behavioral tests. It would be naive to argue from these results that the fosB gene is a "nurturing gene," for example, but these kinds of approaches will be critical in understanding the genetics of behavior. As basic behavioral scientists work toward understanding the neurobiological substrates of behavior, and as the techniques improve for altering the mouse genome, important information can be derived. Eventually it should be possible to decide whether fosB plays a critical role in the hypothalamus in the processes by which mouse mothers learn to nurture their young; that is, whether fosB plays a role in the encoding of memories or in important behavioral switches within the hypothalamus.

Manipulation of the mouse genome will not only contribute significantly to the dissection genes and gene–environment interactions regulating behavior; these are also the types of approaches that may contribute to our understanding of the function of disease vulnerability genes after they are found in humans. With the identification and molecular cloning of disease vulnerability genes in humans, mouse homologues will be sought. This will permit knock-out experiments to study the normal function of these genes, or knock-in experiments aimed at reproducing in the mouse the human mutations that contribute to mental disorders. Transgenic mice overexpressing the relevant genes will also be made. There is no guarantee that a distinct phenotype will be produced in the mouse, an organism neurobiologically quite different from ourselves, but this will be an important place to start. Given the need to understand the pathophysiology of mental disorders, it might also prove necessary to attempt to produce informative transgenic and knock-out models in species more closely related to ourselves.

Clearly, when combined with neuroscience and behavioral neuroscience, manipulation of the genome of mice—and perhaps other organisms—holds great promise for psychiatric research.

Gene–environment interactions underlying neural plasticity. As has been described, even after the overall phenotype of a cell has been determined during development (for some cells within the mammalian nervous system this point may not be reached until well after birth), environmentally induced changes in cellular structure and function occur throughout the life of the cell. These processes permit a mature organism to adapt successfully to a changing environment. Such adaptations have long been recognized for nonnervous tissues, and the most important molecular mechanisms involved have been shown over the years to be altered patterns of protein phosphorylation and of gene expression. Some environmental factors can lead to relatively isolated changes in the expression of particular genes; for example, ingestion of ethanol increases the expression of certain metabolic enzymes in liver cells. In other cases, complex effects on cell structure may occur that depend on changes in the expression of a relatively large number of genes; for example, as seen during hypertrophy of skeletal or heart muscle cells with exercise. In yet other cases, environmental stimuli may trigger cell division and actually alter the total number of cells; for example, exposure to an antigen may lead to clonal expansion of lymphocytes that recognize that antigen (Hyman and Nestler 1993). Within the adult mammalian nervous system neurons are postmitotic; that is, they no longer undergo cell division; however, they appear to exhibit every other type of adaptive change that has been recognized in peripheral tissues. Sensory information, psychotropic drugs, psychological experience, and psychotherapeutic interventions all produce long-term effects on the brain, many of them mediated by alterations in gene expression (Hyman and Nestler 1996).

Molecular mechanisms underlying regulation of gene expression by neural signals. Regulation of gene expression is a ubiquitous cellular mechanism that is central to normal development, homeostasis, and adaptation to the environment. In addition, within the nervous system, gene regulation likely represents a critical mechanism of neural plasticity, subserving, for example, the formation of different types of long-term memory. For psychiatry, the effects of environmental stimuli—including pharmacological agents—on the genome almost certainly play key roles in the pathogenesis of psychiatric disorders and in the slow-onset, long-lived therapeutic effects of antidepressants, antipsychotic drugs, and lithium (reviewed in Hyman and Nestler 1993).

Even in nondividing cells, whether they are truly postmitotic, as in the case of neurons, or merely quiescent, as in the case of glia, the ability to regulate gene expression is necessary for normal maintenance of function and for adaptation to changes in the environment. Proteins, which are the essential building blocks of cells, can only be made by new transcription and translation. Whether receptors, enzymes, or structural elements, proteins are continually turning over within cells and must be replaced. In addition, the ability of cells to adapt to environmental change or to altered patterns of intercellular signaling often depends on their ability to alter the rate at which certain genes are expressed, or even to activate genes not normally expressed within that cell. Thus, for example, when demanded by circumstance, neurons can increase or decrease the number of neurotransmitter receptors being synthesized, increase the production of vital enzymes, or alter the synthesis of structural proteins to make new connections with other neurons.

Transcription

Genes contain two types of functional regions. One region specifies the sequence of the transcribed RNA and hence, in the case of protein-coding genes, the amino acid sequence of the protein product. Genes also contain regulatory regions that determine in which cells, under what circumstances, and at what rate the gene will be expressed. In eukaryotes, transcription of genes that encode proteins is carried out by the enzyme RNA polymerase II and associated regulatory proteins called transcription factors. The process of transcription can be divided into three steps: initiation, mRNA chain elongation, and chain termination. Although regulation may occur at any step in the processes of transcription and translation, transcription initiation appears to be the most significant control point gating the flow of information out of the genome into the synthesis of specific proteins. The regulation of transcription initiation involves two critical processes: positioning of polymerase at the correct start sites of genes, and controlling the efficiency of initiations to produce the appropriate transcriptional rate for the cell (Hyman 1996). These control functions are subserved by short stretches of DNA within genes—called *cis*-regulatory elements—that serve as specific binding sites for the transcription factors that regulate the process (Figure 7–2) (Ptashne 1988). The specific sequences within *cis* elements form high-affinity binding sites for particular transcription factors or for families of related transcription factors with similar DNA-binding properties.

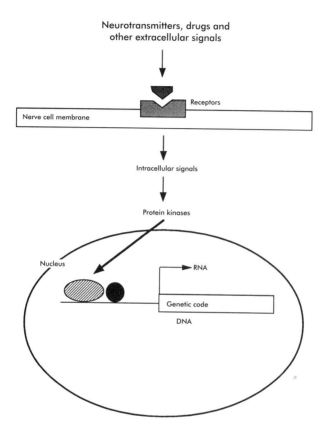

Figure 7–2.   Signal transduction to the nucleus. The schematic shows activation of a neurotransmitter receptor leading to stimulation of cellular signaling cascades (e.g., G proteins, second-messenger synthesizing enzymes, and second messengers) that regulate the activation of protein kinases. Phosphorylation of transcription factors may occur in the nucleus (as shown) or in the cytoplasm, followed by translocation of the now-active factor to the nucleus. Steroid hormone receptors (not shown) represent another type of signaling to the nucleus. These receptors are held in the cytoplasm until a steroid hormone, such as cortisol or estrogen, enters the cell and binds the receptor. Upon ligand binding the receptor translocates to the nucleus to bind DNA, whereupon it can activate or repress gene expression.

Cells contain a large number of transcription factors with markedly different functional and structural properties. Some of these proteins interact with many genes, others with only a small number. Transcription factors can increase or decrease the rate of expression of genes with which they interact;

that is, they can act as transcriptional activators or repressors. The function of *cis*-regulatory elements is to tether the appropriate transcription factors to the correct target genes but not to other genes (Ptashne 1988).

Cis-regulatory elements are generally found within several hundred bases of the start site of transcription but can occasionally be found many thousands of base pairs away. The control region of a gene that is near the start site of transcription is called the promoter. Regulatory elements that exert control at a distance from the start site have been called enhancers, but the distinction between promoter and enhancer elements appears to be artificial from a mechanistic point of view. Promoter and enhancer elements appear to function similarly; both are generally composed of smaller "modular" elements (often 7–12 base pairs in length), each of which is a specific binding site for one or more transcription factors. Studies in which these elements have been deleted or mutated have shown that each gene has a particular combination of *cis*-regulatory elements, the nature, number, and spatial arrangement of which determine the gene's unique pattern of expression, including the cell types in which it is expressed, the times during development in which it is expressed, and the level at which it is expressed in adults both basally and in response to physiological signals.

Regulation of Genes by Neural Signals

Since all cells of an organism contain the same DNA (i.e., a complete copy of the organism's genome), individual genes must contain regulatory elements that permit selective expression of the genes during development and adult life. Differential expression of a common genome is required for the formation of distinct cell types during development (e.g., neuron versus kidney versus liver cells), including the differentiation of thousands of distinct types of neurons found in the brain. Differential gene expression also underlies the unique functional properties of these various cell types. Differential gene expression is established by a number of mechanisms. Some genes contain *cis*-regulatory elements that bind transcriptional repressor proteins; the presence of the repressor proteins in a particular cell type would block expression of those genes in that cell type (Chong et al. 1995). Other genes may have their expression restricted to certain cell types because a critical activator protein is found only in a limited number of cell types. This is exemplified by the pituitary hormones somatotropin and prolactin, which are expressed only in pituitary lactotrophs and somatotrophs because their critical positive activator, a protein called Pit 1, is found only in those two cell types in the adult organism (Nelson et al. 1988). In other cell types the Pit 1 binding site is unoccupied, presumably yielding a transcriptionally silent gene. The sequential expression, during development, of hierarchies of activator and repressor proteins appears to depend on the asymmetric distribution of critical signaling molecules within the embryo that lead to differential gene expression within embryonic cells. Genes that are silent during particular phases of development may become unavailable for subsequent activation by changes in the structure of chromatin, the folded nucleoprotein complex that forms the chromosome. It is not well understood how silent genes can become activated under certain circumstances during the life of a cell. Overall, the mechanisms by which expression of genes is restricted only to appropriate cells is a complex subject that is not yet understood in full detail.

Many—and possibly most—genes contain *cis*-regulatory elements that confer responsiveness to physiological signals. Such *cis* elements are often called *response elements*. Response elements work by binding transcription factors that are activated (or inhibited) by specific physiological signals, such as by second messenger–dependent phosphorylation (Figure 7–2) or steroid hormone binding. It is this type of regulatory mechanism, which transduces physiological signals into changes in gene expression, that is very likely involved in the types of plasticity that are relevant to the etiology and course of psychiatric disorders and the therapeutic actions of psychotropic medications. Regulation of neural gene expression by neurotransmitters, hormones, and drugs can potentially produce long-lasting alterations in virtually all aspects of a neuron's functioning—for example, by altering levels of neurotransmitter-synthesizing enzymes, peptide neurotransmitters, receptors, ion channels, signal transduction proteins, cytoskeletal components within the cells, and other critical neural proteins.

Implications of the Study of Transcriptional Regulation for Psychopharmacology

Transcriptional regulation within the nervous system will prove to be an important frontier in understanding how memories are produced, how the brain changes over time, and how mental disorders come about and change over time. Perhaps the clearest illustration of the need to understand regulated gene expression in the brain, however, comes from psychopharmacology. In contrast to benzodiazepine anxiolytics, most psychiatric drugs—such as antidepressants, antipsychotic drugs, and lithium—work over a period of days to weeks, rather than minutes to hours. Thus, the direct, rapidly occurring effects of these drugs on neurotransmitter reuptake transporters (antidepressants), neurotransmitter receptors (antipsychotic drugs), or other components of the synaptic machinery do not represent their ultimate therapeutic mechanism. Rather, these effects serve as initial stimuli for slower-onset therapeutic actions (Hyman and Nestler 1996). Regulation of gene expression is one of the few known biological mechanisms that could explain continued, progressively developing change over a period of weeks.

Classic pharmacology has established the initial molecular targets for almost all of the psychotropic drugs in common use, both therapeutic agents and drugs of abuse. More recently, most of the genes encoding these target proteins have been cloned. For example, cyclic antidepressants block the norepinephrine and serotonin reuptake transporters, and the selective serotonin reuptake inhibitors block the serotonin reuptake transporter alone with the result that, depending on the drug, norepinephrine and/or serotonin action in synapses is enhanced and prolonged. However, treatment of depressive symptoms lags by weeks or longer. Moreover, for patients to develop therapeutic responses to antidepressants (or, for that matter, to antipsychotic drugs or lithium), the drugs must be taken at adequate dosages with adequate frequency and duration. Antidepressant-induced increases in synaptic norepinephrine and serotonin or neuroleptic blockade of dopamine neurotransmission act as initiating events for longer-term changes in neural functioning. It is the adaptive response of the nervous system to adequate, repeated perturbations mediated via these initial targets that produces the therapeutic responses to antidepressants or antipsychotic drugs or, in the case of the psychostimulants, addiction. These adaptations are rooted in homeostatic mechanisms that exist, presumably, to permit appropriate responses to alterations in the environment and to changes in the internal milieu (Hyman and Nestler 1996). Long-term administration of psychotropic drugs creates perturbations in neurotransmitter function that likely exceed the strength or time course of almost any natural stimulus. The result of such repeated perturbations or initiating events is to usurp normal homeostatic mechanisms within neurons, resulting in adaptations that produce substantial and long-lasting alterations in neural functioning. In the case of antipsychotic drugs, these adaptations are therapeutic; in the case of drugs of abuse, the result is addiction. Based on their time course, it is likely that the most significant adaptations with relevance to behavior involve regulations in gene expression. Although it is beyond the scope of this chapter, candidate mechanisms of drug-regulated gene expression are now being explored in detail, and one of the major goals of psychiatric neuroscience over the next decade is to understand how gene regulation contributes to the mechanism of action of psychotropic drugs as well as to other types of long-term change in the nervous system.

References

Brown JR, Ye H, Bronson RT, et al: A defect in nurturing in mice lacking the immediate early gene, fosB. Cell 86:297–309, 1996

Chong JA, Tapia-Ramirez J, Kim S, et al: REST: a mammalian silencer protein that restricts sodium channel gene expression to neurons. Cell 80:949–957, 1995

Giros B, Jaber M, Jones SR, et al: Hyperlocomotion and indifference to cocaine and amphetamine in mice lacking the dopamine transporter. Nature 379:606–612, 1996

Huntington's Disease Collaborative Research Group: A novel gene containing a trinucleotide repeat that is expanded and unstable on Huntington's disease chromosomes. Cell 72:371–383, 1993

Hyman SE: Regulation of gene expression by neural signals. Neuroscientist 2:217–224, 1996

Hyman SE, Nestler EJ: The Molecular Foundations of Psychiatry. Washington, DC, American Psychiatric Press, 1993

Hyman SE, Nestler EJ: Initiation and adaptation: a paradigm for understanding psychotropic drug action. Am J Psychiatry 153:151–162, 1996

Konig M, Zimmer AM, Steiner H, et al: Pain responses, anxiety, and aggression in mice deficient in pre-proenkephalin. Nature 383:535–538, 1996

Lander ES, Schork NJ: Genetic dissection of complex traits. Science 265:2037–2048, 1994

Nelson C, Albert VR, Elsholtz HP, et al: Activation of cell-specific expression of rat growth hormone and prolactin genes by a common transcription factor. Science 239:1400–1405, 1988

Ptashne M: How eukaryotic transcriptional activators work. Nature 335:683–689, 1988

Risch N, Merikangas K: The future of genetic studies of complex human diseases. Science 273:1516–1517, 1996

Sharp AH, Ross CA: Neurobiology of Huntington's disease. Neurobiol Dis 3:3–15, 1996

Schulman H, Hyman SE: Intracellular signaling, in Fundamental Neuroscience. Edited by Zigmond M, Bloom F, Landis S, et al. New York, Academic Press, 1999, pp 269–316

Swedo SE, Leonard HL, Mittleman BB, et al: Identification of children with pediatric autoimmune neuropsychiatric disorders associated with streptococcal infections by a marker associated with rheumatic fever. Am J Psychiatry 154:110–112, 1997

CHAPTER 8

Functional Brain Imaging

Future Prospects for Clinical Practice

Joseph H. Callicott, M.D.
Daniel R. Weinberger, M.D.

One of the most influential developments in psychiatry during the last quarter of the twentieth century has been the advent of neuroimaging. Although "findings" in psychiatric neuroimaging research, both structural and functional, have been numerous, the most remarkable fact to note as we approach the new millennium may be the paucity of clinical applications. In the general sense of contributing practical information to the diagnosis, treatment, and prognosis of psychiatric illness, neuroimaging (with a few exceptions) currently plays a minor, ancillary role. The most common clinical application remains the identification of structural pathology (e.g., via computerized tomography or magnetic resonance imaging of the brain) during the diagnostic workup of "psychiatric" symptomatology. By identifying potentially reversible "organic" causes for these symptoms, structural neuroimaging has contributed significantly to the treatment of some mental illness, as in the diminution of dementia symptoms following ventricular bypass in normal-pressure hydrocephalus. Furthermore, by suggesting correlations between regional pathology and psychiatric symptoms, structural imaging has also provided important clues about the etiopathogenesis of mental illness, particularly schizophrenia (Liddle 1995; Weinberger 1995).

Although it is a subject of some controversy, it is probably safe to say that no gross "pathognomonic" structural lesions are associated with the major mental illnesses. Whatever anatomical pathology is associated with mental illness, it is likely either to be subtle (e.g., abnormalities at the cellular level or only appreciable grossly in large group averages) or to affect complex functional dynamics, perhaps at the intricate level of cortical processing. Thus, although structural imaging will continue to play a role in clinical practice in terms of differential diagnosis, it is hardly surprising that measuring the size and shape of brain regions without accessing the underlying functional state of these regions has not drastically promoted diagnosis, treatment evaluation, or prognostication. Functional neuroimaging, in contrast, offers the alluring possibility of examining in vivo the machinery of the mind at work (i.e., while producing thought, behavior, and emotion). In this regard, we might still hope for a more fruitful future for these techniques in clinical practice. However, it will be important when approaching brain function to consider the question of which (if any) measurable neurophysiological parameters are likely to generate clinically relevant useful information.

In some sense, our limited understanding of healthy brain function (likely to improve at its current rapid rate) places an unfair burden on any given modality to thoroughly scrutinize mental illness. It is conceivable that the state of technical development is still premature and our knowledge about basic brain function still too limited to address the important clinical questions. Nevertheless, the recent explosion of multiple magnetic resonance imaging (MRI) methodologies has once again raised hopes that clinical applications are just over the horizon. In particular, because these methods are less invasive, are nonradioactive, permit multiple repetitions, and offer improved spatial and temporal resolution, we are now able to obtain reliable individual data rather than simply group-averaged data. But, as MRI findings begin to multiply, there has also been a growing appreciation of the methodological pitfalls accompanying their ostensible promise. Furthermore, while some pitfalls are particular to these newer methods (e.g., magnetic susceptibility artifacts), others are particularly problematic in the populations we study (e.g., increased subject movement during scanning procedures) and thus may thwart any new technology. Even if the technical problems are solved, the challenges of informative experimental design and data interpretation may be daunted by our limited knowledge about brain–behavior relationships. These concerns need to be kept in mind in the discussion that follows.

Numerous prior articles have summarized a dizzying array of psychiatric findings in the more traditional functional neuroimaging fields of positron-emission tomography (PET) and single photon emission computed tomography (SPECT) (Baxter 1991; Berman and Weinberger 1991; Herscovitch 1994; Liddle 1995). Rather than review these findings again, we will attempt to answer these two questions about the future of clinically applicable functional neuroimaging. First, is clinical functional neuroimaging possible? Second, is help really on the way from new technologies? To answer the first question, we will briefly review some recent studies that suggest that current technologies are producing the kind of information that may one day enter the realm of everyday practice. To answer the second question, we will present recent studies from our laboratory using two MRI techniques, proton magnetic resonance spectroscopic imaging (^{1}H-MRSI) and functional magnetic resonance imaging (fMRI). These techniques particularly illustrate the point that while new technology may allow us to refine our understanding of mental illness, wise consumers of this information will need to appreciate the potential problems within these methodologies before they are widely disseminated and applied.

Is "Clinical" Functional Neuroimaging Feasible?

We began this discussion by framing "clinical neuroimaging" in terms of producing practical information regarding the diagnosis and treatment of mental illness. Several questions are worth exploring. Are clinical symptoms, particularly their severity, reflected in measurable neurophysiological parameters? If so, measurement of these parameters will undoubtedly add additional information to the diagnostic process that at the current time rests on the occasionally imprecise identification of clinical symptom patterns. Might treatment response be more accurately gauged by changes in these neurophysiological parameters? If there is a valid link between quantifiable neurophysiology and psychiatric symptoms, the impact of functional neuroimaging on treatment will rest on the ability to correlate measurable changes in these neurophysiological parameters with observable changes in clinical status.

Considerable evidence suggests that quantifiable neurophysiological parameters are reliably accessible via one or a combination of neuroimaging methods. Given the limitations of in vivo work in humans (e.g., invasiveness) and of current technology (e.g., spatial resolution in millimeters is still an order of magnitude larger than the size of individual neurons), we have amassed an impressive array of neurophysiological information. Roy and Sherrington (1890) first demonstrated the interrelationship between neural activity and two quantifiable neurophysiological parameters of blood flow and cerebral metabolism. Since that time, the majority of techniques subsumed under the title "functional neuroimaging" measure these two variables. Concomitantly, information at the cellular level has traditionally been obtained via receptor-specific radioligands, although MRI technologies may expand this work (see below). Electroencephalography, also in its infancy at the turn of the century (Berger 1929), gave rise to the other major family of brain mapping methodologies that have as their common trait the assessment of the brain's electrical activity. Magnetoencephalography, which maps magnetic fields generated by electrical point sources (Reeve et al. 1989), is the latest approach to localizing the origins of brain electrical activity. For reasons of space, these latter techniques will not be covered here, but they are reviewed in detail elsewhere (Lewine and Orison 1995; Rogers 1994).

Cerebral blood flow (CBF) and cerebral blood volume (CBV) are currently quantifiable via SPECT using inhalation of xenon 133 gas or compounds labeled with technetium 99 (e.g., hexamethylpropyleneamine oxime [HMPAO]) (Hartshorne 1995), PET using H_2O^{15} (Herscovitch 1994), and fMRI using either dynamic susceptibility contrast (to measure CBV) (Belliveau et al. 1991; Rosen et al. 1989) or arterial spin-tagging (to measure CBF) (Ye et al. 1996). Blood oxygenation level–dependent (BOLD) fMRI (see below) measures signal changes reflecting a combination of blood flow, blood volume, and oxygen utilization (Ogawa et al. 1990; Turner 1992). Cerebral glucose metabolism is currently assessed using fluorodeoxyglucose F 18 ([18]FDG) PET measurement of regional cerebral glucose metabolism (Huang et al. 1980; Reivich et al. 1979). At the cellular level, a growing and exhaustive list of studies using radiolabeled receptor ligands for SPECT and PET have documented the receptor distribution and pharmacology of several neurotransmitter systems important to neuropsychiatric research, notably the biogenic amines like dopamine (Sedvall et al. 1986). On a similar cellular scale, magnetic resonance spectroscopy (MRS), particularly ^{1}H-MRSI (Sanders 1995), has the capability to measure local concentrations of various chemical compounds (see below) based on small differences in their molecular environments and thus has the potential to provide a wealth of data regarding neuronal metabolic states (Dager and Green 1992). If one expands the definition of neuroimaging to include electrophysiological methods, such as electroencephalography and magnetoencephalography, this list of parameters grows larger still. Thus, we currently have access to a number of quantifiable neurophysiological parameters directly and indirectly reflecting neuronal activity on a variety of spatial and temporal dimensions.

Considerable evidence suggests that various mental illnesses are associated with regionally specific aberrations in these measures. The modern era of neuroimaging began with neuropsychiatric researchers demonstrating these links. Building on the general principles developed by Kety and Schmidt (1945, 1948), Ingvar and Franzen (1974) demonstrated physiological "hypofrontality" (i.e., decreased frontal relative to posterior regional cerebral blood flow [rCBF]) in patients with schizophrenia. Two general strategies for mapping mental illness grew out of this work: attempts to directly correlate symptoms with regional physiological patterns and attempts to illuminate disordered physiological function with cognitive activation tasks. The direct approach is highlighted in studies from Hammersmith, England, in which positive and negative symptoms were differentially correlated with activity in different brain areas (Liddle 1995; Liddle et al. 1992). One weakness of this approach is the variability of the resting state, as illustrated by the fact that the finding of hypofrontality has been inconstant in studies examining patients with schizophrenia at rest (Berman and Weinberger 1991). Although the cognitive activation approach (Weinberger et al. 1986) is a more direct method of probing particular neurophysiological regions or functions—as illustrated by the fact that cognitive activation studies have for the most part shown a failure to activate prefrontal cortex in schizophrenia—factors like poor patient performance on these tests remain potential confounding variables (Weinberger and Berman in press).

Other neuropsychiatric illnesses have been associated with a variety of functional abnormalities. Both PET and SPECT studies have reported progressive temporoparietal hypofunction, as measured by cerebral metabolism and blood flow, in dementia of the Alzheimer's type (Guze et al. 1991). [18]FDG PET has revealed dorsal prefrontal hypofunction in major depressive disorder (Baxter 1991; Baxter et al. 1989), whereas both [18]FDG PET (Baxter et al. 1987) and HMPAO SPECT (Machlin et al. 1991) have suggested abnormalities in orbitofrontal cortex and caudate nucleus/basal ganglia in obsessive-compulsive disorder (OCD) (Baxter 1992; Baxter et al. 1987). In an intriguing modification of the activation paradigm, Rauch, Breiter, and colleagues have demonstrated limbic and paralimbic activation in patients with OCD exposed to phobia-inducing stimuli utilizing PET (Rauch et al. 1994) and BOLD fMRI (Breiter et al. 1996). Thus, it is clear that these functional tests are capable of differentiating ill from healthy populations. But, as has been the case with schizophrenia, these functional studies are most reliable in documenting abnormalities associated with experimentally controlled provocations (Gur et al. 1992) and not in simply placing a patient at rest in a scanning environment, as has been the procedure in traditional medical practice.

For additional reasons, we are not ready to simply place a subject in the machine and generate a diagnosis. As has been the case with structural imaging, no pathognomonic functional pattern has been associated yet with any of these mental illnesses. However, the lack of thoroughly documented normative data and the fact that, until recently, the results mentioned above derive from group-averaged data prevent the assessment of sensitivity or specificity of any given neurofunctional finding. Furthermore, it remains unclear whether the ever-growing list of functional abnormalities are state or trait specific. Ultimately, these neurofunctional tests, although not diagnostic, may have the ability to suggest early signs of illness, perhaps even identify early risk factors, which would be helpful in patient management. For example, in a neuropsychiatric illness with an insidious onset, like Alzheimer's disease, the early identification of focal hypometabolism might clarify further evaluation and treatment alternatives (Haxby et al. 1985).

Since there appears to be at least a gross link between quantifiable neurophysiology and psychiatric symptoms, the impact of functional neuroimaging on treatment may rest on the correlation within subjects between changes in these neurophysiological parameters and observable changes in clinical status. A series of ^{123}I-IBZM SPECT studies has recently been undertaken in our laboratory to begin to examine this correlation. Using ^{123}I-IBZM to measure dopamine D_2 receptor binding potential, Knable et al. (1995) studied a cohort of patients with asymmetric Parkinson's disease and found that the degree of right–left asymmetry in the availability of extracellular dopamine (as reflected in lower IBZM equilibrium binding) in the basal ganglia correlated with the degree of asymmetry in clinical ratings of parkinsonian symptoms (e.g., Abnormal and Involuntary Movement Scale [AIMS], Spearman's rank order $\rho = 0.82$, $P = .0012$). Similarly, Wolf et al. (1996) showed that D_2 receptor binding differences within monozygotic twin pairs discordant for Tourette's syndrome predicted phenotypic differences within the pairs in terms of symptom severity (i.e., tics) $(r = 0.99)$. Finally, Knable and colleagues (1997) examined D_2 receptor binding within schizophrenic patients at two time points during a neuroleptic-free interval. Although group mean values of IBZM binding did not differentiate patients from control subjects or patients over time, consistent with most prior studies, the change over time in IBZM binding within a given patient correlated significantly with the same patient's change over time in negative symptoms as measured by the Scale for the Assessment of Negative Symptoms (SANS) $(r = 0.72$, $P < .05)$. In conclusion, this series of studies in a variety of neuropsychiatric populations suggests that the within-subject correlations between changes in a neurophysiological parameter (here D_2 receptor binding) and clinical symptoms are attainable.

How might one use this relationship to guide treatment? The idea that we can reliably monitor pharmacological manipulations of neurophysiology with functional neuroimaging has been demonstrated in healthy control subjects. Using H_2O^{15} PET, Mattay et al. (1996) administered dextroamphetamine to healthy control subjects performing two abstract reasoning tasks: the Wisconsin Card Sorting Task (WCST), a measure of working memory, and Ravens Progressive Matrices (RPM), a nonverbal intelligence test. The drug did not change rCBF in a fixed, stereotyped manner. Instead, the effect varied depending on the task, as rCBF was altered most in the regions (and presumably the networks) that are specific for each task. Thus, we may be able to measure the same kind of subtle pharmacological effects in patient populations. To some degree, this is already happening. For example, a number of groups have correlated measures of dopamine D_2 receptor occupancy with clinical response to and side effects from antipsychotic drugs (Farde et al. 1992; Klemm et al. 1996; Knable et al. 1997). Having thus assured ourselves that "clinical" functional neuroimaging is feasible, let us turn to the question of new technologies.

Recent Advances in Neuroimaging: Promise and Pitfalls

Two recent neuroimaging tools under development in several centers and extensively used in our laboratory are ¹H-MRSI and fMRI. Preliminary results gathered with these technologies highlight both the improvements in methodology (e.g., resolution) and a trend toward greater integration of structural and functional neuroimaging. However, early experience suggests an awareness of their limitations is necessary before assessing their future in clinical practice.

There continues to be a large gap between our appreciation of the gross anatomical structure of individual brains and our understanding of the neuronal function within these structures. Traditionally, radiotracer studies have defined the measurable parameters in brain function. As detailed above, these techniques allow us to measure rCBF, regional metabolism via glucose consumption, and finally local concentrations of neurotransmitter receptors using radiolabeled compounds. However, the expense, the need for special facilities (e.g., an onsite cyclotron for PET), the issue of radiation exposure, the limited spatial and temporal resolution, and the need for complex algorithms to interpret these data are some of the factors that diminish their clinical usefulness. Furthermore, because these methods rely on group-averaged data and cannot as readily create functional maps for individual patients, their widespread clinical use may always be limited.

In this context, ^{1}H-MRSI is unique. It provides a new kind of information that may link abnormalities of cognitive function and of other complex behaviors with intracellular processes. ^{1}H-MRSI, at least at long echo times, measures the relative concentrations of N-acetyl aspartate (NAA), creatine/phosphocreatine (CRE), choline-containing moieties (CHO), and lactate. The complexity of this information is exemplified by the wide spectrum of intracellular processes represented by these signals. As key metabolites in cellular metabolism, the CRE signal may reflect relative neuronal activity. At the same time, CHO may reflect ongoing turnover of cell wall constituents, like phosphocholine and glycerophosphocholine, and may be a sensitive indicator of astrocytic proliferation (Urenjak et al. 1993). NAA is of particular interest to neuroscientists because it appears to be located exclusively in neurons (Urenjak et al. 1993). As such, NAA may be a measure of neuronal vitality, although it is unclear on what scale NAA reflects state and/or trait characteristics of neurons (Miller 1991). A number of single-voxel ^{1}H-MRSI studies have, for the most part, demonstrated regional pathology in mesial temporal cortex and frontal lobes of patients with schizophrenia (Buckley et al. 1994; Maier et al. 1995; Nasrallah et al. 1994; Renshaw et al. 1995; Yurgelun-Todd et al. 1996a).

A series of experiments in our laboratory by Bertolino and colleagues has extended these early findings to the interface of clinical and basic research, another step that may be required to map mental illness (Mazziotta 1996). Using ^{1}H-MRSI (Duyn et al. 1993), an MRS technique with greater brain coverage and spatial resolution, Bertolino et al. (1996, 1998a, 1998b) found a bilateral reduction in NAA in the hippocampus and dorsolateral prefrontal cortex in three cohorts of patients with schizophrenia (one of which included neuroleptic-naive patients). That these abnormalities were regionally specific and not associated with increases in CHO signals suggestive of gliosis seems consistent with data from prior neuropathological and neuroimaging studies suggesting a neurodevelopmental etiology for schizophrenia (Weinberger 1995). As an exploration of the hypothesis that a developmental insult to prefrontal–temporolimbic connectivity might lead to the pattern of regional neuronal pathology suggested by the NAA findings in schizophrenia, Bertolino et al. (1997) performed ^{1}H-MRSI on a cohort of adult rhesus monkeys that included subjects that had experienced mesial temporal cortex ablations as neonates and subjects that had experienced similar ablations as adults. Remarkably, the monkeys whose lesions occurred neonatally exhibited a significant reduction in prefrontal NAA not shared by the animals whose lesions occurred in adulthood. This finding suggests that the developmental insult has a unique impact on the development and maturation of prefrontal cortex. This may in turn mirror a process in humans wherein an insult during a crucial phase of prenatal development leads to adult psychopathology accompanied by abnormal prefrontal and temporolimbic NAA concentrations. Nevertheless, there are limitations to the methodology, including the unclear role of the metabolites measured, large voxel sizes (and associated partial-volume effects), uncertain effects of subject motion, and variability in the data (Bertolino et al. 1998b). These problems must be overcome before this assay can move into the realm of clinical practice.

Another rapidly developing MRI technique, fMRI, has been touted as a paradigm shift in functional neuroimaging. Although initial work with fMRI involved dynamic tracking of a bolus of paramagnetic contrast agent (e.g., gadolinium), fMRI studies have increasingly exploited signal changes related to the blood oxygenation level–dependent (BOLD) effect. Simply put, the BOLD effect is thought to arise as local blood flow changes caused by neuronal activity alter the local concentration of deoxygenated hemoglobin. Deoxyhemoglobin is paramagnetic; as such it exaggerates local magnetic field inhomogeneities (i.e., T2-star [T2*] effects) causing nuclear spin dephasing and loss of the signal. Since increases in local neuronal activity increase rCBF in excess of oxygen utilization (Raichle et al. 1976), relatively more oxygenated hemoglobin is delivered to the active region, thereby diluting the deoxyhemoglobin present (reducing T2*-induced signal decay) and thus increasing the local fMRI signal (Ogawa et al. 1990, 1992).

As a less invasive, nonradioactive methodology, fMRI also offers improved spatial and temporal resolution, virtually unlimited study repetitions, straightforward registration of functional and anatomic scans, and use of widely available MRI scanners (Levin et al. 1995). These characteristics, particularly the repeatability and noninvasiveness of fMRI, offer the unique potential to generate reliable individual data (Table 8–1). In turn, individual data might allow us to address a number of long-standing issues in functional neuroimaging, including the distinction between state and trait characteristics, the effects of medication, the reliability of findings, and the temporal evolution of adaptation (plasticity) or neuropathology (progression). Our understanding of healthy human brain function will be advanced enormously by studies in novel populations like children (Casey et al. 1995) or at-risk individuals. As suggested by functional studies of phenotypic variability (Wolf et al. 1996), neurophysiological variables may be particularly useful in generating quantifiable characteristics for genetic linkage studies (Benjamin and Gershon 1996; Flint et al. 1995). Finally, the impending development of

Table 8–1. Unique potential of functional magnetic resonance imaging (fMRI) in psychiatry

Within-subject studies

Mapping individual neurophysiology to individual neuropsychology

Characterizing state-dependent variability

Clarifying confounding variables (e.g., medication effects)

Improving reliability of findings

Understanding temporal resolution of neural function (e.g., plasticity)

Studies of novel populations

At-risk subjects

Children

Genetic linkage: physiological correlates of phenotypic variability

Real-time interactive studies: the "physiological interview"

Source. Adapted from Weinberger et al. 1996.

"real-time" functional MRI (Frank et al., in press), in which an investigator has immediate data feedback while the subject is still in the scanner, promises true interactive studies—the "physiological interview."

Although a number of groups have begun applying fMRI to the study of mental illness (Breiter et al. 1996; Renshaw et al. 1994; Schroder et al. 1995; Yurgelun-Todd et al. 1996b), it has been increasingly apparent that failure to systematically control for artifacts renders any such work difficult to interpret (Hajnal et al. 1994, 1995; Weinberger et al. 1996; Weisskoff 1995). Recently, we utilized the three-dimensional fMRI technique—Principles of Echo Shifting with a Train of Observations (Ramsey et al. 1996; VanGelderen et al. 1995)—to study 10 patients with schizophrenia and 10 matched control subjects (Callicott et al. 1998). We used a version of the "n" back working memory task (Cohen et al. 1994; Gevins et al. 1990) specifically designed to probe prefrontal cortex (PFC) function and to generate a signal in contralateral sensorimotor cortex as an "internal" activation standard or quality control. In the initial analysis, we found a predictable lack of PFC activation in patients with schizophrenia (9 of 10 did not activate PFC). At the same time, however, we found what appeared to be a group difference in sensorimotor cortex activation. Closer examination of these data revealed a systematic group difference in signal intensity variance, most likely the result of increased motion by some of the patients during the scan procedure. Subsequently, we matched patients and control subjects for a measure of variance, producing a subsample of six patients and six control subjects. All of these patients and control subjects activated the sensorimotor control region (eliminating the spurious finding), whereas patients (5 of 6) still did not activate PFC. We used this experience to illustrate the need for a systematic approach to the acquisition, analysis, and evaluation of these data (summarized in Table 8–2). These MRI technologies promise much in terms of ease of use, noninvasiveness, and improved spatial and temporal resolution. However, the dependent variables measured (e.g., metabolite "ratios" or the BOLD effect) are not straightforward, like cerebral blood flow, and thus bring the attendant risks of oversimplification until more is understood of their details.

Table 8–2. A structured approach to the evaluation of functional magnetic resonance imaging (fMRI) data

Stage 1: Data acquisition

1. Machine-related artifact: standardized assessment of machine stability (e.g., signal drift, field characteristics)

2. Subject-related artifact

   a. *Physiological variability:*

      i. Assessment of physiological parameters during experiment (e.g., end-tidal CO_2, pulse)

      ii. Use of "gated" pulse sequences

   b. *Movement:* prevention through head immobilization

Stage 2: Data analysis ("quality control")

1. Standardized assessment of motion correction (registration)

   a. Visual inspection for postregistration residual movement (e.g., cine loop)

   b. Examination for "edge artifacts"

   c. Comparison across groups (or time) of motion correction parameters (translation, pitch, roll, yaw)

2. Examination of signal change time course in "activated" voxels

3. Comparison of activation in pathophysiologically neutral region: the "internal activation standard"

4. Comparison across groups (or time) of voxel variance (e.g., pooled standard deviation)

Stage 3: Evaluation of results

1. Use of stringently defined threshold for "activation"

2. Placing activation into context: cautious reification of activation in "new" regions (e.g., hypothesis-driven vs. catalogue approach)

Source. Adapted from Callicott et al. 1998.

Conclusions

Although few clinical applications for functional neuroimaging currently exist, ample evidence suggests that these applications are likely on the way. In the infancy of twentieth-century neuropsychiatric research, a similar crossroads was confronted in applying the early techniques of neuropathology. Researchers were unable to discover clear, discrete neuropathological lesions underlying mental illness. Though some abandoned their search for underlying "biological" causes for these illnesses based on this early failure, history suggests that technological advances and an expanding understanding of brain function opened new chapters for those who persevered. As we have seen, we are capable of accessing a variety of information regarding healthy and diseased brain function. This information is slowly beginning to inform clinical practice. Functional neuroimaging may allow a radical reframing of our understanding of the clinical psychiatric syndromes by identifying neurophysiological phenotypes that may be more "valid" or "reliable" than current classifications based on often difficult-to-quantify and overlapping symptomatology (Callicott et al., in press). Furthermore, these phenotypes may refine our search for the etiopathogenesis of mental illness through genetic linkage studies. In the tradition of the neuropsychologist's testing battery, functional neuroimagers may wield a number of neurophysiological probes— components of a "physiological interview"—which may be a fruitful addition to clinical practice. Finally, as we develop new neuroimaging technologies, we must also avoid pitfalls by controlling, as much as possible, for methodological artifact.

References

Baxter L: PET studies of cerebral function in major depression and obsessive-compulsive disorder: the emerging prefrontal cortex consensus. Ann Clin Psychiatry 3:103–109, 1991

Baxter L: Neuroimaging studies of obsessive-compulsive disorder. Psychiatr Clin North Am 15:871–884, 1992

Baxter L, Phelps M, Mazziotta J, et al: Local cerebral metabolic rates in obsessive-compulsive disorder. Arch Gen Psychiatry 44:211–281, 1987

Baxter L, Schwartz J, Phelps M, et al: Reduction of prefrontal cortex glucose metabolism common to three types of depression. Arch Gen Psychiatry 46:243–250, 1989

Belliveau JW, Kennedy DN, McKinstry RC: Functional mapping of the human visual cortex by magnetic resonance imaging. Science 254:716–719, 1991

Benjamin J, Gershon E: Genetic discoveries in human behavior: small effect genes loom large. Biol Psychiatry 40:313–316, 1996

Berger H: Uber das elektrekephalogramm des menchen. Archiv fur Psychiatrie und Nervenkrankheiten 87:527–570, 1929

Berman KF, Weinberger DR: Functional localization in the brain in schizophrenia, in American Psychiatric Press Review of Psychiatry, Vol 10. Edited by Tasman A, Goldfinger SM. Washington, DC, American Psychiatric Press, 1991, pp 24–59

Bertolino A, Nawroz S, Mattay V, et al: Regionally specific pattern of neurochemical pathology in schizophrenia as assessed by multislice proton magnetic resonance spectroscopic imaging. Am J Psychiatry 153:1554–1563, 1996

Bertolino A, Saunders R, Mattay V, et al: Altered development of prefrontal neurons in rhesus monkeys with neonatal mesial temporo-limbic lesions: a proton magnetic resonance spectroscopic imaging study. Cereb Cortex 7:740–748, 1997

Bertolino A, Callicott J, Ellman I, et al: Regionally specific neuronal pathology in untreated patients with schizophrenia: a proton magnetic resonance spectroscopic imaging study. Biol Psychiatry 43:641–648, 1998a

Bertolino A, Callicott J, Nawroz S, et al: Reproducibility of proton magnetic resonance spectroscopic imaging in patients with schizophrenia. Neuropsychopharmacology 18:1–9, 1998b

Breiter HC, Rauch SL, Kwong KK, et al: Functional magnetic resonance imaging of symptom provocation in obsessive-compulsive disorder. Arch Gen Psychiatry 53:595–606, 1996

Buckley P, Moore C, Long H, et al: ^{1}H-Magnetic resonance spectroscopy of the left temporal and frontal lobes in schizophrenia: clinical neurodevelopmental and cognitive correlates. Biol Psychiatry 36:792–800, 1994

Callicott J, Ramsey N, Tallent K, et al: fMRI brain mapping in psychiatry: methodological issues and a study of working memory in schizophrenia. Neuropsychopharmacology 18:186–196, 1998

Callicott J, Egan M, Bertolino A, et al: Hippocampal N-acetyl aspartate in unaffected siblings of patients with schizophrenia: a possible intermediate neurobiological phenotype. Biol Psychiatry (in press)

Casey BJ, Cohen JD, Jezzard P, et al: Activation of prefrontal cortex in children during a nonspatial working memory task with functional MRI. Neuroimage 2:221–229, 1995

Cohen JD, Forman SD, Braver TS, et al: Activation of the prefrontal cortex in a nonspatial working memory task with functional MRI. Human Brain Mapping 1:293–304, 1994

Dager S, Green R: Applications of magnetic resonance spectroscopy to the investigation of neuropsychiatric disorders. Neuropsychopharmacology 6:249–266, 1992

Duyn J, Gillen J, Sobering G, et al: Multisection proton MR spectroscopic imaging of the brain. Radiology 188:277–282, 1993

Farde L, Nordstrom A, Wiesel F, et al: Positron emission tomographic analysis of central D_1 and D_2 dopamine receptor occupancy in patients treated with classical neuroleptics and clozapine: relation to extrapyramidal side effects. Arch Gen Psychiatry 49:538–544, 1992

Flint J, Corley R, Defries J, et al: A simple genetic basis for a complex psychological trait in laboratory mice. Science 269:1432–1435, 1995

Frank J, Ostoni J, Yang Y, et al: A technical solution for an interactive fMRI examination: application to a physiological interview and the study of cerebral physiology. Radiology (in press)

Gevins A, Bressler S, Cutillo B, et al: Effects of prolonged mental work on functional brain topography. Electroencephalogr Clin Neurophysiol 76:339–350, 1990

Gur R, Erwin R, Gur R: Neurobehavioral probes for physiologic neuroimaging studies. Arch Gen Psychiatry 49:409–414, 1992

Guze B, Hoffman J, Baxter L, et al: Functional brain imaging and Alzheimer-type dementia. Alzheimer Dis Assoc Disord 5:215–230, 1991

Hajnal JV, Myers R, Oatridge A, et al: Artifacts due to stimulus correlated motion in functional imaging of the brain. Magn Reson Med 31:283–291, 1994

Hajnal JV, Bydder GM, Young IR: fMRI: does correlation imply activation? NMR Biomed 8:97–100, 1995

Hartshorne M: Single photon emission computed tomography, in Functional Brain Imaging. Edited by Orison W, Lewine J, Saunders J, et al. St. Louis, MO, CV Mosby, 1995, pp 213–238

Haxby J, Duara R, Grady C, et al: Relationship between neuropsychological and cerebral metabolic asymmetries in early Alzheimer's disease. J Cereb Blood Flow Metab 5:193–200, 1985

Herscovitch P: Radiotracer techniques for functional neuroimaging with positron emission tomography, in Functional Neuroimaging: Technical Foundations. Edited by Thatcher R, Hallet M, Zeffiro T, et al. San Diego, CA, Academic Press, 29–46, 1994

Huang S, Phelps M, Hoffman E, et al: Noninvasive determination of local cerebral metabolic rate of glucose in man. Am J Physiol 238:E69–E82, 1980

Ingvar D, Franzen G: Distribution of cerebral activity in chronic schizophrenia. Lancet 2:1484–1486, 1974

Kety S, Schmidt C: The determination of cerebral blood flow in man by the use of nitrous oxide in low concentrations. Am J Physiol 143:43, 1945

Kety S, Schmidt C: Effects of altered arterial tensions of carbon dioxide and oxygen on cerebral blood flow and cerebral oxygen consumption of normal young men. J Clin Invest 27:484, 1948

Klemm E, Grunvald F, Kasper S, et al: I-123 IBZM SPECT for imaging of striatal D_2 dopamine receptors in 56 schizophrenic patients taking various neuroleptics. Am J Psychiatry 153:183–190, 1996

Knable M, Jones D, Coppola R, et al: Lateralized differences in iodine-123-IBZM up-take in the basal ganglia in asymmetric Parkinson's disease. J Nucl Med 36:1216–1225, 1995

Knable M, Heinz A, Raedler T, et al: Extrapyramidal side effects with risperidone and haloperidol at comparable D_2 receptor occupancy levels. Psychiatry Res 75: 91–101, 1997

Levin J, Ross M, Renshaw P: Clinical applications of functional MRI in neuro-psychiatry. J Neuropsychiatry Clin Neurosci 7:511–522, 1995

Lewine J, Orison W: Clinical electroencephalography and event-related potentials, in Functional Brain Imaging. Edited by Orison W, Lewine J, Saunders J, et al. St. Louis, MO, CV Mosby, 1995, pp 327–368

Liddle P: Brain imaging, in Schizophrenia. Edited by Hirsch S, Weinberger D. London, Blackwood Press, 1995, 425–439

Liddle P, Friston K, Frith C, et al: Patterns of cerebral blood flow in schizophrenia. Br J Psychiatry 160:179–186, 1992

Machlin S, Harris G, Pearlson G, et al: Elevated medial-frontal cerebral blood flow in obsessive-compulsive patients: a SPECT study. Am J Psychiatry 148:1240–1242, 1991

Maier M, Ron M, Barker G, et al: Proton magnetic resonance spectroscopy: an in-vivo method of estimating hippocampal neuronal depletion in schizophrenia. Psychol Med 25:1201–1209, 1995

Mattay V, Berman K, Ostrem J, et al: Dextroamphetamine enhances "neural network-specific" physiological signals: a positron-emission tomography rCBF study. J Neurosci 16:4816–4822, 1996

Mazziotta J: Mapping mental illness: a new era. Arch Gen Psychiatry 53:374–376, 1996

Miller B: A review of chemical issues in ^{1}H NMR spectroscopy: N-acetyl-l-aspartate, creatine and choline. NMR Biomed 4:47–52, 1991

Nasrallah H, Skinner T, Schmalbrock P, et al: Proton magnetic resonance spectroscopy of the hippocampal formation in schizophrenia: a pilot study. Br J Psychiatry 165:481–485, 1994

Ogawa S, Lee T-M, Nayak AS, et al: Oxygenation-sensitive contrast in magnetic resonance image of rodent brain at high magnetic fields. Magn Reson Med 14:68–78, 1990

Ogawa S, Tank DW, Menon R, et al: Intrinsic signal changes accompanying sensory stimulation: functional brain mapping with magnetic resonance imaging. Proc Natl Acad Sci U S A 89:5951–5955, 1992

Raichle MR, Robert L, Grubb J, et al: Correlation between regional cerebral blood flow and oxidative metabolism: in vivo studies in man. Arch Neurol 33:523–526, 1976

Ramsey NF, Kirkby BS, Gelderen PV, et al: Functional mapping of human sensorimotor cortex with 3D BOLD fMRI correlates with $H_2^{15}0$ PET rCBF. J Cereb Blood Flow Metab 16:755–764, 1996

Rauch S, Jenike M, Alpert N, et al: Regional cerebral blood flow measured during symptom provocation in obsessive-compulsive disorder using ^{15}O-labeled CO_2 and positron emission tomography. Arch Gen Psychiatry 51:62–70, 1994

Reeve A, Rose D, Weinberger D: Magnetoencephalography. Applications in psychiatry. Arch Gen Psychiatry 46:573–576, 1989

Reivich M, Kuhl D, Wolf A, et al: The [^{18}F]fluorodeoxyglucose method for the measurement of local cerebral glucose utilization in man. Circ Res 44:127–137, 1979

Renshaw PF, Yurgelun-Todd DA, Cohen BM: Greater hemodynamic response to photic stimulation in schizophrenic patients: an echo planar MRI study. Am J Psychiatry 151:1493–1495, 1994

Renshaw P, Yurgelun-Todd D, Tohen M, et al: Temporal lobe proton magnetic resonance spectroscopy of patients with first-episode psychosis. Am J Psychiatry 152:444–446, 1995

Rogers R: Magnetoencephalographic imaging of cognitive processes, in Functional Neuroimaging: Technical Foundations. Edited by Thatcher R, Hallet M, Zeffiro T, et al. San Diego, CA, Academic Press, 1994, pp 289–297

Rosen B, Belliveau J, Chien D: Perfusion imaging by nuclear magnetic resonance. Magnetic Resonance Quarterly 5:263–281, 1989

Roy C, Sherrington C: On the regulation of the blood supply of the brain. J Physiol 11:85–108, 1890

Sanders J: Magnetic resonance spectroscopy, in Functional Brain Imaging. Edited by Orison W, Lewine J, Saunders J, Hartshorne M. St. Louis, MO, CV Mosby, 1995, 419–467

Schroder J, Wenz F, Schad LR, et al: Sensorimotor cortex and supplementary motor area changes in schizophrenia: a study with functional magnetic resonance imaging. Br J Psychiatry 167:197–201, 1995

Sedvall G, Farde L, Persson A, et al: Imaging of neurotransmitter receptors in the living human brain. Arch Gen Psychiatry 43:995–1005, 1986

Turner R: Magnetic resonance imaging of brain function. American Journal of Physiologic Imaging 7:136–145, 1992

Urenjak J, Williams S, Gadian D, et al: Proton nuclear magnetic resonance spectroscopy unambiguously identifies different neural cell types. J Neurosci 13:981–989, 1993

VanGelderen P, Ramsey NF, Liu G, et al: Three-dimensional functional magnetic resonance imaging of human brain on a clinical 1.5-T scanner. Proc Natl Acad Sci U S A 92:6906–6910, 1995

Weinberger DR: Schizophrenia as a neurodevelopmental disorder: a review of the concept, in Schizophrenia. Edited by Hirsch SR, Weinberger DR. London, Blackwood Press, 1995, pp 293–323

Weinberger DR, Berman KF: Prefrontal function in schizophrenia: confounds and controversies. Philos Trans R Soc Lond B Biol Sci 351:1495–1503, 1996

Weinberger D, Berman K, Zec R: Physiological dysfunction of dorsolateral prefrontal cortex in schizophrenia, I: regional cerebral blood flow evidence. Arch Gen Psychiatry 43:114–124, 1986

Weinberger DR, Mattay V, Callicott J, et al: fMRI applications in schizophrenia research. Neuroimage 4:5118–5126, 1996

Weisskoff RM: Functional MRI: are we moving towards artifactual conclusions? Or fMRI fact or fancy? NMR Biomed 8:101–103, 1995

Wolf S, Jones D, Knable M, et al: Tourette syndrome: prediction of phenotypic variation in monozygotic twins by caudate nucleus D_2 receptor binding. Science 273:1225–1227, 1996

Ye F, Pekar J, Jezzard P, et al: Perfusion imaging of the human brain at 1.5 T using single-shot EPI spin tagging approach. Magn Reson Med 36:219–224, 1996

Yurgelun-Todd D, Renshaw P, Gruber S, et al: Proton magnetic resonance spectroscopy of patients with first-episode psychosis. Schizophr Res 152:444–446, 1996a

Yurgelun-Todd DA, Waternaux CM, Cohen BM, et al: Functional magnetic resonance imaging of schizophrenic patients and comparison subjects during word production. Am J Psychiatry 153:200–205, 1996b

SECTION II

The Practice of Psychiatry

INTRODUCTION

A close scrutiny of how psychiatry was practiced in the United States in each decade since the end of World War II would demonstrate the existence of only one constant, change. In this section, we will elaborate on the varied issues that affect the shape of psychiatric practice today and its likely evolution.

In Chapter 9, Practice Guidelines in Psychiatry and a Psychiatric Practice Research Network, John McIntyre, Deborah Zarin, and Harold Pincus first present a review of the process in which practice (treatment) parameters or guidelines were developed for all of American medicine. They then address the specific activities that have led to the development by the American Psychiatric Association of broadly based psychiatric practice guidelines. The process is presented in a format that national psychiatric societies in other nations could use in developing their own psychiatric practice guidelines.

Having addressed the development of practice guidelines, the authors then describe how the American Psychiatric Association has developed a practice research network (PRN) utilizing the experiences of pediatrics and family practice associations in its establishment. The practice research network allows psychiatry to develop a natural national laboratory based on the practices of a representative sample of psychiatrists to assess the effectiveness of varied treatment approaches. It also allows the discipline to examine change in practice patterns brought about either by economic factors or research in the conduct of practice.

Together, practice guidelines and the practice research network are presented as a way that a national professional society can ensure the quality of professional practice. This can be done by monitoring the conduct of practitioners joined in a practice research network.

In Chapter 10, The Psychiatrist as Psychotherapist, Glen Gabbard reviews the evolving role of psychotherapy as a core skill or competency of psychiatrists. He explores the contemporary reasons for its apparent decline in importance in recent decades. He further argues that to allow psychotherapy to be lost as one of the core therapies of psychiatry could sound the death knell of the specialty.

To elaborate on his argument, Gabbard presents a series of examples wherein a knowledge of psychotherapy is critical in providing competent care even if the major element of care is use of medication or another similar therapy. Gabbard states further that the psychiatrist cannot be an expert in all psychotherapies but must remain knowledgeable in their optimal uses. Gabbard also reviews the residency training necessary in psychotherapy for psychiatric residents.

In Chapter 11, Psychopharmacology in the New Millennium: Emphasis on Depression, by Alan Schatzberg, we are introduced to a review of the current and near-term psychopharmacological approaches to the treatment of depression. Schatzberg uses depression as a model to guide us in developing a conceptual approach the clinician can use to understand psychopharmacologic research. Not surprisingly, when he discusses our current understanding of why it can take antidepressants up to 3 weeks to affect depression, he reconnects us to the earlier presentation of Hyman and our need to understand second-messenger systems in the cell by the use of molecular biology.

Strikingly, Schatzberg notes that neurosciences and thus psychopharmacology alone are not enough to effectively understand and treat our patients and practice psychiatry.

In Chapter 12, A Clinical Model for Selecting Psychotherapy or Pharmacotherapy, Mark Levey addresses the implicit complexity the practicing psychiatrist faces in initiating a treatment employing both approaches. We learn that two quite different theoretical models are used by practitioners who utilize both treatment modalities at one time with one patient. One view sees the joint use of pharmacotherapy and psychotherapy as combining two distinct treatment approaches to address symptoms that have either biological or psychological causality. For example, pharmacotherapy is used for Axis I DSM-IV diagnoses and psychotherapy for Axis II diagnoses. Levey demonstrates that this is, at best, an artificial distinction. He observes that obsessive-compulsive patients treated effectively with either medication or psychotherapy demonstrate comparable brain changes. In light of this, Levey proposes an integrated approach. The clinician assesses the patient and individualizes the treatment to the uniqueness of the patient, not the theoretical framework of the clinician. Levey offers clinical examples of his model. Although he does not discuss this, an example of the combined approach versus an integrated one is when the psychiatrist prescribes medication and a non-physician provides psychotherapy. Following Levey's model, one can distinguish patients for whom this is potentially effective as well as situations in which it is not likely to be helpful to the patient.

In Chapter 13, Studying the Respective Contributions of Pharmacotherapy and Psychotherapy: Toward Collaborative Controlled Studies, Donald Klein explores the difficulty in developing research to understand how these two modalities, when applied concurrently to treatment, work together. If, as our contributors note, behavior can be understood only by using our evolving neuroscience approaches coupled with understanding of the diverse aspects of the human environment that affect behavior, then treatment to change behavior must also link these variables. Psychotherapy as a means of modulating certain variables has a critical role in changing behavior. Klein tells us how much more we need to know and do to understand how to effectively assess joint treatments.

In Chapter 14, Less is More: Financing Mental Health Care for the New Century, Steven Sharfstein reviews the history of mental health care in the United States for the past 150 years. He notes that what have started in the past as reform movements became crude ways to shift the expense of caring for the mentally ill from one governmental jurisdiction to another. First was the asylum movement in the 1850s. This collapsed as a reform and became a means of shifting the cost and care of individuals from local communities to state government. A hundred years later, the community mental health movement used federal dollars to shift costs away from the states. This led to the emptying of state hospitals and the return of patients to the community with a portion of funding from the federal government. Today, Sharfstein points out, managed care uses market forces to further reduce or shift the cost of mental health care.

Sharfstein reviews the development of managed care and addresses the damage it has done to mental health care as well as its current positive contributions and how, if effectively harnessed, it can contribute to quality mental health care.

Sharfstein looks to the future and predicts a development of universal health insurance for all Americans. In this context, we see a vital psychiatry, but one that will need to respond to new challenges of cost effectiveness.

In Chapter 15, The Ethical Conduct of the Psychiatrist, Jeremy Lazarus introduces us to an area where we frequently feel our practice values and code of conduct are long-standing and fixed, only to discover, as we approach the twenty-first century, that they are as fluid and changing as is the rest of our field. Lazarus traces for us the evolution of medical ethics from the Code of Hammurabi in 2000 B.C. to the present. He points out that we are confronted by challenges in each area of our practice. New technologies and science create one set. Clinical demands require a need to affirm the significance of the doctor–patient relationship and to affirm and maintain the essential boundaries between doctor and patient. Yet Lazarus concludes with an echo from Sharfstein that the most profound ethical challenges we face are related to the economics of health care. Can a psychiatrist effectively advocate for his or her patient while appropriately utilizing the fixed resources available for a population? Should such roles be split to avoid conflicts of interest? If we see patients as customers or consumers, will we use business ethics rather than the ethical standards initially described in the Hippocratic Oath? Lazarus' chapter gives us a sobering view of the ethical standards we must maintain and the challenges we face to do it.

CHAPTER 9

Practice Guidelines in Psychiatry and a Psychiatric Practice Research Network

John S. McIntyre, M.D.
Deborah A. Zarin, M.D.
Harold A. Pincus, M.D.

Under the leadership initially of Dr. Melvin Sabshin and currently of Dr. Steve Mirin, the American Psychiatric Association (APA) has for the past two decades firmly and systematically moved the field in the direction of evidence-based psychiatry. Beginning with a criteria-based nomenclature, the APA has developed a rigorous process for the development of practice guidelines. The association has organized a practice research network that is adding substantially to its database. This chapter focuses on these efforts, describing in detail the APA's practice guideline project and reviewing the development of the APA's practice research network.

Practice guidelines are systematically developed strategies of patient care that are developed to assist clinicians (and patients) in clinical decision making (McIntyre and Talbott 1990). Eddy (1990) used the term *parameters* to encompass standards, guidelines, and options. In this framework, standards are instructions that should be followed in essentially all cases. Exceptions to the recommended approach should be rare and require considerable justification. Guidelines are recommendations that should be followed in the large majority of cases. Exceptions are more frequent and require minimal justification. Options are clinical strategies in clinical contexts in which there is no clearly preferred strategy. Using these definitions, the APA chose the term *guidelines* to describe its recommendations in this arena, and that is the term that will be used throughout this chapter.

In the last decade throughout medicine there has been an explosion in the development of practice guidelines. Guidelines are being developed by professional associations, insurance companies, health maintenance organizations (HMOs), provider groups, state governments, and the federal government. Guidelines have become essential to accreditation processes and are beginning to influence educational programs.

There are several reasons for the heightened interest in the development of practice guidelines.

1. There has been an exponential growth in our knowledge base. Physicians even in subspecialty areas experience increasing difficulty staying abreast of the latest research findings, and for the generalist the problem is greatly magnified. Even when one is knowledgeable about the most recent studies, it is not always easy to determine the optimal clinical strategy for an individual patient. The data must be integrated and prioritized to become part of a patient care strategy.

2. In part because of the knowledge explosion and the development of expensive technology, health care costs have risen dramatically, and cost containment has become a pervasive concern. Identifying treatments that are effective as well as those that are not has become an economic imperative.

3. Numerous studies have demonstrated that there is significant regional variation in treatment approaches for a given illness (Chassin et al. 1986; Lewis 1969). National guidelines are one approach to addressing this issue.

4. Increasingly, patients and potential patients participate in the decisions concerning the choice of treatments. This reality necessitates a clear description of treatment options and the evidence supporting the various choices.

Although these reasons have coalesced to account for the recent great upsurge in guideline development, parameters of care have been published for centuries. In American psychiatry such instructions for practice go back to the beginning of the APA in 1844. In 1851, the association approved 26 propositions relative to "the construction of hospitals for the insane" (American Psychiatric Association 1851). In the following year it adopted 14 propositions relative to the organization of these facilities (American Psychiatric Association 1853). Although these nationally approved guidelines or standards were pronouncements by recognized experts, they differ from recent guidelines in that there was no attempt to provide any data that supported the various recommendations. More recent APA works such as the Task Force Reports on Benzodiazepines and Laboratory Tests in Psychiatry include evidence for the recommendations but lack the formal and systematic development process that characterizes the practice guidelines (American Psychiatric Association 1985, 1990).

This historical progression of guideline development in psychiatry is similar to what has happened throughout medicine. Over 50 years ago the American Academy of Pediatrics issued statements on immunization that resemble guidelines. However, in the last decade it became clear that some standardization of guideline development would be useful—guidelines for guidelines! The Institute of Medicine and the American Medical Association (AMA) have both developed a series of principles to be followed in the development of practice guidelines. The AMA's efforts have emerged from the Practice Parameters Partnership begun in 1989, which includes 14 major medical associations, including the American Psychiatric Association (Table 9–1). The partnership receives input from the Practice Parameters Forum, also coordinated by the AMA and representing more than 65 medical specialty organizations and state medical societies. Also regularly participating in the work of the partnership are the American Hospital Association, the Joint Commission on Accreditation of Healthcare Organizations, the Agency for Health Care Policy and Research, and the Health Care Financing Administration. The AMA partnership initially described the following five "attributes" that guidelines should reflect (American Medical Association 1990):

- Be developed by or in conjunction with physician organizations.
- Use reliable methodologies that integrate relevant research findings and clinical expertise.
- Be as comprehensive and specific as possible.
- Be based on current information.
- Be widely disseminated.

In 1996 the partnership added a sixth attribute: guideline development should include outcomes research, goals, and measures.

The Institute of Medicine (IOM) identified eight attributes of good guidelines (Institute of Medicine 1992):

Table 9–1.   Practice Parameters Partnership
American Academy of Family Physicians
American Academy of Ophthalmology
American Academy of Orthopaedic Surgeons
American Academy of Pediatrics
American College of Cardiology
American College of Obstetricians and Gynecologists
American College of Radiology
American College of Surgeons
American Medical Association
American Psychiatric Association
American Society of Anesthesiologists
American Society of Internal Medicine
American Urological Association
College of American Pathologists

- Validity,
- Reproducibility,
- Clinical applicability,
- Clinical flexibility,
- Clarity,
- Multidisciplinary process,
- Scheduled review, and
- Documentation.

The attributes of the Practice Parameters Partnership and the IOM have together essentially set national standards for guideline efforts.

Although physicians and physician organizations are now heavily involved in guideline development and dissemination, there was initially considerable resistance (which continues in muted tones) to the concept of practice guidelines. The major opposition has been based on the concern that guidelines promote "cookbook" medicine—a sterile, oversimplified, and rigid set of prescriptions that do not take into account individual symptoms in patient illnesses and that ignore subtleties in clinical work and the concept of the "art of medicine" ("Legislated Clinical Medicine," 1990). There are also concerns that guidelines will limit innovations in practice and increase professional liability exposure. In psychiatry, a process that is evidence-based and open and that has involved a large number of clinicians (see below) has decreased some of these concerns, and most psychiatrists have experienced the completed guidelines as being flexible and appropriately attending to the many variables in the expression of illness and the strategies for care. However, there remains a valid concern that the guideline process might diminish clinical innovation, retarding the development of novel approaches to patient care. Well-developed guidelines minimize this possibility by not overstating the evidence from research or clinical consensus and by clearly identifying the areas of relative uncertainty. At this time the impact of guidelines on professional liability exposure remains unclear. At least one study reports that guidelines are more frequently used by plaintiffs' attorneys than defense attorneys (Hyams et al. 1995). However, there are significant data to the contrary, including the significant (25%) decrease in anesthesiologists' professional liability insurance premiums and similar reductions in obstetricians' and gynecologists' premiums when guidelines were accepted by their national association ("OBGYN Premiums Decrease Drastically," 1993; Garnick et al. 1991). In fact, there are pilot programs in some jurisdictions (e.g., Maine) in which compliance with guidelines can be used only as an affirmative malpractice defense. Although the debate on this issue continues, the prediction that guidelines will result in decreased professional liability exposure seems to be increasingly favored. Further protection for the clinician results from a clear qualifying description of the intent and limitations of the guidelines. Each APA guideline has a clearly worded "statement of intent" serving this purpose (see below).

American Psychiatric Association Practice Guideline Project

In 1989, the APA Assembly approved an action paper urging the association to develop practice guidelines. Subsequently, the APA Board of Trustees established, within the Council on Research, the Steering Committee on Practice Guidelines to oversee the project. The steering committee and the Council on Research have developed a process document that formalizes the development of each guideline and puts into operation the principles described above. The process comprises eight stages:

- Topic selection,
- Work group appointment,

- Evidence definition,
- Draft development,
- Review process,
- Dissemination and implementation,
- Evaluation, and
- Revision.

Topic Selection

The steering committee selects topics for practice guidelines according to the following criteria: 1) degree of public importance (prevalence and seriousness of the condition), 2) relevance to psychiatric practice, 3) availability of information and relevant data, 4) availability of work already done that would be useful in the development of a practice guideline, and 5) extent to which increased psychiatric involvement in the area would be helpful for the field.

Appointment of a Work Group

Following topic selection, a 6- to 8-member work group is appointed. Work group members must be in active clinical practice and are chosen because of their expertise in the area that is the focus of the guideline. Some are primarily involved in academic or research efforts, but all must be involved in the care of patients. All are asked to declare that there are no conflicts of interest that would affect their ability to maintain objectivity concerning the guideline recommendations. If there is a potential bias or the appearance of a conflict of interest, the conflict is reviewed by the work group chair and the steering committee chair, and a decision is made regarding the participation of that member. All work group members are committed to the guideline development process described by the steering committee and influenced by the IOM and AMA criteria noted above. Work group members are informed that a significant commitment of time is required for the process, which generally takes 2 years.

Determining the Scope and Developing an Outline

Once a topic has been selected, the standard outline is customized, as appropriate. The first step in this process is determining the scope of the outline.

The guideline on bipolar disorders included a discussion of disease definition, specific treatment approaches, formulation of an individual treatment plan, and clinical factors influencing treatment. However, treatment of patients with bipolar II disorder was not covered. Similarly, the schizophrenia guideline covers the issues mentioned above, but not schizoaffective disorder. By further defining the scope of the guideline, the transition from evidence tables to draft guidelines is made more clear and can move more swiftly.

Evidence Defined

At the heart of good guideline development is the delineation of the evidence supporting treatment strategies. The evidence is derived from two sources: research studies and clinical consensus. The literature review process is explicitly described in each guideline and identifies the basic search strategy, sources used, criteria for selecting publications, review methods, and methods for cataloging reported outcomes. Evidence tables are created to aid the work group in writing the guideline. Generally the evidence tables are not part of the published guidelines. Evidence-based guidelines should explicitly describe the nature of the supporting evidence. The APA process uses the following coding system to describe the type of evidence being cited:

A. *Randomized clinical trial.*   A study of an intervention in which subjects are prospectively observed over time; there are treatment and control groups; subjects are randomly assigned to the two groups, and both the subjects and the investigators are "blind" to the assignments.
B. *Clinical trial.*   A prospective study in which an intervention is made and the results of that intervention are tracked longitudinally; the study does not meet the standards for a randomized clinical trial.
C. *Cohort or longitudinal study.*   A study in which subjects are prospectively observed over time without any specific intervention.
D. *Case–control study.*   A study in which a group of patients is identified in the present and information about them is pursued retrospectively or backward in time.
E. *Review with secondary data analysis.*   A structured analytic review of existing data; for example, a meta-analysis or a decision analysis.
F. *Review.*   A qualitative review and discussion of previously published literature without a quantitative synthesis of the data.
G. *Other.*   Textbooks, expert opinion, case reports, and other reports not included above.

Despite the great advances in our research knowledge base, many questions crucial for clinical decision making must be answered by consensus of expert clinicians. Organizing this input and shaping its focus is a major challenge in guideline development. A new tool, a Practice Research Network (described below), will eventually be able to provide some of the necessary answers in a generalizable and systematic manner.

Development of a Draft

The work group, assisted by staff in the Office of Research, then begin the arduous task of writing the guideline, integrating the data into clinical strategies. The work group uses the "process document," which contains many of the items discussed in this chapter, as a starting point for understanding guideline development and as a resource document throughout the ensuing process.

Review Process

The development of APA guidelines is an iterative process, with multiple drafts each being reviewed by increasing numbers of experts and clinicians. The first draft is reviewed by the steering committee (approximately 20 individuals), whereas draft 3 is reviewed by several hundred members of the association and other organizations. Although the work group itself is composed only of APA members, reviewers include experts from other mental health disciplines, patient and patient advocate organizations, and organizations of nonpsychiatric physicians and other health care professionals. The restriction of the steering committee and the work groups to members of the APA has led to some criticism. Other guideline efforts—such as that of the Agency for Health Care Policy and Research (AHCPR)—include multidisciplinary panels (as recommended by the IOM), which have the advantages of providing diverse points of view and minimizing the potential for discipline-specific biases. However, a major advantage of the APA process is that the completed guideline is approved by the Assembly and the Board of Trustees, which greatly increases its acceptability by APA members. At the present time it would be very difficult to obtain the approval of multiple mental health organizations, and if it were possible, the time required would certainly be much greater.

Dissemination and Implementation

Effective dissemination of the guideline is critical to its achieving significant impact. Each APA guideline is published by the *American Journal of Psychiatry* and subsequently by the American Psychiatric Press, Inc. However, a number of studies have concluded that simply publishing guidelines does not change physician behavior (Asaph et al. 1991; Greco and Eisenberg 1993). For example, Lomas and colleagues in Ontario, Canada (Lomas et al. 1991), studied the impact of an obstetrical guideline on vaginal deliveries after cesarean section. A major aim of the guideline was to increase the frequency of attempting vaginal delivery in women who had a prior cesarean delivery. The Society of Obstetricians and Gynecologists of Canada strongly supported the guideline, sent it to each member of the academy, and urged its use. Follow-up was then done after 24 months. Discouragingly, there was no significant change in the obstetricians' behavior in the hospitals in which the physicians received feedback after audit; that is, the same rates of trial of labor and vaginal birth continued. However, in the intervention hospitals there was a significant change in direction encouraged by the guideline. In these intervention hospitals, "opinion leaders"—recognized excellent clinicians highly regarded by their peers—organized special sessions to review and discuss the guideline and its implications. Another major dissemination strategy is to incorporate the guideline into teaching programs at all levels: medical student, residency, and continuing education. Questions concerning the APA guidelines are now included in the Psychiatric Residents in Training Examination (PRITE), and the guidelines are to be the primary source for recertification conducted by the American Board of Psychiatry and Neurology. Furthermore, the APA process itself aids in dissemination by involving several hundred persons in the development of the guideline, thus providing a nucleus on which to build dissemination strategies. Also, as noted above, approval of a guideline by the association carries significant weight and significantly increases its acceptance by members of the association. Similarly, in a survey of internists, Tunis et al. (1994) found that the internists were much more likely to accept guidelines developed by their professional associations than guidelines developed by others, especially insurance companies.

Defining effective dissemination strategies will be one of the most important issues in the guideline arena over the next several years. The New York State Psychiatric Association, in collaboration with the APA, the RAND Corporation, the National Alliance for the Mentally Ill (NAMI), and the National Depressive and Manic-Depressive Association (NDMDA), studied the effectiveness of dissemination strategies for the APA major depressive disorder guideline. One of the strategies involves the use of opinion leaders, similar to what was described above in the Lomas study. Similar approaches are being considered in other parts of the country and for other guidelines. Interactive computer programs and other dissemination strategies influenced by the knowledge of how psychiatrists learn will also be explored. The district branch structure of the APA may offer some advantages in designing and promoting local initiatives in the dissemination and implementation stages of guideline development.

Although the guidelines are developed primarily to assist clinicians, there are two other audiences to be considered in guideline dissemination: policy makers and patients. Policy makers must be targeted so they will be influenced by the reality that there are specific treatments for specific psychiatric disorders, and there is substantial evidence that these treatments work. Guidelines concretize these arguments and as a result can affect policy-level discussions, including those on reimbursement. In psychiatry, where myths and stigma abound, this influence is crucial. In addition, the process of developing guidelines makes information gaps apparent, thus laying out an agenda for research. In fact, a section of the guidelines on future research directions is specifically intended to suggest policy directions for research funding and development.

It is also a high priority that patients and families have information about treatment options. Patients are increasingly seeking information; when it is readily available, compliance with treatment is improved and the doctor–patient relationship is strengthened. In collaboration with patient and patient advocacy organizations, the APA guideline project develops patient brochures that present the guidelines in considerable detail.

Evaluation

Evaluation is an essential aspect of guideline development and in a quality improvement framework should lead to improvement in the content of the guideline as well as the development process. There are four major parameters along which guidelines should be measured: reliability/validity, utilization, psychiatrist behavior, and patient outcomes. Clearly, guidelines should accurately reflect the research literature and the existing clinical consensus. The process should be reliable, meaning that another group focusing on the same data and using a similar process will arrive at similar recommendations. Furthermore, the recommendations must speak to the issues that clinicians need to have addressed. The material must be presented in a manner clinicians find useful, and the recommendations must be in a form that can be easily incorporated into clinical practice. Some assessment must occur as to whether in fact clinicians actually use the guidelines, and if not, what modifications might increase their use. The desirability of a high rate of use is to actually influence clinicians' behavior in the targeted areas of the recommendations. Studies such as the New York State project described above help to assess whether this objective is being met. Since the ultimate purpose of guidelines is to have a positive impact on patient care, evaluation of guidelines must eventually include measuring patient outcomes. This objective has resulted in the AMA Practice Parameter Partnership recently adding the sixth attribute for guidelines described in the initial section of this chapter, namely that guideline development should include outcomes research, goals, and measures.

Revision

Because of the rapid growth in our knowledge base and to incorporate changes suggested by the evaluation processes described above, guidelines should be revised at regular intervals. In the APA project it is planned that guidelines will be revised at intervals no longer than 5 years. If there is insufficient data to warrant a revision of the entire guideline, a more focused revision will be done within 5 years and a complete revision within 10 years.

Content

Influenced by the principles described above, the APA has developed a standard format for guidelines.

Each guideline begins with a Statement of Intent. The first paragraph of the statement is as follows: "This practice guideline is not intended to be construed or to serve as a standard of medical care. Standards of medical care are determined on the basis of all clinical data available for an individual case and are subject to change as scientific knowledge and technology advances and patterns evolve. These parameters of practice should be considered guidelines only. Adherence to them will not ensure a successful outcome in every case nor should they be construed as including all proper methods of care or excluding other acceptable methods of care aimed at the same results. The ultimate judgment regarding a particular clinical procedure or treatment plan must be made by the psychiatrist in light of the clinical data presented by the patient and the diagnostic and treatment options available."

The second paragraph characterizes those involved in the development of the guideline and describes the process for dealing with potential and perceived conflicts of interest.

It is hoped that this clearly stated intent of the guideline will minimize misinterpretation or misuse of the guideline.

The guideline itself consists of eight sections:

I.   Executive Summary
II. Disease Definition, Epidemiology, and Natural History
III. Treatment Principles and Alternatives
IV. Formulation and Implementation of a Treatment Plan
V.   Clinical Features Influencing Treatment
VI. Research Directions
VII. Individuals and Organizations That Submitted Comments
VIII. References

Each of these sections is described briefly below.

I. Executive Summary.   This section provides an overview of the guideline with major recommendations succinctly presented. In this section and throughout the guideline each recommendation is weighted by the following levels of endorsement:

1. *Recommended with substantial clinical confidence.*   These recommendations are usually based on several well-controlled clinical trials that reported similar findings or that represent key principles of clinical psychiatric care with broad expert consensus.
2. *Recommended with moderate clinical confidence.*   These recommendations are usually based on a few positive studies or on less consistent data from many sources.
3. *May be recommended on the basis of individual circumstances.*   These recommendations usually have not been adequately tested or have conflicting reports about efficacy but are consistent with expert opinion and with accepted principles of treatment.

The executive summary is not intended to stand by itself, and in the summary the reader is explicitly encouraged to consult the relevant portions of the guideline for more information concerning the recommendations.

II. Disease Definition, Epidemiology, and Natural History. This section begins with a brief discussion of diagnoses using the current DSM-IV (American Psychiatric Association 1994) criteria, the differential diagnoses, and appropriate diagnostic procedures. Also included in this section is a limited review of epidemiological data and aspects of the natural history of the disorder, with emphasis on issues with important treatment implications.

III. Treatment Principles and Alternatives. This is the largest section and generally constitutes about half of the guideline. Specific treatment approaches are described, including indications, safety, efficacy, and alternative treatment strategies. The supporting data from both research studies and clinical consensus are included.

The treatments are grouped into three broad categories: A) psychiatric management, B) psychosocial interventions, and C) somatic interventions. The meaning of the term *psychiatric management* evolved during the writing of the first six guidelines. It includes approaches and techniques that had previously been included in the concept of "supportive psychotherapy." It includes aspects of the doctor–patient relationship and issues important in developing a therapeutic alliance. Conceptually, the recommendations in this area can be thought of as emanating from three levels of specificity: 1) principles and techniques that are important for all physicians, 2) principles and techniques that are important for psychiatrists, and 3) principles and techniques that are important for psychiatrists treating all patients with this particular disorder. The components of psychiatric management for bipolar disorder include 1) establishing and maintaining a therapeutic alliance; 2) monitoring the patient's psychiatric status; 3) providing education regarding bipolar disorder; 4) enhancing treatment compliance; 5) promoting regular patterns of activity and wakefulness; 6) promoting understanding of and adaptation to the psychosocial effects of bipolar disorder; 7) identifying new episodes early; and 8) reducing the morbidity and sequelae of bipolar disorder.

IV. Formulation and Implementation of a Treatment Plan.
This section assists the psychiatrist in moving from the data presented in Section III to making decisions for the individual patient. Whereas Section III is organized by treatment, this section is organized by the patient—perhaps in a given phase of the illness. For example, in the bipolar disorder guideline, many effective treatments are described in Section III. Section IV delineates how to select among them for a particular patient in each phase (i.e., manic, depressive, maintenance).

V. Clinical Features Influencing Treatment. This section addresses psychiatric, general medical, demographic, and other psychosocial variables that influence treatment. Comorbidities are considered in this section. Research has demonstrated that a large percentage of patients have more than one illness (Kessler et al. 1994). This reality presents a major challenge in writing guidelines that are relevant and specific for patients with multiple disorders. In the APA guideline only those aspects of the comorbid disorder that have specific treatment implications for the patient with the disorder being addressed by the guideline are considered. For further details about the treatment of the comorbid psychiatric disorder, the reader is referred to the appropriate guideline for that disorder. This section also includes ethnic, cross-cultural, gender, age, and socioeconomic issues that may be relevant to the formulation of a treatment plan.

VI. Research Directions. A significant benefit of developing practice guidelines is the identification of gaps in our knowledge base that impede the formulation of clear and specific treatment recommendations. In terms of the APA process a goal is to be able to describe more Level I recommendations. In this section of the guideline, the research that is necessary to achieve this goal is identified. Ideally, this section will influence policy decisions concerning research funding and priorities.

VII. Individuals and Organizations That Submitted Comments. As noted above, a large number of individuals and organizations receive a draft of the guideline and are encouraged to review, comment, and provide specific recommendations. In this section of the guideline the individuals and organizations who provided substantial suggestions are listed.

VIII. References. In this section the coding system described above is noted and is followed by the coded references.

Using the principles and following the format described above, the APA (as of the end of 1996) has approved and published the guidelines listed in Table 9–2.

Listed in Table 9–3 are guidelines currently being developed and their anticipated date of publication. Other topics being considered for development as guidelines are posttraumatic stress disorder, obsessive-compulsive disorder, somatoform disorders, and other personality disorders.

National and International Collaboration

In addition to the work with the AMA's Practice Parameter Partnership and Forum focusing especially on process issues, the APA is also collaborating with others on content issues. The American Academy of Child and Adoles-

Table 9–2. American Psychiatric Association published practice guidelines

Topic	Initial publication	Anticipated update
Eating disorders	February 1993	1999
Major depressive disorder	April 1993	1999
Bipolar disorder	December 1994	2000
Substance use disorders	November 1995	2000
Psychiatric evaluation	November 1995	
Nicotine dependence	September 1996	2001
Schizophrenia	April 1997	2002
Alzheimer's and other dementias	May 1997	2002
Panic disorder	May 1998	2003

Table 9–3. American Psychiatric Association practice guidelines in development

Topic	Anticipated publication
Delirium	Spring 1999
Geriatric care	Fall 1999
Human immunodeficiency virus (HIV)	Spring 2000
Borderline personality disorder	Fall 2000

cent Psychiatry has published a number of guidelines beginning in 1991. The leadership of the APA and the Academy projects work closely together to avoid duplication and to support each other's efforts. The Royal Australian and New Zealand College of Psychiatrists published the first practice guidelines in psychiatry beginning in 1981, and many other countries are developing evidence-based guidelines. The APA has established dialogue with several of these countries to promote collaborative efforts on guideline development. For example, the Royal College of Psychiatrists in the United Kingdom, following extensive consultation, has initiated a practice guidelines program in large part modeled on that of the APA.

Practice Research Network

As the practice guidelines project evolved, it became increasingly clear that there are a number of limitations in our existing knowledge base.

1. There are significant gaps in the research data on many key clinical issues facing psychiatrists. For example, if a patient has major depressive disorder and an antidepressant appears warranted, but the disease does not respond to the first antidepressant prescribed, what data are available to help the clinician select a second antidepressant?
2. Frequently, there are questions about the generalizability of the research data that do exist—are the patients seen by most psychiatrists in their daily practices similar to patients who are subjects in traditional research protocols? Most randomized clinical trials are conducted in tertiary care centers with rarefied patient referral patterns. A single exclusion criterion of the absence of comorbid psychiatric disorders (which is very common in most randomized clinical trials) by itself eliminates a large number of patients.
3. There is no national systematic assessment of clinical experience. Although the practice guidelines process incorporates broad clinical input throughout the development of drafts, there is no assurance that this input accurately and objectively represents the full range of clinical experience. As evidence-based guidelines were being developed, the recognition of these gaps in the knowledge base led to an exploration of how these gaps could be addressed. At the same time it was clear that it would be most helpful to have a national research and monitoring system that would help inform major policy debates about health care services, including access and reimbursement issues.

Both of these major objectives can be met by the establishment of a practice research network (PRN). A PRN is a group of practicing clinicians who cooperate to collect data and to conduct research studies on a variety of clinical and service delivery issues. There are a number of networks in medicine. The Ambulatory Sentinel Practice Network (ASPN) was developed by the University of Colorado and the American Academy of Family Physicians in 1981. It currently has 718 national members. The American Academy of Pediatrics developed the Pediatric Research in Office Settings (PROS) in 1986. Currently 1,254 pediatricians in 418 practices make up the network.

In 1993, the APA established a national practice-based research network of psychiatrists who collaborate to collect data and conduct clinical and health services research. The APA PRN serves as a "national psychiatric research laboratory" to strengthen and expand the clinical services and health services research base in psychiatry so that psychiatric treatments and outcomes of care for persons with mental disorders can be improved.

One of the primary goals of this initiative is to bridge the gap between current clinical research and the practical needs of clinicians and patients (Zarin et al. 1993). The network's "observational" or "naturalistic" research design will facilitate this by assessing the effectiveness of psychiatric treatments provided in routine practice rather than the efficacy of treatments under optimal circumstances. The network is designed to collect ongoing data regarding clinical status, treatments provided, and outcomes (Davies et al. 1994).

The APA views the network as a valuable opportunity to engage members in clinically meaningful research with important policy implications, particularly in light of the rapid changes in the organization, financing, delivery, and management of psychiatric care. Modeled after other well-established research networks, the APA PRN has adapted time-tested methods and structures used in other networks to the clinical psychiatric setting, while simultaneously developing innovative strategies that help ensure continuous practice participation and successful study implementation.

By 2000, the APA PRN will consist of 1,000 APA members representative of American psychiatry and the range of public and private psychiatric treatment settings. Currently, 750 APA members make up the network. Members must spend at least 15 hours per week in direct "face-to-face" care; this requirement ensures that members are substantially engaged in treating patients. The network provides a nationally representative sample of psychiatrists, settings, patients, and treatments to provide statistically significant subsamples for most factors of interest (Zarin et al. 1997).

Measurement Methods

On a regular basis, core data characterizing the network membership, their practices, and patient caseloads are being collected. These data will be used to plan and assess the feasibility of specific network studies; to analyze study-specific findings, eliminating the need to collect this type of denominator data and basic descriptive information for each study conducted under the network; and to systematically track trends and changes in the network membership, psychiatric treatment settings, patients, and treatment patterns. The network's annual core data are developed using two data collection instruments: a core network member instrument and a core patient-level instrument.

The network member instrument characterizes network members and their practices, providing data on demographic characteristics, training and certification, professional activities, patient care workload, and practice settings as well as aggregate demographic and diagnostic data on their patient caseloads. This instrument is also implemented in a randomly selected, nationally representative sample of the APA membership, enabling the comparison of the network members to American psychiatry as a whole (Zarin et al. 1998). The core patient-level instrument gathers more detailed data characterizing a randomly selected sample of each network member's patients and the treatments they receive. The core patient-level database enables the network and other mental health researchers to study and analyze a wide range of issues related to psychiatric treatment patterns. Using this database, we will be able to examine combinations of treatments provided to patients with different clinical and sociodemographic characteristics.

To study specific clinical services and health services issues, the network will utilize "study-specific" instruments and measures. As study topics are developed and variables of interest identified, existing psychiatric research instruments will be reviewed to determine whether they will meet the needs of the particular study, and new instruments will be developed.

Data collection is carried out by network members submitting paper-based data through the mail. As the scope of the network's data collection efforts expands and more instruments are developed, more cost-efficient methods will be implemented. The network will also conduct patient follow-up to collect longitudinal data from the patient perspective. These and other issues are currently being reviewed by the PRN's staff and scientific advisory committee.

Conclusion

Together the APA Practice Research Network and the practice guideline project promote and enhance the dissemination and practice of evidence-based psychiatry. By contributing to the scientific information knowledge base for the revision of DSM-IV and for new and revised practice guidelines, the PRN represents a significant step forward in bridging the gaps in the current clinical and health services research base in psychiatry. Both the APA's PRN and practice guidelines projects provide clinically useful and generalizable information that physicians will need to practice medicine as we enter the twenty-first century.

References

American Medical Association, Office of Quality Assurance: Attributes to Grade the Development of Practice Parameters. Chicago, IL, American Medical Association, 1990

American Psychiatric Association: Diagnostic and Statistical Manual of Mental Disorders, 4th Edition. Washington, DC, American Psychiatric Association, 1994

American Psychiatric Association, Standing Committee: Report on the Construction of Hospitals for the Insane. American Journal of Insanity 8 (July):79–81, 1851

American Psychiatric Association, Standing Committee: Report on the Organization of Hospitals for the Insane. American Journal of Insanity 10 (July):67–69, 1853

American Psychiatric Association, Task Force on the Use of Laboratory Tests in Psychiatry: Tricyclic antidepressants—blood level measurements and clinical outcome: an APA task force report. Am J Psychiatry 142:155–162, 1985

American Psychiatric Association: Benzodiazepine Dependence, Toxicity and Abuse: A Task Force Report of the American Psychiatric Association. Washington, DC, American Psychiatric Association, 1990

Asaph JW, Janoff K, Wayson K, et al: Carotid endarterectomy in a community hospital: a change in physicians' practice patterns. Am J Surg 161:616–618, 1991

Chassin M, Brook R, Park R, et al: Variations in the use of medical and surgical services by the Medicare population. N Engl J Med 314:285–290, 1986

Davies AE, Doyle MA, Lansky D, et al: Outcomes assessment in clinical settings: a consensus statement on principles and best practices in project management. Jt Comm J Qual Improv 20:6–16, 1994

Eddy D: Practice policies—what are they? JAMA 263:877–880, 1990

Garnick DW, Hendricks AM, Brennan TA: Can practice guidelines reduce the number and cost of malpractice claims? JAMA 266:2856–2860, 1991

Greco PJ, Eisenberg JM: Changing physician practices. N Engl J Med 329:1271–1274, 1993

Hyams AL, Brandenberg BA, Lipsitz SR, et al: Practice guidelines and malpractice litigation: a two-way street. Ann Intern Med 122:450–455, 1995

Institute of Medicine, Committee on Clinical Practice Guidelines: Guidelines for Clinical Practice: From Development to Use. Edited by Field MJ, Lohr KN. Washington, DC, National Academy Press, 1992

Kessler RC, McGonagle KA, Zhao S, et al: Lifetime and 12-month prevalence of DSM-III-R psychiatric disorders in the United States. Results from the National Comorbidity Survey. Arch Gen Psychiatry 51:8–19, 1994

Legislated clinical medicine (editorial). Lancet 335:1004–1006, 1990

Lewis CE: Variations in the incidence of surgery. N Engl J Med 281:880–885, 1969

Lomas J, Enkin M, Anderson GM, et al: Opinion leaders vs audit and feedback to implement practice guidelines. Delivery after previous cesarean section. JAMA 265:2202–2207, 1991

McIntyre J, Talbott J: Developing practice parameters. Hospital and Community Psychiatry 41:1103–1105, 1990

OBGYN premiums decrease drastically. AMA News, February 2, 1993, p 31

Tunis SR, Hayward RS, Wilson MC, et al: Internists' attitudes about clinical practice guidelines. Ann Intern Med 120:956–963, 1994

Zarin DA, Pincus HA, McIntyre JS: Practice guidelines (editorial). Am J Psychiatry 150:175–177, 1993

Zarin DA, Pincus HA, West JC, et al: Practice-based research in psychiatry. Am J Psychiatry 154:1199–1208, 1997

Zarin DA, Pincus HA, Peterson BD, et al: Characterizing psychiatry with findings from the 1996 National Survey of Psychiatric Practice. Am J Psychiatry 155:397–404, 1998

CHAPTER 10

The Psychiatrist as Psychotherapist

Glen O. Gabbard, M.D.

Psychiatrists occupy a unique niche among the medical specialties. They are the integrators par excellence of the biological and psychosocial in both diagnosis and treatment. That integration is a critical component to the provision of optimal clinical care. Without it the patient is fragmented into either a "mind" or a "brain." Moreover, in a practical sense, the specialty of psychiatry is at risk of disappearing if we consign ourselves to a reductionistic approach to patient care. If psychiatry became identified with prescribing psychotropic medication as the exclusive treatment, we could easily be replaced by internists, primary care practitioners, or neurologists. If we eschewed the biological and became identified with the practice of psychotherapy alone, we could easily be replaced by other mental health professionals trained in nonmedical disciplines at less cost than that incurred in educating psychiatrists.

From this perspective it is imperative that psychotherapy continue to be taught in psychiatric residency training as a core skill of the psychiatrist. Similarly, in a health care marketplace preoccupied with the lowering of costs, even if it means suboptimal care, psychotherapy must remain one of the fundamental treatment modalities practiced by psychiatrists. In this chapter I will identify forces working against the practice of psychotherapy within psychiatry and describe a rationale for retaining psychotherapy as a core skill of psychiatrists.

From Psychotherapists to Psychopharmacologists

In the 1940s and 1950s, the core identity of the psychiatrist was clearly that of the psychoanalytic psychotherapist, if not a fully trained psychoanalyst. The psychiatrist today is much more likely to be relegated to the role of providing psychotropic medication, with psychotherapy regarded as a relatively minor aspect of training and practice. This sea change can be accounted for by examining three major influences: advances in neuroscience, competition in the psychotherapy marketplace, and the impact of managed care.

Advances in Neuroscience

In the 1950s the psychiatrist had a limited therapeutic armamentarium, and so most interventions were by necessity psychotherapeutic. The extraordinary growth in new psychotropic drugs in the 1960s, 1970s, 1980s, and 1990s was associated with remarkable advances in basic neuroscience research. Neuroscience investigations have led to a greater understanding of the role of genetic influences in psychiatric disorders while also facilitating the development of new diagnostic tools, such as brain-imaging techniques. As a result, many psychiatrists increasingly came to see psychiatric illness as having a predominantly biological etiology and requiring psychopharmacological treatments.

Competition in the Psychotherapy Marketplace

In parallel with the explosion of neuroscience research, a host of other mental health professionals have appeared, many of whom define themselves as psychotherapists. Whereas psychiatrists were once the primary practitioners of psychotherapy, they are now in the minority. The 1987 National Medical Expenditure Survey (Olfson and Pincus 1994a, 1994b) determined the volume and distribution of psychotherapy visits by provider specialty and setting. It was calculated that 79.9 million outpatient psychotherapy visits had taken place in calendar year 1987. Psychologists were the most frequent providers of psychotherapy, accounting for 31.6%. Other mental health professionals were second at 25.2%, and psychiatrists were third at 23.9%.

In the November 1995 *Consumer Reports* survey of 2,900 individuals who saw a mental health professional, similar trends were identified ("Mental Health: Does Therapy Help?" 1995). Of this group 37% saw psychologists,

22% saw psychiatrists, 14% visited social workers, 9% saw marriage counselors, and 18% saw other mental health professionals. This survey also reported that the consumers found no differences in treatment effectiveness between psychiatrists, psychologists, and social workers.

The Impact of Managed Care

One aspect of the competition among mental health professionals for patients requiring psychotherapy has been seized by the managed care industry—namely, that nonpsychiatrists charge lower fees than psychiatrists as a general rule. A routine occurrence in today's managed care climate is that a psychiatrist is told that he or she can only see a patient for a 15- or 20-minute medication check. If the psychiatrist argues that psychotherapy is needed in addition to medication, the managed care company will frequently refer the patient to another mental health professional who may charge less than half the fee of the psychiatrist. Even in cases where psychiatrists may be allowed to provide psychotherapy under managed care scrutiny, the reimbursement for a 50-minute hour of psychotherapy may be considerably less than that for an hour filled with three or four medication appointments. Hence, psychiatrists may respond to this financial incentive by encouraging the delegation of psychotherapy to nonmedical practitioners while restricting their own practice to patients needing psychopharmacology appointments.

The Pendulum Swings Back

In recent years there have appeared signs that the pendulum may have swung so far to the neuroscience end of the psychiatric continuum that it is now making its way back toward the middle. The neuroscience revolution has produced a somewhat paradoxical development (Gabbard and Goodwin 1996). The overreliance on psychopharmacological treatments has underscored their limitations. Moreover, neuroscience research has reached a level of sophistication that allows it to serve as a bridge between the genetic and the environmental on the one hand, and between the psychopharmacological and the psychotherapeutic on the other. The discovery that gene expression is not static—but rather is influenced in an ongoing way by interactions with the environment—has led to a corresponding interest in the influence of psychosocial treatments on illnesses that are thought to have strongly biological underpinnings.

For example, schizophrenia, long regarded as a "brain disease," is a disorder with some of the most compelling evidence that psychosocial treatments are effective. Patients with schizophrenia have much lower rates of relapse when a specific form of family therapy is added to the maintenance dose of antipsychotic medication (Falloon et al. 1982, 1985; Hogarty et al. 1986, 1987; Köttgen et al. 1984; Leff et al. 1982, 1985; Tarrier et al. 1988, 1989). Based on the observation that high levels of expressed emotion (high EE) in the families of schizophrenic patients predicted relapse following hospital discharge, clinicians and researchers found that working with families to modify certain components of expressed emotion prevented relapse. Specifically, in this approach the family therapist teaches the family about the role of criticism, intrusiveness, and emotional overinvolvement in overwhelming the patient and in leading to a return of symptoms and a need for rehospitalization.

A careful examination of the impressive outcomes reported by Hogarty et al. (1991) suggest that family therapy has an impact on relapse equivalent to that of antipsychotic medication. Approximately 80% of patients with schizophrenia will relapse 1 year after leaving the hospital if they receive no treatment. That percentage is reduced by half if antipsychotic medication is added. When family therapy is added to the medication regimen, the relapse rate was reduced in half once again. In other words, only 20% of the patients relapsed during the first year following discharge.

The advantage of combining psychotherapeutic and psychopharmacological approaches is becoming clearer and clearer as clinical trials of these two-pronged approaches are reported in the literature. Luborsky et al. (1993) looked at 17 studies that allowed a comparison of brief psychodynamic therapy with other forms of psychotherapy. Although they found that in most cases dynamic therapy was no better or worse than other forms of psychotherapy, there were some important exceptions. Most significant in this context is that they found a distinct advantage when pharmacotherapy and psychotherapy were combined. Better outcomes were achieved than either psychotherapy or pharmacotherapy alone.

In a well-designed study of combined treatments of depression (Weissman et al. 1979), a clear advantage for combining interpersonal therapy (IPT) and antidepressants was found in the treatment of 96 primarily female depressed outpatients compared with the outcomes for either pharmacotherapy or psychotherapy alone. Medication acted more rapidly than the psychotherapy and appeared to have its effect primarily on vegetative symptoms, whereas psychotherapy appeared to influence interest and mood preferentially. As this study suggests, combining psychotherapy and medication enhances the breadth of the patient's response (Hollon and Fawcett 1995). There is also some evidence that the addition of psychotherapy may reduce subsequent risk of relapse to a greater degree.

The positive effects of combining behavior therapy and medication in the treatment of anxiety disorders are also clear. Mattick et al. (1990) did a meta-analytic study showing that the combination of imipramine and behavior therapy was more effective on symptoms of depression, phobia, and anxiety than either modality alone. Telch et al. (1985) found that patients receiving imipramine plus exposure showed a significantly greater decrease in the frequency of panic attacks compared with groups receiving either imipramine alone or exposure alone. Similarly, several studies suggest that a combination of a serotonin reuptake inhibitor and behavior therapy increases both short- and long-term improvements as well as producing more rapid response in patients with obsessive-compulsive disorder (Cottraux et al. 1990; Marks et al. 1980, 1988).

Inherent in much of the research demonstrating the advantage of combined approaches over either modality alone is the notion is that psychotherapy works by affecting the brain. This observation has been validated by highly sophisticated research using positron emission tomography (PET). Baxter et al. (1992) found that fluoxetine and behavior therapy have virtually the same effects on the brains of patients with obsessive-compulsive disorder (OCD). In a subsequent report (Schwartz et al. 1996), nine patients with OCD were studied with PET before and after 10 weeks of behavioral and cognitive treatment; the six who were responders had significant bilateral decreases in glucose metabolic rate in the caudate nucleus.

Similarly, the old distinction between "reactive" and "endogenous" depression is no longer regarded as useful. All depression has biological and psychological components. Indeed, research is now suggesting that even severe depressions may respond well to cognitive therapy alone (Persons et al. 1996), again suggesting that chemical changes in the brain can be reversed by psychotherapeutic interventions.

These studies and others have underscored the fact that traditional distinctions between "biologically based" disorders and "psychologically based" disorders are becoming meaningless. To say that the former require medication and the latter require psychotherapy is not well grounded in empirical data. This conclusion leads us to a central point: *Psychotherapy is just as much a medical treatment as pharmacotherapy, in that both affect the brain.*

This point of view has been elaborated in an official Position Statement on Medical Psychotherapy by the American Psychiatric Association (APA) published in the November 1995 issue of the *American Journal of Psychiatry* (Clemens 1995). The statement was written by Norman Clemens, M.D., in consultation with the American Psychiatric Association Committee on the Practice of Psychotherapy. It was subsequently approved by the APA Assembly and the APA Board of Trustees in the same year of its publication. In this statement the following argument is presented:

> As physicians, psychiatrists add unique and vital dimensions to psychotherapy that limited licensed practitioners do not have: medical standards of ethics and professional responsibility for life-and-death decisions, comprehensive grounding in medical diagnosis and treatment, the capacity to integrate complex psychopharmacology with psychotherapy and social rehabilitation, and in-depth knowledge of human biology, general medical conditions, and their interaction with psychiatric illness and mental phenomena. Psychiatrists are thoroughly grounded in human emotional development and the life cycle. Provision of both psychotherapy and medication management by the same treating psychiatrist provides high-quality, comprehensive, and accountable care. However, psychiatrists are also in an optimal position to prescribe and perform psychotherapy as the sole treatment modality. Psychiatrists in organized systems must be free to conduct psychotherapy with their patients without financial or other disincentives. (Clemens 1995, p. 1700)

This statement is a beginning effort by psychiatrists to articulate their unique position among mental health professionals. There are certainly many clinical psychologists, social workers, and other mental health professionals who are highly skilled psychotherapists—perhaps even more skilled in psychotherapy than many psychiatrists coming out of training programs today where psychotherapy is underemphasized. This lack of exposure to psychotherapy training limits residents' understanding of the unique niche that the psychiatrist occupies in the simultaneous provision of both psychotherapy and pharmacotherapy. Unfortunately, in many residency training programs, the integration of the two modalities is not emphasized. Often, the teaching of pharmacotherapy and psychotherapy occur independently in the curriculum without stressing the unique challenges involved in integrating the two approaches.

Psychiatrists may be particularly needed to provide combined treatments for both severely disturbed patients and those with complex problems in which biological and psychological factors converge. Compliance is an enormous problem with bipolar and schizophrenic patients, for example, and one person attending to the psychological issues around compliance as well as the psychopharmacological issues may maximize the adherence to the treatment plan. Also, with severe Axis II conditions such as borderline personality disorder, there is great potential for a splitting process to occur when the pharmacotherapist and the psychotherapist are two separate individuals. One clinician who can deal with the variety of transferences connected with both the medication and the psychotherapy is probably the optimal arrangement.

This arrangement may be more cost-effective in the long run as well. If combining the functions in one person serves to prevent relapse, expenditures will be reduced by fewer hospitalizations. Moreover, there is a hidden cost in the time that it takes two different individuals to communicate about the treatment plan, a cost that is not reimbursed by insurance companies and not paid by the patient, hence discouraging professionals from collaborating.

Although this argument has a commonsense appeal, psychiatry has been hampered by lack of data. Outcome studies rarely pit one mental health discipline against another. Also, there is virtually no literature comparing psychotherapy and pharmacotherapy conducted by one clinician to an arrangement whereby the two modalities are conducted by separate clinicians. The research on cost-effectiveness parallels the efficacy research. Whereas many studies point to a beneficial economic impact of psychotherapy (Gabbard et al. 1997), few shed any light on the cost-effectiveness of one person performing both functions. Ironically in the United States, companies that manage mental health benefits (managed care companies), and who are carefully monitoring costs, may be the first source of such data in favor of combining functions. Preliminary data suggest that with certain severe disorders, it makes financial sense to have a psychiatrist do both the psychotherapy and the pharmacotherapy (Goldman et al. 1998).

In discussing issues of cost, however, we must avoid a narrow perspective that cheaper is always better. As Wells and Sturm (1995) have stressed, cost-effectiveness should be construed as meaning *high value*. For example, in their research sponsored by the RAND Corporation, they noted that fewer dollars were spent if primary care practitioners treated depressed patients. However, the diagnosis of depression was frequently missed, and the patients who were diagnosed were undertreated and so they continued to have many functional impairments. By spending 20%–30% more for the involvement of mental health specialists, the effectiveness of care was quadrupled as measured by functional improvement. Counseling or psychotherapy was a key component of the treatment provided by the specialists. The researchers concluded that providing ineffective treatment does not make sense just because it is inexpensive.

Future Roles of Psychiatrists

As we contemplate psychiatry in the twenty-first century, we can envision a variety of roles for the psychiatrist, all of which may be enhanced by knowledge and skills in psychotherapy.

Supervision and Consultation to Other Therapists

In health care delivery systems, the trend is definitely toward the delivery of psychotherapy by nonpsychiatrists. Psychiatrists will continue to function in supervisory and consultative roles, however, and a knowledge of psychotherapy will be crucial to assisting nonmedical therapists with difficult clinical problems.

Management of Delivery Systems

Many psychiatrists currently function in the role of clinical administrator in hospital, partial hospital, and outpatient settings. This trend is likely to continue into the next century, and psychiatrists must understand the psychodynamics of groups and institutions for optimal functioning in a clinical administrative role.

Somatic Treatments

Pharmacotherapy occurs (or at least *should* occur) within a therapeutic relationship. Attention to issues such as the therapeutic alliance are just as important in prescribing medication as they are in psychotherapy. Issues of noncompliance often can best be understood in terms of psychodynamic constructs such as transference, countertransference, and resistance. Careful attention to the meaning of the medication to the patient may also shed light on the patient's reluctance to take medication as prescribed. As the APA Practice Guidelines for Depression (American Psychiatric Association 1993) suggest, psychotherapeutic management is essential for the treatment of all depressed persons, regardless of the modality used. The same principles apply to other somatic treatments, such as electroconvulsive therapy.

Direct Provision of Combined Psychotherapy and Pharmacotherapy

This unique province of psychiatrists will probably become more and more crucial as adverse experiences accumulate when other arrangements are tried. Over the next several years more and more data will illuminate which illnesses especially require a psychiatrist to conduct both treatment modalities to provide optimal care and reasonable cost-effectiveness.

Expertise in Specific Forms of Psychotherapy

A subgroup of psychiatrists today have developed special expertise in psychoanalysis by virtue of analytic training. These psychiatrists are often sought out for consultation with particularly difficult cases, and many of them analyze patients who have been treatment failures when other modalities were used. Other psychiatrists have become expert in cognitive therapy, behavior therapy, interpersonal therapy, group therapy, marital therapy, or family therapy. These areas of superspecialization will continue to flourish into the twenty-first century just as certain psychiatrists develop special expertise in specific psychopharmacological agents.

Core Psychotherapeutic Skills Essential in Psychiatric Residency Training

Given this future picture of the diversity of psychiatric practice, psychotherapeutic training appears to be an essential component in the creation of a well-rounded and highly skilled psychiatrist. I would suggest that a set of core psychotherapeutic skills as outlined below should be a fundamental part of every psychiatric residency program.

Clinical Interviewing/Rapport/Empathy

The model of a 15- or 20-minute medication check so prevalent in managed care systems places extraordinary time pressure on the clinician. This pressure may lead to a hurried interaction in which the psychiatrist attempts to elicit the major descriptive characteristics of the illness, particularly the target symptoms for which the medication is prescribed. Lack of attention to rapport and the building of a therapeutic alliance often result in poor compliance with the prescribed treatment. Similarly, failures to empathize with the patient's internal experience may leave the patient feeling misunderstood and dissatisfied. A key component of good clinical interviewing is actively engaging the patient as a collaborator in the process of identifying the problems and thinking through the optimal treatment. This always takes into account that the clinician is treating a *person*, not just an illness. These skills are often not well taught in medical school, and one cannot assume natural talents in this area among psychiatric residents.

Brief and Extended Psychodynamic Therapy

Sitting in a room with another person over a long period of time and trying as best you can to understand how that individual's mind works is a unique learning experience. The nuances of transference, countertransference, and resistance can best be understood in this setting as they unfold over time and are carefully monitored by the beginning psychotherapist in supervisory hours with an experienced therapist. Developmental issues in adult patients can also be best appreciated with the luxury of time. However, while extended psychodynamic therapy is a skill in and of itself with which all residents should be familiar, optimal teaching involves a process of generalizing what is learned in the crucible of the psychotherapeutic drama to other settings in clinical psychiatry (Gabbard 1997). Residents should learn that the unconscious is not an abstraction but is directly observable in terms of slips of the tongue, enactments within the transference, and nonverbal behavior. Similarly, psychoanalysts and psychoanalytic therapists who teach dynamic therapy in most residency training programs should stress that the principles of psychoanalytic thinking can be applied to a *focal issue* when extended therapy is reduced to the brief therapy settings of managed care.

Despite the economic climate, some residents will find themselves practicing extended dynamic therapy after they leave the residency. Many patients feel constrained by the limitations placed on psychotherapy by managed care firms. These companies may advertise themselves as providing 20 to 30 sessions per year but in fact limit any one psychotherapy process to six or eight sessions through intensive utilization review. Patients with economic means frequently obtain psychotherapy on their own after benefits are restricted. Additionally, successful professionals often wish to bypass their managed care system entirely and pay out of pocket for extended psychotherapy so that they have an opportunity for detailed examination of long-standing, unconscious patterns that are problematic at work or in relationships and maintain confidentiality while undertaking this exploration.

In some cases psychiatrists may need to lower their customary fees to treat patients in psychotherapy outside the managed care systems. This tradeoff may not be so bad. I teach residents that sacrificing a small amount of income for a more satisfying and intellectually stimulating day at the office may be well worth it.

Cognitive Therapy and Behavior Therapy

Cognitive therapy and behavior therapy have been extensively validated by solid empirical research. Cognitive-behavior therapy (CBT) is a well-established treatment for depression that was determined to be efficacious for patients with unipolar depression in the National Institute of Mental Health (NIMH) Treatment of Depression Collaborative Research Program (Elkin et al. 1989). In many quarters there is increasing emphasis on teaching and practicing empirically validated treatments. Many patients with obsessive-compulsive disorder, for which behavior therapy and a selective serotonin reuptake inhibitor are the treatments of choice, are unable to find psychiatrists trained in behavior therapies who can administer both treatments. Although these therapies are often administered by nonpsychiatrists, residents should be well acquainted with them because of the potential to be involved in a consultative or supervisory arrangement with the therapists. Moreover, residents often may find themselves prescribing medication for someone who is also receiving behavior therapy or cognitive therapy.

Interpersonal Therapy

Interpersonal therapy (IPT) evolved between the late 1960s and the early 1980s. Klerman and Weissman (1982) developed IPT based on the work of Adolph Meyer, who emphasized that psychosocial and interpersonal experiences occurring within a comprehensive psychobiological model of psychopathology were highly significant. Four areas are targeted by the interpersonal therapist: unresolved grief, social role disputes, social role transitions, and interpersonal deficits. IPT was conceived as a brief psychotherapy for unipolar major depression and was also demonstrated in the NIMH Treatment of Depression of Collaborative Research Program to be highly effective (Elkin et al. 1989). As with dynamic therapy and cognitive therapy, manuals are available that will assist residents in learning the technique. Newer applications of IPT to other diagnostic entities, such as eating disorders and substance abuse, are rapidly evolving.

Group Dynamics and Group Psychotherapy

Many residencies offer an experiential seminar in group dynamics, in which the residents meet over a period of weeks with a group expert to experience how individuals may behave differently in group settings. They also gain a firsthand account of common group dynamics, such as Bion's three basic assumptions: dependency, fight/flight, and pairing (Bion 1961; Rioch 1970). Groups are powerfully regressive, and the trainees can also become familiar with primitive anxieties that many of their patients will experience. The principles learned in group dynamics will be invaluable in the psychiatrist's future roles in health care systems and institutions. The apparently irrational forces at work in hospitals, outpatient settings, and other delivery systems become less mystifying when one is thoroughly grounded in group theory. In addition, of course, residents should be exposed to didactic seminars in group psychotherapy techniques and have the opportunity to actually function as a group therapist in the course of their 4-year training. Group therapy is a highly cost-effective modality in an age of great cost consciousness, and one can anticipate that more and more patients will receive psychotherapeutic interventions through groups.

Family and Marital Therapy

Psychopathology does not develop in a vacuum. Families are often intimately involved in the pathogenesis of illness. In addition, interactions with the family may either improve or exacerbate preexisting illnesses. Illnesses often serve specific functions for marital and family systems, and this perspective may be crucial in many situations to improve the symptoms of an individual. Psychiatry has often been accused of being a bit myopic by focusing on the individual while neglecting the broader systems in which they live. This sensitivity to family and marital dynamics should also extend to the cultural system, the broader network or community in which the families live. All residents should have experiences as a family therapist and/or a marital therapist in the course of their residency program while also receiving didactic instruction in seminars on the topic.

Conclusions

Psychiatry must maintain a central role for psychotherapy, in both training and practice. To lose this dimension of psychiatry would very likely sound the death knell for the future of the specialty. The principles learned in psychotherapy practice will serve the clinician well, regardless of the psychiatric activity in which he or she is engaged. Even when psychotherapeutic interventions are not explicitly called for, the understanding of what is going on within the patient or within a treatment system enriches the psychiatrist's everyday experience in the workplace. Much that is obscure becomes understandable.

The core psychotherapeutic skills addressed in this chapter are considered the bare minimum for the generalist. Those psychiatric residents who take a special interest in psychotherapy will undoubtedly want to have a treatment experience of their own, whether psychotherapeutic or psychoanalytic, to gain a greater understanding of their own complex defenses, internal object relations, cognitive schema, and so forth. Self-understanding may be a critically important factor in preventing boundary violations and other harmful actions growing out of countertransference that is inadequately understood.

One potential obstacle that may interfere with securing a firm place within psychiatry for psychotherapy is fighting among ourselves. In dealing with managed care companies and policymakers in government, psychiatrists can undermine their cause by devaluing some psychotherapies while singing the praises of others. There is much to be gained by presenting psychotherapeutic treatments as a group of modalities with common characteristics that can be scientifically deployed based on the diagnosis and characteristics of a given patient.

One of the most compelling and fascinating aspects of psychiatry as a medical specialty is that it is pluralistic in terms of treatment approaches and conceptualizations of psychopathology. One individual cannot master all aspects of psychiatry, and continued diversity in terms of special areas of expertise is essential for the field. The future psychiatrist does not need to know how to administer every treatment expertly. He or she should know enough of the fundamentals about that treatment to know when it is indicated and when referral to a colleague is necessary. One of these areas of expertise that will continue to be needed is the psychiatrist whose primary identity is that of a psychotherapist. The rationale for this continued role has been laid out in the foregoing discussion. It is now up to the profession to make sure that this special niche does not disappear because of disuse atrophy.

References

American Psychiatric Association: Practice guideline for major depressive disorder in adults. Am J Psychiatry 150(suppl 4):1–26, 1993

Baxter KR, Schwartz JM, Bergman KS, et al: Caudate glucose metabolic rate changes with both drug and behavior therapy for obsessive-compulsive disorder. Arch Gen Psychiatry 49:618–689, 1992

Bion WR: Experiences in Groups and Other Papers. New York, Basic Books, 1961

Clemens N: Position statement on medical psychotherapy. Am J Psychiatry 152:1700, 1995

Cottraux J, Mollard E, Bouvard M, et al: A controlled study of fluvoxamine and exposure in obsessive-compulsive disorder. Int Clin Psychopharmacol 5:17–30, 1990

Elkin I, Shea T, Watkins JT, et al: National Institute of Mental Health Treatment of Depression Collaborative Research Program: general effectiveness of treatments. Arch Gen Psychiatry 46:971–982, 1989

Falloon IRH, Boyd JL, McGill CW, et al: Family management in the prevention of exacerbations of schizophrenia: a controlled study. N Engl J Med 306:1437–1444, 1982

Falloon IRH, Boyd JL, McGill CW, et al: Family management in the prevention of morbidity of schizophrenia: clinical outcome of a two-year longitudinal study. Arch Gen Psychiatry 42:887–896, 1985

Gabbard GO: Training residents in psychodynamic psychotherapy, in Acute Care Psychotherapy: Diagnosis and Treatment. Edited by Sederer LJ, Rothschild AJ. Baltimore, MD, Williams & Wilkins, pp 481–491, 1997

Gabbard GO, Goodwin FK: Integrating biological and psychosocial perspectives, in American Psychiatric Press Review of Psychiatry, Vol 15. Edited by Dickstein LJ, Riba MB, Oldham JM. Washington, DC, American Psychiatric Press, 1996, pp 527–548

Gabbard GO, Lazar SG, Hornberger J, et al: The economic impact of psychotherapy: a review. Am J Psychiatry 154:147–155, 1997

Goldman W, McCulloch J, Cuffel B, et al: Outpatient utilization patterns of integrated and split psychotherapy and pharmacotherapy for depression. Psychiatr Serv 49:477–482, 1998

Hogarty GE, Anderson CM, Reiss DJ, et al: Family psychoeducation, social skills training, and maintenance chemotherapy in the aftercare treatment of schizophrenia, I: one-year effects of a controlled study on relapse and expressed emotion. Arch Gen Psychiatry 43:633–642, 1986

Hogarty GE, Anderson CM, Reiss DJ: Family psychoeducation, social skills training and medication in schizophrenia: the long and the short of it. Psychopharmacol Bull 23:12–13, 1987

Hogarty GE, Anderson CM, Reiss DJ, et al: Family psychoeducation, social skills training, and maintenance chemotherapy in the aftercare treatment of schizophrenia: two-year effects of a controlled study on relapse and adjustment. Arch Gen Psychiatry 48:340–347, 1991

Hollon SD, Fawcett J: Combined medication and psychotherapy, in Treatments of Psychiatric Disorders, 2nd Edition, Vol 1. Edited by Gabbard GO. Washington, DC, American Psychiatric Press, 1995, pp 1221–1236

Klerman GL, Weissman MM: Interpersonal psychotherapy: theory and research, in Short-Term Psychotherapies for Depression. Edited by Rush AJ. New York, Guilford, 1982, pp 88–106

Köttgen C, Sonnichsen I, Mollenhauer K, et al: Group therapy with families of schizophrenic patients: results of the Hamburg Camberwell Family Interview Study III. International Journal of Family Psychiatry 5:83–94, 1984

Leff J, Kuipers L, Berkowitz R, et al: A controlled trial of social intervention in the families of schizophrenic patients. Br J Psychiatry 114:121–134, 1982

Leff J, Kuipers L, Berkowitz R, et al: A controlled trial of social intervention in the families of schizophrenic patients: two-year follow-up. Br J Psychiatry 146:594–600, 1985

Luborsky L, Diguer L, Luborsky E, et al: The efficacy of dynamic psychotherapies: is it true that "everyone has won and all must have prizes"? in Psychodynamic Treatment Research: A Handbook for Clinical Practice. Edited by Miller NE, Luborsky L, Barber JP, et al. New York, Basic Books, 1993, pp 497–516

Marks IM, Stern RS, Mawson D, et al: Clomipramine and exposure for obsessive-compulsive rituals. Br J Psychiatry 136:1–25, 1980

Marks IM, Lelliott P, Basoglu M, et al: Clomipramine, self-exposure and therapist-aided exposure for obsessive-compulsive rituals. Br J Psychiatry 152:522–534, 1988

Mattick RP, Andrews G, Hadzi-Pavlovic D: Treatment of panic and agoraphobia. J Nerv Ment Dis 178:567–576, 1990

Mental health: does therapy help? Consumer Reports, November 1995, pp 734–739

Olfson M, Pincus HA: Outpatient psychotherapy in the United States, I: volume, costs, and user characteristics. Am J Psychiatry 151:1281–1288, 1994a

Olfson M, Pincus HA: Outpatient psychotherapy in the United States, II: patterns of utilization. Am J Psychiatry 151:1289–1294, 1994b

Persons JB, Thase ME, Crits-Cristoph P: The role of psychotherapy in the treatment of depression: review of two practice guidelines. Arch Gen Psychiatry 53:283–290, 1996

Rioch MJ: The work of Wilfred Bion on groups. Psychiatry 33:56–66, 1970

Schwartz JM, Stoessel PW, Baxter LR, et al: Systematic changes in cerebral glucose metabolic rate after successful behavior modification treatment of obsessive-compulsive disorder. Arch Gen Psychiatry 53:109–113, 1996

Tarrier N, Barrowclough C, Vaughn C, et al: The community management of schizophrenia: a controlled trial of a behavioral intervention with families to reduce relapse. Br J Psychiatry 153:532–542, 1988

Tarrier N, Barrowclough C, Vaughn C, et al: Community management of schizophrenia: a two-year follow-up of a behavioral intervention with families. Br J Psychiatry 154:625–628, 1989

Telch MJ, Agras WS, Taylor CB, et al: Combined pharmacological and behavioral treatment for agoraphobia. Behav Res Ther 23:235–335, 1985

Weissman MM, Prusoff VA, DiMascio A, et al: The efficacy of drugs and psychotherapy in the treatment of acute depressive disorders. Am J Psychiatry 136:555–558, 1979

Wells KB, Sturm R: Care for depression in a changing environment. Health Aff 14:78–89, 1995

CHAPTER 11

Psychopharmacology in the New Millennium

Emphasis on Depression

Alan F. Schatzberg, M.D.

In the past few decades, psychopharmacology has had a major impact on both psychiatry and psychiatric patients. More effective, better tolerated, and safer agents have supplanted our first-generation treatments, and new treatment strategies are emerging almost daily. Moreover, biological research is leading to new theoretical constructs of pathophysiology with the aim that over the next two decades different and more effective pharmacological approaches to both the treatment and prevention of psychiatric disorders will emerge for use in clinical practice. In this chapter, I discuss what the practice of psychopharmacology may be like in the twenty-first century, emphasizing the arena of antidepressant drug development as a model. I describe the likely practice in the early part of the next century and then speculate on how psychopharmacology might appear later in the twenty-first century.

Current Status and Near-Term Advances

Currently available antidepressants act primarily by blocking the reuptake of monoamines, inhibiting their degradation, or interfering with their binding to specific receptors. The introduction of selective serotonin reuptake inhibitors (SSRIs) in 1988 into the United States revolutionized pharmacological therapy for a number of depressive, anxiety, and eating disorders. There are now five SSRIs on the United States market—fluoxetine, paroxetine, sertraline, fluvoxamine, and citalopram. These drugs differ from their predecessor tricyclic antidepressants (TCAs) by selectively and potentially inhibiting the uptake of serotonin into presynaptic neurons with little effect on blocking norepinephrine reuptake. The TCAs are primarily noradrenergic in their effect. Moreover, the SSRIs exert virtually no effect on blocking muscarinic acetylcholine, α_1, or histamine-1 (H_1) receptors and thus do not produce the panoply of side effects that are seen commonly with the TCAs, for example, dry mouth, constipation, orthostatic hypotension, or sedation (Potter et al. 1995; Tollefson 1995). These pharmacological differences have accounted for efficacy of the SSRIs over a wider range of conditions (major depression, dysthymia, obsessive-compulsive disorder, premenstrual dysphoria, etc.) as well as a more favorable side-effect profile.

In the early part of the twenty-first century, we will likely still be using SSRIs for many of our patients. Citalopram, an SSRI that is commonly used in Scandinavia, has recently become available in the United States. Citalopram is thought to produce less sexual dysfunction than do other SSRIs, although data on this are limited. In Europe, it is available in parenteral form. Otherwise it is largely similar to the other SSRIs.

Subsequent to the release of the SSRIs, three new antidepressants have been introduced in the United States. Venlafaxine is a mixed norepinephrine/serotonin uptake blocker that also exerts little in the way of anticholinergic, antihistaminic, or α_1-blocking effects. The drug's side-effect profile is similar to that of the SSRIs with the exception of its causing increased blood pressure in some patients at high doses (Golden et al. 1995). After its release, venlafaxine gained wider acceptance with psychiatrists, who have found the agent effective in specific situations and have learned to dose the drug conservatively when initiating treatment to prevent nausea and other side effects. A new extended-release formulation has made the drug even easier to use. Venlafaxine has attracted considerable attention in the past 2 years because of trials that suggest that it may be more effective than some SSRIs in treating patients with melancholic or endogenous depressions (Clerc et al. 1994) and that it may be effective in those patients whose symptoms have failed to respond to other medications (Nierenberg et al. 1994). This experience suggests that noradrenergic uptake blockade may be important in the treatment of more severe depressive disorders. A new antidepressant, reboxetine, is a pure norepinephrine uptake blocker that, unlike TCAs, has no anticholinergic effects. Controlled trials in Europe suggest that it may have more potent effects than does fluoxetine in more severely depressed patients (Massana 1998).

Over the next 5 years, we are likely to have a better sense of the relative advantage of using noradrenergic agents in specific situations. At this time, there is an intense debate as to whether SSRIs produce as much effect as do the older TCAs in geriatric and severely depressed patients (Roose et al. 1994; Schatzberg 1996/1997). Although a discussion of the debate is beyond the scope of this chapter, the psychopharmacologist of the early twenty-first century will have a better understanding of the maximal gain to be expected from SSRIs versus that from TCAs or other noradrenergic agents in more severely depressed or elderly patients. We may then have a hierarchy of treatments based on severity of depression. For example, a particular SSRI might be used preferentially in a patient with mild-to-moderate depression, whereas a TCA-like agent or reboxetine or venlafaxine at higher doses might be prescribed for a more severely depressed patient.

Nefazodone is primarily a serotonin-2 ($5\text{-}HT_2$) receptor blocker. It has weak effects on blocking serotonin and norepinephrine reuptake. The drug exerts little or no antihistaminic or anticholinergic effects. It is, however, a weak α_1 blocker. Side effects include sedation, nausea, and dizziness. The medication appears to be calming, and some clinicians use it preferentially in patients whose depressions are characterized by pronounced anxiety. A recent trial suggests that, in contrast to the SSRIs, sexual function is not worsened by exposure to this agent (Feiger et al. 1996).

Mirtazapine is a European drug that is primarily an α_2 antagonist. This effect results in release of norepinephrine and indirectly in increased serotonin activity at the $5\text{-}HT_{1A}$ receptor. The drug is a potent antihistamine and is quite sedating initially. Some clinicians have found that the drug is less sedating at higher doses (15–30 mg/day) than at 7.5 mg/day. To date, mirtazapine has seen limited use in the United States such that it is difficult to describe its ultimate range of applications.

Bupropion has been on the United States market for several years. It is a norepinephrine reuptake blocker with mild dopamine-blocking effects as well. Its release was initially delayed because of seizures in bulimic patients. However, clinical trials and experience to date have not indicated that the drug is particularly epileptogenic. Bupropion has little effect on muscarinic acetylcholine, H_1, or α_1 receptors and thus generally has a favorable side-effect profile. Increasingly, the drug has been used in combination with the SSRIs to decrease SSRI-induced sexual dysfunction or to bring out an antidepressant response in patients whose symptoms are not responding to the SSRI alone. An extended-release formulation of bupropion is now available.

A number of reports indicate that the addition of dopaminergic agents to SSRIs may help to overcome the anergia that some patients experience with SSRIs. Bromocriptine, methylphenidate, and dextroamphetamine have all been used successfully in this regard. Missing from our armamentarium today is a potent dopaminergic antidepressant. As indicated above, bupropion has weak dopaminergic properties. A number of years ago, nomifensine, a mixed norepinephrine/dopamine uptake blocker, appeared briefly on the United States market but was withdrawn worldwide by the manufacturer because of Guillain-Barré–like reactions in Europe. Many patients, however, responded well to this drug because of its energizing properties. The development of effective, nonaddicting dopaminergic agents would be a major step forward for antidepressant therapy. Unfortunately, we know of no such agents currently under study in the United States.

Deprenyl (selegiline) is a monoamine oxidase B (MAO-B) inhibitor that is used as an adjunct in the treatment of Parkinson's disease and by itself has also been studied as an antidepressant. However, it appears to be effective only at very high doses (Sunderland et al. 1994), in which case it loses selectivity for inhibiting MAO-B and its potential advantage for avoiding interactions with certain foodstuffs. Selegiline does not yet appear to be the dopaminergic agent that the field would appreciate.

Special Populations

As described above, the field has begun to consider whether severity (and perhaps age) has an effect on drug selection. This type of thinking points to a need to go beyond categorical classifications and to incorporate other data (e.g., age and gender) and a more dimensional approach to assessing symptoms and severity in depression before ultimately selecting specific treatments. Three such areas among others are becoming foci for investigation and ultimately will change how we treat depressed patients.

Gender

Over the past few years psychopharmacology has begun to address whether men and women differ in their responses to psychotropic agents and to pay more attention to gender-specific disorders such as postpartum depression and late luteal phase dysphoria.

For many years, medicine in general has overlooked the possible effects of gender on response to drug treatment. Unfortunately, drug development has focused on males in both lower animals and humans, with drug testing in rodents and mice being carried out in males to avoid possible confounds of the estrous cycle (Schatzberg 1997). Moreover, the thalidomide tragedy of decades ago resulted in further limitations on exposing women of childbearing potential to investigational psychotropic agents. The result has been that many agents have reached the market without having been evaluated in younger women. This state of affairs has changed dramatically over the past few years, in part because of political initiatives that led to the passing in 1993 of the Women's Health Equity Act. This reform mandated, among other things, the testing of medications in younger women and the study of how new agents might interact with female gonadal hormones.

Recently, research on SSRIs has resulted in the uncovering of possible differences between men and women in their responses to antidepressants. In a large-scale study comparing sertraline with imipramine in chronic major depression and so-called double depression, the dropout rate was significantly higher in women treated with imipramine than with sertraline (S. Kornstein, A. F. Schatzberg, and M. E. Thase, et al., "Gender Differences in Treatment Response to Sertraline Versus Imipramine in Chronic Depression," submitted for publication, 1999); Schatzberg et al. 1995). This was not the case for men. Moreover, women showed greater antidepressant responses with sertraline (particularly those who were premenopausal). In contrast, men responded better to imipramine than to the SSRI. These data suggest that women tolerate these two classes of agents differently. In another study on dysthymia, women responded significantly better to sertraline than to imipramine (Halbreich et al. 1995). These data suggest that the SSRIs may be better tolerated by and be more effective in women than are the TCAs. Moreover, studies pointing to the efficacy of fluoxetine in late luteal phase dysphoria (Steiner et al. 1995) indicate that the SSRIs may be helpful for women with a wide range of mood problems.

The psychopharmacologist of the early twenty-first century will undoubtedly have to be more gender sensitive with regard to drug selection and prescription. This will require a greater sensitivity to the types of symptoms that women patients may experience, how the symptoms vary during the menstrual cycle and around the menopause, and the potential interactions with gonadal hormones. To achieve this shift, training of residents and those at the postgraduate level will need to incorporate more information about specific gender-based symptoms of dysphoria as well as the effects of gender on drug response.

Agitation

Recently we reported (Schatzberg et al. 1996) that in depressed patients with severe agitation the addition of divalproex sodium may be extremely helpful in controlling motoric restlessness and in aiding an antidepressant response. The use of this agent has also uncovered a potential need for defining other dimensions—for example, agitation and affective instability—in approaching the depressed patient (Schatzberg et al. 1996).

Some individuals with pronounced symptoms of major depression and agitation will meet criteria for mixed mania while many others will not. Of those who do not, some may have histories suggestive of mild elation or overactivity but whose symptoms fall short of meeting criteria for bipolar disorder or cyclothymia. For depressed patients, one might begin to develop dimensions of agitation and history of relative affective instability to guide drug selection. Patients whose scores on these dimensions are high could be candidates for adjunctive or combination treatments, for example, divalproex sodium with an antidepressant. This would also move the field beyond drug selection based largely on categorical diagnoses—for example, major depressive disorder—to one in which the initial categorical definition is supplemented with dimensional data to select optimal single drug or combination strategies. This will require further development of our classification nomenclature but ultimately will bring us closer to how clinical practice is conducted. It also may support efforts to identify genes that underlie psychiatric disorders by bringing in behavioral dimensions (rather than categorical syndrome definitions) that could prove to be more closely linked to specific genes.

Ethnicity

The United States is becoming more ethnically diverse daily. Research efforts are under way to determine differences among ethnic groups in pharmacokinetic and pharmacodynamic properties of specific agents. Much of the research today is focusing on how specific ethnic groups "handle" and respond to antipsychotic agents, but it is likely that such data will affect all psychopharmacological practice. Thus, in the twenty-first century, the psychopharmacologist will need to routinely incorporate data about ethnicity into his or her practice.

New Antidepressant Strategies

Biological and pharmacological research are providing us with a number of insights regarding potential new treatment approaches. As indicated above, to date, our treatment of depression has revolved around agents that exert effects on monoamine reuptake or receptor activity. Many of our current agents are variations on a specific theme (e.g., serotonin reuptake blockade), and, as such, agents within one class are remarkably similar to each other in both therapeutic effect and side reactions. To move to another plane, agents will have to be developed that work on subreceptor components of monoamine systems or that exert effects on other neurochemical or neuroendocrine systems. These approaches offer new opportunities for drug development and will become the cornerstones of psychopharmacology in the next millennium.

Hypothalamic-Pituitary-Adrenal Axis

More than two decades ago, a number of research groups reported that hypothalamic-pituitary-adrenal (HPA) axis overactivity was a biological feature of depression (Sachar et al. 1970). Initial reports emphasized increased frequency of pulses of cortisol release, disruption of 24-hour diurnal rhythm, and increased excretion of urinary free cortisol or its precursors. Subsequently, depressed patients were reported to more commonly escape challenge with the synthetic glucocorticoid dexamethasone than were control subjects. Although the exact sensitivity and specificity of the dexamethasone suppression test (DST) in depression and its melancholic subtype have been the subject of debate (Arana et al. 1985), it is clear that many patients demonstrate disruption and overactivity of the HPA axis even though they may suppress their cortisol secretion when challenged with dexamethasone.

More importantly perhaps, research on the DST has led to a reassessment of the role that HPA axis overactivity may play in the pathogenesis of depression or in its symptom expression. The axis includes three major components: *corticotropin-releasing hormone* (CRH), a brain peptide that stimulates the pituitary to release *adrenocorticotropic hormone* (ACTH), which stimulates the adrenal to release *cortisol*. Cortisol provides feedback inhibition on the release of both CRH and ACTH.

Nemeroff's and Gold's groups have elegantly described increased CRH activity in depression, with some reports showing elevated CRH levels in the cerebrospinal fluid (Banki et al. 1987) and others reporting blunted ACTH responses to CRH administration (Gold et al. 1986). Thus, overactivity of central CRH has become a major hypothesis of the biology of both depressive and anxiety disorders because in lower animals central administration of CRH appears to produce signs (e.g., diurnal rhythm variation) suggestive of depression in humans.

CRH overactivity has become the possible target of drug development—specifically, agents that would act as antagonists at central CRH receptor sites. Early agents, such as αhelical CRH, have limited permeability across the blood-brain barrier and thus were not likely to produce much positive effect. More recently, agents with better distribution properties have been developed, and these agents may prove to be of use clinically. Research on these agents is about to be started in humans and offers great promise. In addition, researchers have begun to study the application of antisense strategies to block the translation of CRH messenger RNA into protein synthesis. Such strategies would also block the ultimate CRH overdrive in response to stress. The use of these types of agents would obviously need to avoid shutting down the HPA axis completely and inducing addisonian states. Theoretically, this should be possible because activity of the HPA axis is stimulated by other peptides in addition to CRH. Trials with one prototypic CRH antagonist are about to begin.

Should untoward stress responses with CRH overactivity prove to be key initiators of the biology of depression, CRH antagonists could be used to help deal with key developmental milestones or particularly stressful periods in individuals who are particularly vulnerable to developing depressive episodes. This could transform the psychopharmacology of depression from a discipline of treating depressive and other disorders to one of preventing their development. The identification of individuals at risk would most likely depend on a genetic marker for the risk of developing CRH overactivity, a marker that does not yet exist. Still, should research continue on this hypothesized tack, psychopharmacology in the year 2010 would be considerably different than that of today. It would incorporate elements of molecular biology and genetics not only to develop new compounds but potentially to identify individuals at risk for developing psychiatric disorders who might benefit from preventive treatment.

The overactivity of the HPA axis has been a focus for other research initiatives. Our group has hypothesized that overactivity of the HPA axis may result in altered central dopamine activity and the development of cognitive disturbance and delusions in depressed patients. One approach to treatment might be using agents that block cortisol synthesis or cortisol receptors. There are several recent reports on the antidepressant effects of agents such as ketoconazole and metyrapone (Murphy et al. 1991; Thukore and Dinan 1995). These studies report responses in some 50% of patients with non-delusional depression. Recently, our group has initiated a crossover study of mifepristone, the progesterone and glucocorticoid antagonist, in delusional depression. These strategies, should they prove of utility and convenience, would change our approaches to treating severely depressed patients, particularly those with psychosis.

Second-Messenger Systems

Although TCAs and SSRIs are primarily characterized by their effects on monoamine uptake, it is likely that downstream postsynaptic receptor effects account for their antidepressant activity. Generally, these agents block re-uptake immediately in animal models, but their clinical antidepressant effects usually require 2–3 weeks of treatment. This discrepancy suggests that mono-amine reuptake is required for clinical response, but that by itself it does not account for patients' responding.

This line of investigation began with the observations by Sulser and colleagues that antidepressants downregulated postsynaptic β-adrenergic receptors (Sulser et al. 1978) and those by de Montigny and Aghajanian (1978) that antidepressants increased the sensitivity of postsynaptic 5-HT_{1A} receptors. Although these were exciting and important findings, these effects, although they occurred after reuptake blockade, still occurred relatively early in comparison with known clinical response times. Also, pharmacological strategies to directly challenge these receptors did not produce more rapid or more complete antidepressant responses. In regard to the 5-HT_{1A} receptor, the agents used (e.g., buspirone and gepirone) may be only partial agonists such that their binding may not be potent or complete enough to effect the hoped for pharmacological and clinical responses. An exciting lead rests with the agent flesinoxan, a more complete 5-HT_{1A} agonist that has been shown to have antidepressant and anxiolytic effects in early clinical trials. This type of agent could produce more rapid responses in both depressed and anxious patients.

Over the past decade, research has continued to move away from the synapse itself (with its receptors) to so-called second-messenger systems. These systems control activity within the cell, the propagation of impulses down the neuron, and even the configuration of the receptors themselves.

Serotonin and norepinephrine receptors are frequently coupled via guanine nucleotide (G) stimulatory or inhibitory proteins to intracellular cyclic adenosine monophosphate (cAMP) systems. Neurotransmitters may also be linked to inositol phosphate second-messenger systems. Over time, antidepressants result in increased cAMP activity, which then results in myriad important intracellular biological effects. The delay to increased activity of such second-messenger systems and their subsequent effects is thought to account in part for the slow clinical responses to antidepressants. The identification of the key proteins involved in the so-called downstream effects and the genes that control them will allow development of treatment strategies or drugs that could affect these various subsystems without acting as agonists or reuptake blockers. Such agents might act more broadly and could be more effective in that they might reestablish normal activity regardless of whether the defect is seen in norepinephrine or 5-HT neurons. This type of approach will result in agents that belong to pharmacological classes that may not yet be described. Second-messenger system research has been helped by the rapid development of molecular biology, which has allowed us to begin to understand how drugs affect important genes that control a host of intracellular processes. Such genes may play key roles in determining not only receptor configuration and number but also whether specific neurons are susceptible to degeneration secondary to hypercortisolism.

Sapolsky and colleagues (1985) have eloquently described that stress and hypercortisolism result in degeneration of neurons and glucocorticoid receptors in the hippocampus. Clinically these findings may be ominously relevant since our group and others have reported that ventricular enlargement is seen in depressed patients with psychosis or in those with overactivity of the HPA axis (Rothschild et al. 1989) and that sustained relative hypercortisolism is associated with poor 1-year outcome on measures of social functioning in depressed patients (Rothschild et al. 1993).

Recently, findings on intracellular genetic processes, the effects of antidepressants, and neuronal protection have been elegantly woven together by Duman et al. (1997) at Yale to develop a new hypothesis of the biology of depression and how antidepressants work. cAMP activity results in increases in protein kinase activity, which then results in the phosphorylation of specific intracellular proteins. One particular transcription factor, cAMP response element binding protein (CREB), appears particularly to be increased by chronic antidepressant therapy. CREB in turn increases concentrations of specific nerve growth factors (NGFs), which is important for maintaining neuronal integrity and supporting the growth of neurons. Should the key mechanism of action of antidepressants be an increase in CREB and NGF activity, such findings would offer important leads into development of new drugs that could stabilize the cell and prevent the degeneration that results from chronic stress. Such agents would probably be radically different from what we use today in that they would likely avoid binding to monoaminergic receptors and instead act more directly on CREB and NGF.

Identity of the New Psychopharmacologist

The changes in drug development that are likely to occur will result in alterations in the identity of the psychopharmacologist in the twenty-first century. We are likely to move to a much more scientifically driven pharmacology in which drug development is based on hypotheses regarding pathophysiology and genetics, and drug selection is based on both clinical and biological profiles of patients. Such profiling may rely on brain imaging and genetics as tools for optimizing drug selection. Thus, the pharmacologist of the future will have to move from the simpler monoamine neurotransmitter models to more complex constructs involving neural systems and molecular pharmacology/biology. Aspects of this type of approach can already be seen in cancer therapy and will be repeated in psychopharmacology. Thus, medical students and residents in psychiatry will need to have well-honed skills in basic areas of neuroanatomy/neural circuitry, molecular biology, psychoneuroendocrinology, and molecular pharmacology to maximize their practice efforts.

Of particular worry to some is that an emphasis on basic biology will compromise our humanistic interests and bent. This is not likely to occur soon. Although we will have a greater sense of what biological processes are involved, environmental influences also will no doubt play strong roles in determining whether an individual becomes ill and then how a disorder may express itself. Thus, a blending of knowledge regarding environment and biology will likely be needed. Today, we hypothesize about dysregulated monoamine systems that may be genetically based but that have occurred in response to one or more psychosocial stressors. We then develop treatment strategies that include elements of psychotherapy and psychopharmacology. It is hoped that in the next century such approaches will have a stronger scientific basis and we will have better rationales for selecting treatments. The pharmacologist of the twenty-first century will be a better scientist but he or she need not be less of a compassionate healer or, as I expect, a preventer of disease development.

Indeed, the identification of important risk genes will begin to allow physicians to identify those specific interpersonal and environmental factors that are most likely to exert untoward effects and ultimately to develop treatment strategies that will incorporate both pharmacology and psychosocial treatment. Part of the pharmacologist's role will probably be to consult on or lead a team devoted to disease management or prevention. Should specific genes provide us with clues as to who will become ill and when, the pharmacologist will need to be able to design specific strategies for preventing disease expression. These strategies may include elements of drug prescription (e.g., CRH antagonists) as well as environmental manipulation. Ultimately, some disorders could be prevented or cured by gene therapy. Such approaches will most likely mean that the pharmacologist in the twenty-first century will be positioned even more centrally than he or she is today.

References

Arana GW, Baldessarini RJ, Ornsteen M: The dexamethasone suppression test for diagnosis and prognosis in psychiatry. Arch Gen Psychiatry 42:1193–1204, 1985

Banki CM, Bissette G, Arato M, et al: Cerebrospinal fluid corticotropin-releasing factor–like immunoreactivity in depression and schizophrenia. Am J Psychiatry 144:873–877, 1987

Clerc GE, Ruimy P, Verdean-Palles J: A double-blind comparison of venlafaxine and fluoxetine in patients hospitalized for major depression and melancholia. Int Clin Psychopharmacol 9:139–143, 1994

de Montigny C, Aghajanian GK: Tricyclic antidepressants: long term treatment increases responsivity of rat forebrain neurons to serotonin. Science 202:1303–1306, 1978

Duman RS, Heninger GR, Nestler EJ: A molecular and cellular theory of depression. Arch Gen Psychiatry 54:597–606, 1997

Feiger A, Kiev A, Shrvastava KK, et al: Nefazodone vs sertraline in outpatients with major depression: focus on efficacy, tolerability, and effects on sexual function and satisfaction. J Clin Psychiatry 57 (suppl 2):53–62, 1996

Gold PW, Loriaux DL, Ray A, et al: Responses to corticotropin releasing hormone in the hypercortisolism of depression and Cushing's disease: pathophysiologic and diagnostic implications. N Engl J Med 314:1329–1335, 1986

Golden RN, Bebchuk JM, Leatherman ME: Trazodone and other antidepressants, in Textbook of Psychopharmacology. Edited by Schatzberg AF, Nemeroff CB. Washington, DC, American Psychiatric Press, 1995, pp 195–213

Halbreich U, Rush AJ, Koran L, et al: Prediction of response of patients with dysthymic disorder to treatment with antidepressants, in Scientific Abstracts, 34th Annual Meeting of the American College of Neuropsychopharmacology, San Juan, Puerto Rico, 1995, p 241

Massana J: Reboxetine versus fluoxetine: an overview of efficacy and tolerability. J Clin Psychiatry 59 (suppl 14):8–10, 1998

Murphy BEP, Dhar V, Ghadirian AM, et al: Response to steroid suppression in major depression resistant to antidepressant therapy. J Clin Psychopharmacol 11:121–126, 1991

Nierenberg AA, Feighner JP, Rudolph R, et al: Venlafaxine for treatment-resistant unipolar depression. J Clin Psychopharmacol 14:419–423, 1994

Potter WZ, Manji HK, Rudorfer MV: Tricyclics and tetracyclics, in Textbook of Psychopharmacology. Edited by Schatzberg AF, Nemeroff CB. Washington, DC, American Psychiatric Press, 1995, pp 141–160

Roose SP, Glassman AH, Attia E, et al: Comparative efficacy of selective serotonin reuptake inhibitors and tricyclics in the treatment of melancholia. Am J Psychiatry 151:1735–1739, 1994

Rothschild AJ, Benes F, Hebben N, et al: Relationships between brain CT scan findings and cortisol in psychotic and nonpsychotic depressed patients. Biol Psychiatry 25:535–550, 1989

Rothschild AJ, Samson JA, Bond TC, et al: Hypothalamic-pituitary-adrenal axis activity and one-year outcome in depression. Biol Psychiatry 34:392–400, 1993

Sachar E, Hellman L, Fukushima D, et al: Cortisol production in depressive illness. Arch Gen Psychiatry 23:289–298, 1970

Sapolsky RM, Krey LC, McEwen BS: Prolonged glucocorticoid exposure reduces hippocampal neuron number: implications for aging. J Neurosci 5:1222–1227, 1985

Schatzberg AF: Introduction, the dynamics of sex: gender differences in psychiatric disorders. J Clin Psychiatry 58 (suppl 15):3–4, 1997

Schatzberg AF: Treatment of severe depression with selective serotonin reuptake inhibitors. Depression and Anxiety 4:182–189, 1996/1997

Schatzberg AF, Kornstein S, Keitner G, et al: Gender and treatment response in chronic depression, in Scientific Abstracts, 34th Annual Meeting of the American College of Neuropsychopharmacology, San Juan, Puerto Rico, 1995, p 247

Schatzberg AF, DeBattista C, DeGolia S: Valproate in the treatment of agitation associated with depression. Psychiatric Annals 26 (suppl):S470–S473, 1996

Steiner M, Steinberg S, Stewart D, et al: Fluoxetine in the treatment of premenstrual dysphoria. N Engl J Med 332:1529–1534, 1995

Sulser F, Vetalani J, Mobley P: Mode of action of antidepressant drugs. Biochem Pharmacol 27:257–261, 1978

Sunderland T, Cohen RM, Molchan S, et al: High dose selegiline in treatment resistant older depressive patients. Arch Gen Psychiatry 51:607–615, 1994

Thukore HH, Dinan TG: Cortisol syntheses inhibition: a new treatment strategy for the clinical and endocrine manifestations of depression. Biol Psychiatry 37:364–368, 1995

Tollefson GD: Selective serotonin reuptake inhibitors, in Textbook of Psychopharmacology. Edited by Schatzberg AF, Nemeroff CB. Washington, DC, American Psychiatric Press, 1995, pp 161–182

CHAPTER 12

A Clinical Model for Selecting Psychotherapy or Pharmacotherapy

Mark Levey, M.D.

Although medication and psychotherapy are routinely combined in most psychiatric practices (Sullivan et al. 1993), there are ongoing questions about how to best conceptualize the combination of interventions, and also about the best practical strategy for combining them in different situations. The majority of psychiatrists have taken the position that medication is a better treatment for some aspects of psychiatric illness, whereas psychotherapy is better for others. This has led to a two-track view of combining the interventions, in which each one has a different specific therapeutic target in the illness of a given patient. Some authors (Cooper 1985; Ostow 1990) have even conceptualized two illnesses in the same patient, one responsive to medication and the other to psychotherapy. In recent years, however, there has been a call for an integrated or unified approach, as contrasted with the combined (two-track) approach. In an integrated approach, the psychiatrist would develop a single, comprehensive, overall goal for the therapeutic endeavor, and the selection of interventions would be based on their effectiveness in furthering this overall goal of the treatment. This approach could ideally provide the psychiatrist with more flexibility, especially in situations where medication and psychotherapy can both address the same therapeutic targets. This approach would also provide an organized way to evaluate the complex interaction of psychotherapy and pharmacotherapy when both are used with the same patient. The stumbling block to this approach has been difficulty in defining overall goals for treatment, beyond symptom alleviation, that are acceptable to pharmacotherapists and to psychotherapists of different schools. However, by using the knowledge gained from the clinical effectiveness of different interventions, as well as from brain research and research in human development, to redefine our understanding of pathology and treatment in nondoctrinaire ways, we may now be in a position to articulate broadly acceptable overall treatment goals.

What I do in this chapter is summarize the literature on combining medication and psychotherapy, highlighting the issues that have been the focus of debate and the different solutions that have been proposed. I then review the arguments for and against trying to develop overall goals for treatment that could become the basis for an integrated, as opposed to a combined, approach in the use of psychotherapy and medication. Finally, I present an example of a nondoctrinaire, overall goal for the treatment of patients with anticipatory anxiety and demonstrate how such a goal would provide a way to choose among different interventions, evaluate their effectiveness, and offer an organized basis for changing tactics if the initial interventions were not fully successful.

Review of the Literature

There has been some question about whether medication and psychotherapy should be combined in a single treatment. Those who question the wisdom of combining the two interventions point out that each requires a different stance toward the patient (Docherty et al. 1977). The psychopharmacologist tends to view the patient as having an illness that requires cure and tends to focus on symptomatic relief as the goal of treatment. The psychotherapist tends to view the patient more as a person communicating distress that needs to be understood and strives to uncover and learn more about the patient (Hyland 1991). The goals of psychotherapy often include reworking underlying distress in addition to relieving the symptoms. This difference has led to warnings that trying to combine medication and psychotherapy ·will create confusion for the therapist and the patient, rendering both interventions ineffective. This is reminiscent of similar warnings about the dangers of combining interventions from different schools of psychotherapy which also differ from each other in their focus on symptom relief or on underlying problems. I return to this point below.

Many studies have implicitly accepted an either/or view by focusing on evaluating which of the two interventions was more effective for a given condition. However, studies that have looked at the effect of combining both interventions have failed to reveal any actual negative interactions (Rounsaville et al. 1981). In fact, although good research in the area of combined therapy is difficult to design and evaluate (Elkin 1988a, 1988b), the research that has been done, both with schizophrenic patients (Hogarty et al. 1991) and with depressed patients (Weissman et al. 1979), seems to indicate that combined treatment is more effective. However, there remain no clear guidelines to follow to most effectively combine these modalities. In current practice, the basis for combining them tends to be pragmatic. Often it is the orientation of the psychiatrist that determines the choice of intervention. Sometimes failure of one modality can lead to trying the other, and economic considerations, particularly in this time of limited economic resources which has created managed care, can also determine the choice (Hunt 1990).

In the effort to develop a theoretical basis for combining interventions, most psychiatrists have considered a two-track model, where psychotherapy and medication each have different specific targets. This model first evolved in thinking about the treatment of patients with schizophrenia. Before the advent of neuroleptics, dynamic and milieu therapy were the mainstays of treatment. When neuroleptics were developed, they were initially seen as stabilizing florid symptoms, thereby permitting the psychotherapy to be more effective. Later, as controlling the symptoms became equated with treating the illness, neuroleptics became the mainstays of treatment, and psychological treatments were viewed as ineffective. Most recently the research has indicated that combined treatment is more effective than medication alone, but the psychotherapy is focused on helping the patient and the family manage the psychosocial aspects of the chronic illness (Hogarty et al. 1991). The medications relieve the symptoms, and the therapy helps the patient to organize his or her life in a more effective manner (an ongoing difficulty created by the illness, but one that is not automatically alleviated even with successful medication for the psychotic symptoms).

Ostow (1962) proposed an analogous dual view in thinking about affective illness, defining separate domains for medication and psychotherapy. Writing from a traditional psychoanalytical viewpoint, he defined the domains as energy and dynamics. Although, in his view, effectively regulating "psychic energy" with medications may aid psychotherapy by enabling the patient to focus on dynamic issues, he emphasized (Ostow 1990) that changing the dynamics in successful therapy does not necessarily preclude an ongoing need for medication to "stabilize the energy." Ostow views the difficulty with energy (or affect) regulation as essentially a biological problem and the dynamic (personality) issues as psychological problems. Other psychiatrists (Loeb and Loeb 1987) have expressed similar views for patients with depression and other affective disorders, including mania and recurrent panic and anxiety. It would seem to follow that the biological problems should be approached with a biological intervention and the psychological problems with a psychological intervention. A similar suggestion about how to differentiate the respective targets of medication and psychotherapy has been to use medications as the treatment for Axis I disorders and psychotherapy for Axis II. By conceptualizing separate targets for interventions, the psychiatrist can implement a complex treatment, with biological and psychological interventions each having a specific role.

However, in spite of the efforts to clearly differentiate the targets of medication and psychotherapy, the two-track model is less clear-cut for patients with depression and other affective disorders than it is for patients with schizophrenia, because both psychotherapy and medication can be effective treatments for the affective symptoms themselves. Additional recent findings, from both clinical practice and biological research, indicate that the overlapping of effectiveness of biological and psychological interventions is even more far-reaching than has been previously believed. The recent work demonstrating that positron-emission tomography (PET) scans of patients with obsessive-compulsive disorder undergo the same changes when they are effectively treated with either behavior therapy or medication, and do not change when either treatment is not clinically effective, is a living demonstration of similar biological effects of psychotherapy and medication (Baxter et al. 1992). Kandel (1983) has written of psychotherapy as a biological intervention. Post (1992) describes psychosocial events triggering gene expression, further blurring the line between the psychological and the biological. From the other direction, Kramer (1993) gives many examples of newer medications being effective treatments for the very characterological and social problems that have traditionally been the province of psychotherapy. Wylie and Wylie (1987) give a case example of the use of phenelzine to aid in the development of the experience of the transference. Both in this case and in Kramer's examples, the target of both psychotherapy and medication is a pattern of relationships, not a clearly defined Axis I symptom.

Nevertheless, Ostow, as well as others (Cooper 1985), believe that a two-track (or two-illness) model is applicable. Cooper even extends the two-track view to the affective symptoms themselves and differentiates be-tween mood changes that are not motivated and therefore nonpsychological, which require the use of medications, and motivated mood changes, which re-spond to psychological interventions. Even Ostow, however, despite his two-track orientation, describes certain masochistic characters who seem to have two sets of problems, but who do not need psychotherapy for the second when medications work for the first.

As a result of this overlapping of effectiveness, the separation of targets for the different interventions is somewhat artificial, and the two-track approach does not help the psychiatrist decide which intervention to use in cases where both may be effective for the same target. This is reflected in the literature, where there has not been a consensus about how to choose between medica-tions and psychotherapy when targeting the same symptoms. Some have sug-gested that one should use medications first to give rapid relief. Others give the opposite suggestion, saying that one should establish an alliance before prescribing medication (Brockman 1990). Still another suggestion has been to use psychotherapy if it works and, if not, then try medication (Dewan 1992). In practice, the choice of intervention tends to be strongly influenced by the ideological preference of the individual psychiatrist.

A second limitation of the two-track model is that the two interventions in-teract with each other in complex ways. So, combining them adds to the com-plexity of the therapeutic situation; it is not simply a matter of using two unrelated interventions. The two-track model, with each intervention being seen as having its own target, does not provide a framework for understanding the inevitable interaction and its effect on the treatment. There is always a psychological meaning to the medication which can sometimes affect the therapy significantly, and, conversely, the effectiveness of the medication de-pends to some extent (greater or lesser in individual cases) on the state of the therapeutic relationship. In this sense, pharmacotherapy is combined therapy (Elkin 1988a) because the psychopharmacologist is also a kind of psychother-apist (Goldhamer 1983; Gutheil 1982).

There is widespread agreement in the literature about the importance of the therapeutic alliance in promoting medication compliance and effective-ness and on the importance for effective treatment of recognizing the psycho-logical meaning of the medication. Gutheil makes the point that the patient is most effectively medicated when attention is paid to forming an alliance and including the patient as a participant. He and others (Adelman 1985; Hausner 1986) point out that there are transference implications of prescribing medi-cation, and that the medication can be experienced as a transitional object, standing for the relationship with the therapist. Awareness of these factors can help the physician understand otherwise puzzling reactions, since the psychological meaning of the medication can tend to either nullify or enhance its pharmacological effects.

Brockman (1990) has discussed the complexity of these issues when working with borderline patients. With these patients, taking medication can be a regressive experience, activating fantasies of both terrifying assault and overvalued hope. So, while the pharmacology is aiding the ego, the psychological meaning may be stimulating a powerful regression. There is no clear boundary between issues of medication and issues of transference. Sometimes the interpretive work that may be necessary to enable a patient to tolerate medication and secure a trusting working alliance involves revealing and exploring primitive fantasies, which is more sophisticated therapy than simply providing support and education.

Nevins (1990) adds that the effects of the medication can also have a meaning. The changes that the medication induces often confront the patient with the requirement for psychological work to integrate what is happening to him or her. Hyland (1991) notes that medication can alter therapeutic issues by putting the patient in a different state. He underlines the fact that we do not know if the changes brought about by the two modalities are actually similar or different, but that the relationship between the two needs to be examined on a case-by-case basis.

This blurring of boundaries in terms of targets of intervention and modes of action has led many to underline the necessity of individualizing the treatment. The importance of considering the individual patient, not simply the diagnosis, is cited repeatedly in the literature. Psychotherapy research indicates that only 10% of outcome variance is due to differences in techniques, whereas therapist and particularly patient characteristics account for 90% of the variation in outcome (Beitman 1987). Many argue, therefore, that the patient's view of his or her own situation and the patient's view of which approaches he or she can best use should be important factors in choosing psychotherapeutic interventions and in deciding when to use medications as well. This orientation was clearly articulated by Sarwer-Foner (1989) when he contrasted a public health model with an individualized treatment model. In his view, psychiatric medications are more like morphine than like penicillin because context has a big impact on the effectiveness of the medication and because psychiatric medications are effective in alleviating symptoms and are not specifically curative of the disease. In the absence of a specifically curative procedure, a scientifically adequate public health model that would permit a formalized, standard mass treatment approach to a diagnostic entity is not possible. Psychiatric illness, from schizophrenia to the neuroses, requires, rather, an individualized, tailored treatment approach.

For some psychiatrists, individualizing the treatment is not a sufficient response to the complexity, because they believe that the blurring of boundaries indicates that the two-track viewpoint is basically flawed. Beitman (1981) believes that seeing medication and psychotherapy as disparate interventions obscures the overriding effect of the therapeutic relationship. Hoffman (1990) agrees that the two-track model creates a false dichotomy and leads to compartmentalization, creating a reluctance to treat supposedly psychological problems with medication (a biological intervention) and a tendency to equate less severe illness with psychological illness, in spite of the fact that there is no basis for dichotomizing an illness such as depression on the basis of severity. Marcus (1990) suggested a distinction be made between the *combination* of medication and psychotherapy (a two-track view) and the *integration* of medication and psychotherapy (a unified model). The crucial difference between a two-track and a unified model is that in the unified model the patient and psychiatrist would develop an explicit, comprehensive, overall goal for the therapy, an integrated view of what the treatment is trying to accomplish, which would provide a defined context for any subgoals included in the treatment. In a unified model, medication and psychotherapy would be viewed as tools that interact in positive or negative ways in promoting the overall goal of the treatment.

The proponents of an integrated approach believe that it would provide a more accurate representation of our developing understanding of how psychiatric treatment is effective. An integrated approach would acknowledge that there are different effective approaches to the same target—that we cannot define etiology by treatment. By explicitly recognizing overall goals beyond symptom relief, such an approach would enable us to look at the effects of any intervention on the treatment as a whole, not just its effect on its designated target, and choose interventions on this basis rather than simply their effect in terms of symptom relief. We would also be able to assess the synergistic and antagonistic effects of combined interventions in terms of their effect on the overall goal.

Perhaps the most important advantage of the unified approach, however, is that it would represent a step toward truly integrating our new knowledge of the mind and brain by developing new and deeper understandings of both psychopathology and psychiatric treatment. The categories we use to conceptualize psychopathology and to understand problematic patterns have always been strongly determined by the effectiveness of interventions, both biological and psychological. Panic became a discrete diagnosis, a particular pattern, only when we had a specific medication to effectively treat it. As Kramer

(1993) has pointed out, the success of serotonin reuptake inhibitors in directly promoting self-esteem, self-confidence, and freedom from guilt begins to change the way we understand and think about those characteristics. In regard to psychotherapeutic treatment, knowing that exposure is crucial in treating phobias may lead us to examine different successful treatments for phobia to discover if, in fact, various treatments all promote exposure in different ways, even if they do not define their interventions in that way. To genuinely use the new findings that are emerging in psychiatric research, we need to generate models that expand the current sectarian biological versus psychological paradigms, and to do that we need to redefine the goals of treatment in nondoctrinaire ways.

At this point, however, there are still people who favor a two-track rather than a unified model (Cooper 1985; Kantor 1990; Karasu 1982, 1990a; Marcus 1990; Ostow 1990). The proponents of both the two-track and unified models agree on several things. They all agree that the complexity of the interaction of the two interventions needs to be taken into account, that factors beyond DSM-IV diagnosis (American Psychiatric Association 1994) need to be integrated into treatment planning, and that it is crucial to individualize the treatment. The proponents of the two-track model believe this can best be done by using different models, such as a biological and dynamic, in combination. Each model can be applied when appropriate. What is necessary is that the therapist have a view of the patient as a whole and be free to take an individualized approach with each patient. Karasu (1990b) takes this position in exploring the treatment of depression. Although he sees medication and psychotherapy having different effects in depressed patients (medications dealing with vegetative effects and symptoms, and psychotherapy dealing with relationships and social adjustment), he subsumes them both under the umbrella of an overall individualized approach to each patient's needs. Marcus develops an overview from his particular dynamic orientation and is able to use it to conceptualize the interaction of medication and psychotherapy.

The question of the possibility of and need for developing a comprehensive, unified therapeutic goal, which divides the proponents of the two-track and unified models, is the same question that is being debated by those who have been trying to integrate different psychotherapeutic approaches with one another. In fact, as Beitman (1981) has stated, combining medication and psychotherapy can be viewed as a special case of combining interventions from different theoretical origins. So, it is informative to look at how this question is being dealt with in the psychotherapy integration literature.

Technical Eclecticism Versus Theoretical Integration

Psychotherapy literature shows the debate between the proponents of technical eclecticism and proponents of theoretical integration. The major disagreement has revolved around the possibility and desirability of agreeing upon comprehensive therapeutic goals. Technical eclecticism refers to a nontheory-based, pragmatic strategy of selecting the most promising treatment procedures from various therapy orientations and testing their efficacy in specific treatment contexts (Wolfe 1989). Beutler (1989), a proponent of systematic eclecticism, says that it is impossible to determine meaningful goals that a range of therapists would agree upon, because the goals of therapy simply reflect the values of the therapist. Therefore, the systematic eclectic is interested only in the question of how to accomplish a given goal most effectively. What are the diagnostic, patient, environmental, therapist, and interaction variables that predispose a patient to be differentially responsive to different treatment approaches?

The proponents of the two-track approach to combining medication and psychotherapy essentially describe a systematic eclectic approach. They define a treatment with multiple goals, each one approached by the most effective intervention. The universal goal implicit in this approach is symptom relief, which can be accomplished by either psychotherapy, pharmacotherapy, or both, whichever is shown to be more effective. For the "school" of pharmacotherapy, symptom relief is *the* given goal, and it is the measuring rod by which the effectiveness of interventions are judged. However, there is room in the two-track approach for additional goals that can vary from patient to patient and therapist to therapist. Most of the therapists who have supported a two-track view have a complex overall view of the patient which involves several therapeutic goals. In fact, as I illustrate in the last section of this chapter, even the proponents of pharmacotherapy generally have implicit goals beyond simple symptom relief. However, these authors believe that constructing comprehensive widely agreed upon therapeutic goals across schools of psychotherapy is not possible, and, as long as the therapist considers the use of different interventions, including medication and psychotherapy, to effectively achieve his or her diverse goals, such a general integration is also unnecessary.

The proponents of theoretical integration, on the other hand, believe that the articulation of unified goals for therapy in a broadly acceptable, non-doctrinaire way is both necessary and possible. Arkowitz (1989) believes that understanding why and how different therapies work is crucial because that knowledge can generate theories of psychopathology which can refine our understanding of what to change, not just how to change it. This resonates with Kramer's position, previously stated, that the effectiveness of new interventions is leading us to redefine the patterns we see. The increasing overlap of the targets for medication and psychotherapy, with medications having effects beyond symptom relief and new psychotherapies being effective in rapidly alleviating symptoms, necessitates a more comprehensive overall model of treatment to enable the psychiatrist to choose between interventions. This is true in regard to choosing between different effective psychotherapeutic interventions, as well as choosing medication or psychotherapy. It would be useful for a therapist to have an integrated way to consider the varying effectiveness of seeming dichotomies such as a subject-subject versus a subject-object orientation to the patient, trying to understand versus promoting action, understanding behavioral contingencies versus understanding dynamic conflict, and to be able to use different stances with the same patient comfortably regardless of which orientation a therapist's particular school espouses. Even how to listen, either for the facts of the story, or for an empathic sense of the other's experience, or for symbolic and displaced references is a choice the therapist has to make (Beitman 1987). Each of these modes can be valuable, but knowing when to use each one requires an integrated sense of what you as a therapist are trying to accomplish and how you plan to go about doing it.

In addition to arguing for the importance of an integrated, unified view of therapy, the proponents of theoretical integration also insist that it is possible to achieve. Goldfried (1980) has pointed out that most psychotherapy schools have grand theories of human motivation, human functioning, and human pathology, and that these are impossible to integrate at the grand level. However, at the level of clinical strategy, or principles of change, he believes that there are important commonalities that can be distilled. For example, what different schools of therapy present as clinical goals in themselves (recognizing one's automatic thoughts, understanding the origin and function of one's fears, or becoming more directly in touch with one's emotional life) can be viewed as different means to similar clinical ends, that is, changing one's expectations and one's self and one's world view. Likewise, specific techniques of different schools can be viewed as particular examples of more general principles of change, that is, promoting new experiences, reframing problems, exposing oneself to what has been feared, and obtaining new information. Overtly articulating these common clinical goals and principles of change can clarify what therapy is trying to accomplish in a nondoctrinaire way and can provide a fresh perspective on how people change.

The early efforts in the direction of psychotherapy integration focused on trying to find the factors common to all psychotherapies (Frank 1976; Marmor 1985). Frank viewed all psychiatric patients as suffering from demoralization as manifested by anxiety, depression, resentment, and feelings of isolation. In his view, all psychotherapies work by relieving the demoralization through the provision of a relationship that the patient values, a rationale explaining the problem to the patient, and a ritual that the therapist and patient engage in to alleviate the problem. This model is consistent with the work demonstrating the importance of the therapeutic relationship for the effectiveness of both pharmacological and psychotherapeutic interventions and suggests using the relief of demoralization as the measure of the relative or combined effectiveness of these interventions. Their effectiveness in relieving psychiatric symptoms is, of course, an important part of their effectiveness in relieving demoralization; however, symptom relief per se becomes subsumed under a more comprehensive therapeutic goal—one that explicitly articulates what the symptom relief has always been implicitly expected to accomplish.

More recently, both Beitman (1987) and Basch (1995) have also developed general models of psychotherapy by reframing the goals of treatment in ways that cut across the seeming theoretical differences of the many schools of therapy. Beitman uses time and the stages of therapy to define general mini-goals for all therapies. Therapy is divided into engagement, pattern search, pattern change, and disengagement. Each stage is characterized by certain expectable goals, content, and techniques for achieving the goals, as well as by expectable transferences, resistances, and countertransferences. The goal of engagement is to develop a relationship in which the therapist is trusted and gains a position of influence with the patient. Pattern search is looking for patterns that, if changed, will alleviate the patient's suffering. Pattern change involves changing these patterns, including giving up the old pattern, initiating new patterns, and practicing the new patterns. Disengagement is concerned with ending the relationship in such a way that the gains are maintained. Although different schools of therapy tend to be characterized by the kinds of patterns they search for and the techniques they favor for changing them, a therapist using this organizational model is free to be guided by the patient in deciding which sort of patterns and change techniques are most effective with each individual case.

This model can provide a structure for integrating medication and psychotherapy that can help a therapist decide which intervention to use through an awareness of what he or she is trying to accomplish beyond symptom removal. For example, medication can be used early in therapy to establish the therapist's credibility by demonstrating his or her expertise and capacity to bring symptom relief. However, it can create problems early in therapy if it is experienced by the patient as an expression of lack of interest by the therapist. So, the crucial early question is not simply will a particular medication diminish anxiety, but rather the question is whether diminishing anxiety with the medication will be a positive experience for the patient and whether it will help establish the psychiatrist as a helpful, reliable, trustworthy person and consolidate a position of influence. Later, medication may be used with a different subgoal in mind, either as a tool to discover patterns (such as using a mood stabilizer to help establish the diagnosis of a mood disorder) or to help change a pattern once a pattern has been discovered. If the pattern in question is, for example, the individual's sense that he or she cannot manage himself or herself effectively, then medication will be useful if it is experienced as a help with his or her self-control, and it can be counterproductive if it is experienced as proof that he or she cannot develop self-control, even though it may alleviate anxiety or depression. By knowing what one is trying to accomplish in the context of the overall treatment, and knowing the individual patient, the therapist can decide if medication will be useful in moving the treatment forward.

Basch has a different model based on developmental theory, but his model also cuts across established therapeutic schools by defining general therapeutic goals phenomenologically. His model can be viewed as a detailed elaboration of Frank's demoralization hypothesis. Basch sees behavior as fundamentally a striving for competence, promoting a situation where one is reasonably well adapted to the environment, yet meeting one's own needs. He describes a developmental spiral, where one makes a decision, implements it with behavior, finds that to be competent, and experiences pleasure in functioning and a rise in self-esteem. When a patient comes into therapy, that spiral is not working effectively, and restoring competent functioning is the goal of treatment. Basch understands the chief complaint as being a confused report of how the patient ceased to function competently and lost self-esteem. During the diagnostic process, the therapist determines what is interfering with good functioning and what to do about it.

A model like Basch's can provide a bridge from a two-track view of medication and therapy to a unified view, by shifting the therapeutic goals from symptom alleviation and character change to the more comprehensive goal of restoring competent functioning, which encompasses both. Medications have a pharmacological effect on symptoms, but their utility in restoring a sense of competence may also relate to the meaning of taking the medication, or the behaviors that the patient engages in as a result of being on the medication, or all of the above. It is how medication affects the treatment in all of these areas that the psychiatrist evaluates.

Although many psychiatrists might not subscribe to alleviating demoralization or restoring competence as universally valid overall therapeutic goals, the general approach of defining broadly acceptable, nondoctrinaire therapeutic goals is a promising one. At this point in time, this approach may be even more powerful with a limited rather than a general focus. To illustrate this I present a conceptual model for patients with anticipatory (stimulus-dependent) anxiety. This model operationally defines what we have come to know about the pathology and effective change procedures for anticipatory anxiety, while at the same time enabling the psychiatrist to take individual differences in patients systematically into account through attention to the therapeutic relationship and resistances. As a result, it becomes possible to use medication as well as multiple psychotherapeutic interventions in an organized way in the treatment by assessing whether and how they promote the general goal.

A Conceptual Model for Anticipatory Anxiety

Anxiety, which was generally viewed by dynamic psychiatry as the signal of a problem, is viewed by descriptive psychiatry as a problem in its own right. Which orientation to assume is the first choice that a psychiatrist must make with a given patient. The situation has, however, been further complicated by the fact that anxiety is no longer regarded as a unitary process. Panic and phobias, for example, have different established treatments, and panic and generalized anxiety respond to different medications. In addition, Kandel (1983) has demonstrated a different molecular basis for anticipatory and chronic anxiety on a cellular level. When one is faced with different forms of anxiety, the general strategy has been to characterize different anxiety syndromes by using descriptive criteria (e.g., panic, phobia, social phobia) and investigate which particular kind of medication or brand of psychotherapy, or combination, is most effective in treating the particular syndrome. The assumption behind this approach has been that the form of the anxiety, the DSM-IV diagnosis, is the most important determiner of effective treatment.

Effective symptomatic treatments for different anxiety syndromes have been developed with this approach, but the clinical situation is often complex. The anxiety response itself is an involuntary biologic response, part of the primary motivational system of humans. However, anxiety is also a learned response. As the brain picks out what predictably and reliably occur together, it can learn to be anxious about almost any situation. Exactly how this learning occurs has been differently conceptualized by behaviorism, psychoanalysis, cognitive psychology, and social learning theory. What has become increasingly clear is that biological factors, trial and error learning, cognitive learning, interpersonal attachment, and unconscious processes are all operative in clinical anxiety disorders, and principles of their interaction are not well understood (Curtis 1985a). In a second article, Curtis (1985b) suggests a two-track approach to this complexity, indicating that one can usually treat Axis I anxiety disorders and get symptomatic improvement and can use psychotherapy if this does not work well enough or if there is also an Axis II problem.

A unified approach would take into account the possibility that the anxiety and the Axis II problem are related. This approach would spell out what would be expected to happen in the treatment if the anxiety itself were the problem, and what could happen that would indicate that the anxiety was part of a larger picture that needed to be addressed. This can be accomplished by articulating a therapeutic goal that defines improvement qualitatively not just quantitatively, but does it in a way that descriptive and dynamic psychiatrists can both agree upon. One could then organize and evaluate interventions based upon the pursuit of that goal.

I suggest that the overall goal in treating a patient who suffers from counterproductive, anticipatory anxiety is to lessen the anxiety, have the patient successfully confront what he or she is afraid to experience (whether it is thoughts, feelings, situations, activities, fantasies, or some combination), find out in the process that the danger is not as great as was feared, and effectively learn from this that he or she has the ability to cope with what was feared, and, therefore, no longer has to be afraid and restrict his or her life. This goal includes decreasing the intensity of the affective response, but also promoting new behaviors, having the behaviors reinforced through success, and having the successes change the patient's actual functioning as well as the patient's view of his or her self and the world, thereby restoring a sense of competence.

This goal is consistent with the general ideas of Frank, Basch, and Beitman. It details the steps in dealing with the "demoralization" created by anxiety and restoring competence. The goal is anchored by the solid evidence that exposure is crucial in eliminating anticipatory anxiety and promoting new learning, but that it is not always enough. The goal provides a way to recognize when anxiety is the problem and when it is part of a larger problem. Because the therapy is not a success until the exposure is effective, the demoralization is alleviated, and competency, a sense of mastery, and self-esteem are restored, the therapist can evaluate whether simply decreasing the anxiety is enough. On the other hand, once the goal is met in full, the treatment can be considered to be a success however this was achieved. Therefore, the therapist is free to individualize the choice of interventions based on the preferences and strengths of the particular patient and can recognize when the intervention has been sufficient.

To individualize the intervention most effectively, the therapist also needs to understand what is maintaining the anxiety. Biological, developmental, and situational factors may all be involved in maintaining anxiety, and the clinician needs to determine what is particularly problematic for a given patient and which factors can be most effectively addressed (Table 12–1). For example, the intensity of the anxiety response itself, a biological factor, may create a problem by precluding new learning. Learned avoidance (behavioral inhibition) may be a problem, preventing the "unlearning," that is, learning that a situation is no longer dangerous. Repression, a kind of learned avoidance of thinking and feeling, can also prevent unlearning. Cognitive distortions about the self and about reality may be a problem because the patient creates a dangerous reality to which he or she then responds with anxiety. Although the cognitive distortions may have arisen from faulty learning, once they have become filters mediating new experiences, even objectively neutral experiences can be interpreted in ways that seem to confirm the reality of the danger. Unconscious conflict, where mutually contradictory important wishes, needs, and fears present a danger to the patient's well-being, can be problematic and maintain anxiety in some patients. The experience of anxiety itself may be threatening, creating a fear of fear. In such a case, any situation that can lead to failure or anxiety is dangerous, because the experience of anxiety is intolerable. For some people, reality factors, that they may or may not be aware of, can maintain anxiety. Interactions with other people or the expectations of others may maintain anxiety. Finally, anxiety may be a response to a realistic

Table 12–1.   Factors maintaining anxiety

Primary dysfunction of nervous system

Avoidant behavior that prevents unlearning

Cognitive distortions creating seeming danger

Inability to tolerate anxiety

Unconscious conflict and disavowed meanings

Inadequacy in confronting adaptive tasks

Actual environmental stressors

appraisal of a lack of skills, information, or psychological capacity, which actually renders the patient unable to cope with a situation or task.

For many patients, several of these factors are involved. Goldstein and Chambless (1978), for example, characterized patients with true agoraphobia as dealing with low self-sufficiency, stimulus-independent (biologically based) panic, and a fear of fear, an inability to tolerate anxiety, all of which needed to be addressed for effective treatment. With the overall goal in mind, the clinician can think about which factors to address, what he or she is specifically hoping to accomplish thereby, and how any particular intervention relates to the overall treatment.

If the initial assessment suggests a normative view that the anxiety is the problem and that the patient is ready to benefit from facing his or her fears, then one would start by trying to decrease the anxiety and promote exposure, anticipating that the patient would cooperate, and expecting that the exposure would be a positive experience and that the learning from the positive experiences would naturally lead to a sense of mastery and a change in the patient's view of himself or herself and the world. Exposure itself is an effective way to decrease anxiety (Marks 1978); however, it can be difficult to induce people to try it, and it is sometimes difficult to discover the precise anxiety cues to which to expose the patient. So, for some patients, diminishing the anxiety by other means may be a precondition for clarifying the anxiety-inducing cues and for effectively promoting exposure.

Because both medication and psychotherapy can be used to decrease anxiety directly, the choice would be based upon individual characteristics and preferences of the patient. Medication makes sense when the problem is conceptualized as a biological difficulty with the anxiety response system itself. Using medication to diminish anxiety may be sufficient treatment if the patient can then expose his or her self to what he or she has feared, learn from that exposure, and change his or her behavior and view of the world. In other cases, medication may be part of getting a person ready to engage in exposure and psychotherapy, especially if a high degree of initial anxiety is a prohibiting factor. Medication may also help promote exposure in a psychological way by giving some patients a sense of control of their anxiety which can build self-confidence and enable them to risk exposure. Whether medication simply diminishes anxiety or achieves other aspects of the overall goal as well (as with patients who change their basic view of themselves and the world while on Prozac [Kramer 1993]) can be evaluated in each case to see if further interventions are necessary.

However, medication is not the only way to diminish anxiety. Psychotherapy can also be used to diminish anxiety and promote exposure. Support and encouragement by a therapist, if the therapist is valued, will diminish anxiety. Relaxation techniques can also do it. At times, cognitive explanations of what is going on and why, or simply putting into words what is threatening can have the same effect. Finding ways to reframe the experience of anxiety that make it less threatening (even, with some people, explaining that they cannot control it) can diminish anxiety.

When the immediate therapeutic goal is to diminish the anxiety, medication and psychotherapy may be interchangeable for many patients. However, for some patients, depending on their expectations, previous experience, and character structure, one or the other approach may be more effective. Similarly, many patients, once they begin to expose themselves to the anxiety-arousing stimuli, find that their anxiety decreases, and they begin to engage in new ways of thinking, feeling, and acting. However, with other patients, these normative expectations turn out not to apply, and, although their anxiety may be diminished, the exposure either does not occur or is not successful.

Some patients will sabotage the exposure, and the psychiatrist has to understand why. It may be that the particular intervention is unacceptable to the patient. Perhaps the patient has a different intervention that he or she requires or prefers. The intervention has to make sense to the patient. The patient may not have the understanding or psychological skill to make use of some interventions effectively. If these factors do not explain the ineffectiveness of the attempt at exposure, then the therapist needs to consider the possibility of a countermotive, a resistance (Table 12–2).

One source of resistance can be the patient's need to hold onto the anxiety itself because the anxiety is serving an important psychological function for the patient, such as binding an unconscious conflict or avoiding potential self-punitive reactions. The more centrally important the fear is to the patient's psychological makeup and functioning, the greater the possibility that this may be a factor.

A second source of resistance can be the patient's realization that he or she is not yet ready to successfully accomplish the exposure. In these situations, the therapist has to help the patient become ready by making a successful outcome more likely. This may be addressed by teaching interpersonal skills where necessary, helping patients develop the capacity to effectively understand and manage the reactions they may get from others, or helping the patient change his or her environment so it is more understanding and supportive.

Medication as well as psychotherapy may be useful in enabling people to recognize or to overcome their resistance. I had one patient who had been in

Table 12–2. Sources of resistance

Intervention not acceptable to the patient

Anxiety is solution to unconscious conflict

Anxiety prevents intolerable possible failure

Anxiety provides other secondary gain

Existence of psychological deficits

Lack of environmental support for change

Inability to learn from new experiences

Unwillingness to learn from new experiences

therapy for a while and felt that it was not helping him to become more relaxed, less self-critical, and happier. Although he felt that he was somehow constitutionally incapable of being less negative and self-critical, when I suggested a trial of Zoloft to see if that would help, he was horrified at the thought of becoming happy on the medication. It was at that point that he could begin to recognize that he was motivated to stay in the emotional state he complained of and that we needed to understand and deal with why and how it was important to him before any therapeutic regimen would have a chance to succeed.

Medication may also help to overcome resistance by enabling patients to effectively manage situations that they could not manage when off medication. Medication's usefulness in this regard depends upon how it is experienced by the patient. If the patient believes that the medication is enabling him or her to master a situation that he or she could not master before and helps build their self-confidence, then it is helping to achieve the therapeutic goal. If being medicated is experienced as proof that the patient cannot handle a situation, then medication can actually undermine the therapeutic goal, even if it diminishes the anxiety and helps to promote exposure. By keeping the therapeutic subgoals in focus, the psychiatrist can evaluate the effectiveness of medication in each individual therapy.

Finally, there are circumstances in which patients expose themselves to the anxiety-provoking situations and manage them successfully, but find that their anxiety is not eliminated and their view of themselves and the world does not change. Their sense of competence is not restored and their demoralization is not relieved. In these cases, the therapist and patient have to work together to explore how and why change is avoided. It may be that the patient does not recognize the significance of the positive experiences; the success may be discounted by thinking things such as it was just luck, it was not really me, I cannot keep this up, etc. At times, this reaction may be unmotivated. It may be the result of passivity in the new experience, or because medication is getting the credit, or because the way anxiety had been dealt with became a barrier to unlearning it.

For example, one patient began to let himself meet new people, which frightened him terribly. He dealt with the fear by trying to be pleasing. He found himself accepted and was making friends. However, he kept experiencing the acceptance as a result of his going out of his way to please people and not be himself. So, the positive experiences did not alter his basic feeling of being unacceptable and did not alleviate his anxiety in future situations. In cases like this, once the interference is understood, the successful experience can often be restructured in a way that lets it sink in.

For other patients, the discounting of success is motivated. They are afraid to change in the ways that they also desire to change. These situations can occur whether the primary positive change is the result of psychotherapy or of medication. When the failure to learn from the positive changes is motivated, then the psychiatrist cannot simply talk the patient into seeing and accepting the positive changes. Instead, the importance of maintaining the status quo needs to be understood and addressed.

One patient, whom I had seen for several years, continued to be very anxious before coming into sessions. He did not think of me as threatening, denied any negative experiences with me, and was vague about what he anticipated. He suggested that he had had bad experiences with his parents, so he expected something vaguely bad with me. However, his several years of good experiences with me had not made any difference. As we continued to focus on this, he finally realized that when he experienced me as accepting he would undo it by telling himself that I was really thinking badly of him, but I was hiding it because therapists are supposed to be supportive. So, although he had objectively positive experiences with me, he had found a way to discount them and not learn from them that I (and the world) was safer than he thought. He was then able to realize that he was motivated to see me as dangerous and that maintaining his anxiety with me was serving an important protective function and helping him to maintain a safe distance. That led to new memories of times he had trusted his mother and been caught with his guard down. So, seeing the world as safe was itself a danger he needed to avoid.

By keeping in mind the overall goal in treating patients with anticipatory anxiety, the psychiatrist is in a position to recognize and respond to whatever interferes with its achievement. Interventions can be evaluated by their effectiveness in promoting this goal in each patient. Whether to use medication, insight, cognitive restructuring, behavior modification, or any other technique depends upon the particular difficulties the patient is having with anxiety as well as the type of interventions to which the patient is most open.

Summary

Medication and psychotherapy can be considered as interventions to be combined with each other or to be integrated with each other. When they are combined, each is directed at a different therapeutic target. Medication is generally targeted at symptom alleviation, whereas additional psychotherapeutic goals tend to be defined by the terms and values of a particular school of therapy. A combined model can be used as long as the therapist has an overall view of the particular patient and is free to individualize the treatment approach. However, an integrated model, where the treatment is organized by a comprehensive, nondoctrinaire, overall goal beyond symptom relief, is potentially more flexible, and it can also help to refine our understanding of psychopathology and psychiatric treatment. When the overall goal is met, the treatment can be considered a success, and interventions can be organized and evaluated in terms of their effectiveness in promoting the overall goal and the subgoals it includes. This chapter provides an illustrative example of how such a model can be used in the treatment of patients with anticipatory anxiety. By developing nondoctrinaire clinical goals in various areas of psychiatric treatment, we can eventually create a conceptual structure that enables us to use medication and different psychotherapies in thoughtful and complementary ways, even as new uses for medication and new therapies are developed.

References

Adelman SA: Pills as transitional objects: a dynamic understanding of the use of medication in psychotherapy. Psychiatry 48:246–253, 1985

American Psychiatric Association: Diagnostic and Statistical Manual of Mental Disorders, 4th Edition. Washington, DC, American Psychiatric Association, 1994

Arkowitz H: The Role of Theory in Psychotherapy Integration. Journal of Integrative and Eclectic Psychotherapy 8:8–16, 1989

Basch MF: Doing Brief Psychotherapy. New York, Basic Books, 1995

Baxter LR, Schwartz JM, Bergman KS, et al: Caudate glucose metabolic rate changes with both drug and behavior therapy for obsessive-compulsive disorder. Arch Gen Psychiatry 49:681–689, 1992

Beitman BD: Pharmacotherapy as an intervention during the stages of psychotherapy. Am J Psychother 35:206–214, 1981

Beitman BD: The Structure of Individual Psychotherapy. New York, Guilford, 1987

Beutler LE: The misplaced role of theory in psychotherapy integration. Journal of Integrative and Eclectic Psychotherapy 8:17–22, 1989

Brockman R: Medication and transference in psychoanalytically oriented psychotherapy of the borderline patient. Psychiatr Clin North Am 13:287–295, 1990

Cooper AM: Will neurobiology influence psychoanalysis? Am J Psychiatry 142:1395–1402, 1985

Curtis GC: Anxiety and anxiety disorders. Psychiatr Clin North Am 8:159–168, 1985a

Curtis GC: New findings in anxiety. Psychiatr Clin North Am 8:169–175, 1985b

Dewan MJ: Adding medications to ongoing psychotherapy: indications and pitfalls. Am J Psychother 46:102–110, 1992

Docherty JP, Marder SR, Van Kammen DP, et al: Psychotherapy and pharmacotherapy: conceptual issues. Am J Psychiatry 134:529–533, 1977

Elkin I, Pilkonis PA, Docherty JP, et al: Conceptual and methodological issues in comparative studies of psychotherapy and pharmacotherapy, I: active ingredients and mechanisms of change. Am J Psychiatry 145:909–917, 1988a

Elkin I, Pilkonis PA, Docherty JP, et al: Conceptual and methodological issues in comparative studies of psychotherapy and pharmacotherapy, II: nature and timing of treatment effects. Am J Psychiatry 145:1070–1076, 1988b

Frank JD: Restoration of morale and behavior change, in What Makes Behavior Change Possible? Edited by Burton A. New York, Brunner/Mazel, 1976, pp 73–90

Goldfried MR: Toward the delineation of therapeutic change principles. Am Psychol 35:991–999, 1980

Goldhamer PM: Psychotherapy and pharmacotherapy: the challenge of integration. Can J Psychiatry 28:173–177, 1983

Goldstein AJ, Chambless DL: A reanalysis of agoraphobia. Behavior Therapy 9:47–59, 1978

Gutheil TG: The psychology of psychopharmacology. Bull Menninger Clin 46:321–330, 1982

Hausner R: Medication and transitional phenomena. International Journal of Psychoanalysis and Psychotherapy 11:375–398, 1986

Hoffman J: Integrating biologic and psychologic treatment: the need for a unitary model. Psychiatr Clin North Am 13:369–372, 1990

Hogarty GE, Anderson CM, Reiss DJ, et al: Family psychoeducation, social skills training, and maintenance chemotherapy in the aftercare treatment of schizophrenia, II: two-year effects of a controlled study on relapse and adjustment. Arch Gen Psychiatry 48:340–347, 1991

Hunt W: A psychoanalyst does psychopharmacology. Psychiatr Clin North Am 13:323–331, 1990

Hyland JM: Integrating psychotherapy and pharmacotherapy. Bull Menninger Clin 55:205–215, 1991

Kandel ER: From metapsychology to molecular biology: explorations into the nature of anxiety. Am J Psychiatry 140:1277–1293, 1983

Kantor SJ: Depression: when is psychotherapy not enough? Psychiatr Clin North Am 13:241–254, 1990

Karasu TB: Psychotherapy and pharmacotherapy: toward an integrative model. Am J Psychiatry 139:1102–1113, 1982

Karasu TB: Toward a clinical model of psychotherapy for depression, 1: systematic comparison of three psychotherapies. Am J Psychiatry 147:133–147, 1990a

Karasu TB: Toward a clinical model of psychotherapy for depression, 2: an integrative and selective treatment approach. Am J Psychiatry 147:269–278, 1990b

Kramer PD: Listening to Prozac: A Psychiatrist Explores Antidepressant Drugs and the Remaking of the Self. New York, Viking, 1993

Loeb FL, Loeb LR: Psychoanalytic observations on the effect of lithium on manic attacks. J Am Psychoanal Assoc 35:877–902, 1987

Marcus ER: Integrating psychopharmacotherapy, psychotherapy, and mental structure in the treatment of patients with personality disorders and depression. Psychiatr Clin North Am 13:255–263, 1990

Marks IM: Behavioral psychotherapy of adult neurosis, in Handbook of Psychotherapy and Behavioral Change. Edited by Garfield SL, Bergin AE. New York, Wiley, 1978

Marmor J: The psychotherapeutic process: common denominators in diverse approaches, in The Evolution of Psychotherapy. Edited by Zeig J. New York, Brunner/Mazel, 1985, pp 266–274

Nevins DB: Psychoanalytic perspectives on the use of medication for mental illness. Bull Menninger Clin 54:323–339, 1990

Ostow M: Drugs in Psychoanalysis and Psychotherapy. New York, Basic Books, 1962

Ostow M: On beginning with patients who require medication, in On Beginning an Analysis. Edited by Jacobs TJ, Rothstein A. New York, International Universities Press, 1990, pp 201–227

Post RM: Transduction of psychosocial stress into the neurobiology of recurrent affective disorder. Am J Psychiatry 149:999–1010, 1992

Rounsaville BJ, Weissman MM, Klerman GL: Do Psychotherapy and Pharmacotherapy Conflict? Arch Gen Psychiatry 38:24–29, 1981

Sarwer-Foner GJ: The psychodynamic action of psychopharmacologic drugs and the target symptom versus the anti-psychotic approach to psychopharmacologic therapy: thirty years later. Psychiatric Journal of the University of Ottawa 14:268–278, 1989

Sullivan M, Verhulst J, Russo J, et al: Psychotherapy vs. pharmacotherapy: are psychiatrists polarized? Am J Psychother 47:411–423, 1993

Weissman MM, Prusoff BA, DiMascio A, et al: The efficacy of drugs and psychotherapy in the treatment of acute depressive episodes. Am J Psychiatry 136:555–558, 1979

Wolfe BE: Introduction: the meaning of integration. Journal of Integrative and Eclectic Psychotherapy 8:7, 1989

Wylie HW, Wylie ML: An effect of pharmacotherapy on the psychoanalytic process. Am J Psychiatry 144:489–492, 1987

CHAPTER 13

Studying the Respective Contributions of Pharmacotherapy and Psychotherapy

Toward Collaborative Controlled Studies

Donald F. Klein, M.D.

Evaluating Treatment

In this chapter, I critically review the literature concerning the respective contributions and relative merits of pharmacotherapy and psychotherapy in the treatment of mental disorders. The grounds for continued rational doubt about studies contrasting psychotherapeutic and pharmacotherapeutic effects are reviewed because almost all comparative therapeutic studies and research summaries are fatally flawed by failings in study administration, sample definition, study design, and treatment execution. Therefore, firm conclusions concerning relative merits are rarely warranted. My second major point is that such flaws are not inevitable because critical collaborations between pharmacotherapists and psychotherapists using improved experimental designs yield substantive conclusions.

Psychotherapy, pharmacotherapy, and their combination are the major modes of psychiatric treatment. *Psychotherapy* and *pharmacotherapy* are

This work was supported in part by Public Health Service Grant MH-30906, Mental Health Clinical Research Center–New York State Psychiatric Institute.

abstractions, encompassing hundreds of divergent procedures and goals. Nevertheless, their relative merits and respective contributions have been incessantly debated. Such debated issues comparing modes of treatment—in the era of cost control and managed care—immediately affect hiring and income. Issues of professional identity and self-esteem heighten this debate's emotional impact because criticizing claims to special competence incites emergency reactions in those criticized.

For pharmacotherapy, following preclinical safety evaluation, studies of volunteers establish safety and tolerability in humans (phase I). Phase II, the first open treatment of patients, is crucial for identifying therapeutic indications. Our grasp of psychiatric pathophysiology is so limited that every major class of psychotropic drugs has been serendipitously discovered by unsystematic phase II open trials. Late phase II and phase III definitively establish specific efficacy by placebo-controlled experimentation, often augmented by a standard reference drug comparison (Laska et al. 1994).

Unlike pharmacological agents, psychotherapy has usually been openly, unsystematically studied. Empirical observations of apparent effectiveness led to theoretical developments justifying these practices but did not proceed to systematic case series or adequately controlled trials. As psychotherapy, initially dominated by psychoanalytic theory, expanded rapidly, the schisms of Jung, Adler, and others made it evident that alternative views of psychoanalytic observations were possible. Furthermore, each new school claimed therapeutic superiority.

Unfortunately, systematic phase II requirements were not met. Accumulating a well-diagnosed, substantial, consecutive patient series in which the patients' symptomatology and impairments were independently, self-, and therapist-described before and during treatment and at the point of dropout, termination, or treatment completion, and then independently followed up has had only recent tentative beginnings. Therefore, arguments about relative merits of treatment continued in the absence of relevant clinical data.

The general assumption of therapeutic efficacy was seriously questioned by Eysenck's conclusion (1952) that the specific effectiveness of psychotherapy was not supported by research evidence and that psychoanalysis might be toxic. Eysenck asserted that psychotherapists erroneously assumed that the untreated would do badly but that studies of untreated neurotic patients showed equivalent or superior spontaneous improvement rates to the treated patients. Attempts to prove Eysenck wrong led to endless inconclusive debate concerning the sample comparability, measures, etc. The need for comparative clinical trials became plain, but the necessary design and control requirements were not critically applied.

Views of Psychopathology
and Treatment

Alternative, conflicting views of appropriate treatment are paralleled by conflicting psychopathological theories (Klein and Rabkin 1984). For instance, psychopathology has been attributed to conditioned reflexes, learned maladaptive attitudes and distorted cognitive maps, unconscious conflicts, early trauma, and maladaptive biological vulnerabilities. These theories, respectively, justify behavior therapy, cognitive therapy, psychodynamic therapy, abreactive techniques, and somatic therapies.

Debatable Therapeutic Priorities

The controversy concerning therapeutic priorities heats up for the modal outpatient, plagued by anxieties, fears, panics, and somatic and depressive complaints and impairments. Science, to date, casts little illumination. Some conclude that psychotherapies do not differ and are not even superior to a credible placebo, whereas others firmly deny this. Medications are usually superior to placebo, yet psychotherapies have been shown to be superior to pharmacotherapy in comparative trials (Antonuccio et al. 1995). It is not surprising that the bewildered clinicians tend to ignore the issue by dismissing the patients studied as irrelevant (particularly in their lack of comorbidity) to those they treat, the treatments studied as not up to their standards, and the treatment comparisons as far too superficial and global.

How Might Psychotherapy and
Pharmacotherapy Differ?

Psychotherapy and pharmacotherapy may each affect different sorts of patients or produce different effects in similar patients. These treatments also may differ in speed of onset, maintenance of benefit after stopping treatment, acceptability, prophylactic effects, sleeper effects, stimulation of environmental engagement, cost/benefit values, and degree of training needed by the professional who applies the treatment. Numerous other possible differences exist, but few of these questions have been addressed with any adequacy, although rational clinical practice needs these answers.

Adequacy of Treatment Studies: Types of Validity

Kazdin (1992) neatly categorizes experimentally answerable questions. The central question is to what extent can the intervention, rather than extraneous influences, be considered to account for the results, changes, or group differences? One can simply give the new treatment to a series of suitable patients, as in early phase II. However, the changes may not be the result of the intervention, because some patients spontaneously improve, some respond to the caring atmosphere, etc. Simple before-and-after comparisons are inadequate. Properly controlled studies make it unlikely that causal efficacy can be attributed to anything other than treatment.

Seemingly better than the historical control group is the concurrent no treatment control group; however, that is rarely a feasible option. Instead, the randomized waiting list control group is used; however, this is not a *no treatment* but a *deferred treatment* control group.

Critelli and Neumann (1984) state that the ready acceptance of waiting list control subjects is deeply puzzling because comparing a therapy-treated group against a waiting list control group incurs an artifactual bias in favor of treatment. Treated patients justify their investment of time and effort by considering themselves improved. Waiting list patients experience the opposite experimental demand to downplay positive changes, thus justifying their waiting list status. Furthermore, untreated patients may be compelled into self-treatment or covertly use psychotherapeutic agents. A waiting list control group thus poorly approximates the "natural history" of the disease.

Placebo Control: Construct and External Validity

Construct validity addresses the question, given that the intervention was responsible for change, what specific aspect of the intervention was the causal agent? Construct validity is impossible to establish without credible placebo control.

In pharmacotherapy, the prime question is whether an agent is specifically useful. One establishes group comparability by randomization, diminishes biased reporting with double-blinded or independent evaluation, and provides all patients with an equivalent amount of caring interaction by giving pill placebo case management to those denied the experimental agent. A placebo lacks the active ingredient. In pharmacology, it is simple to remove the active ingredient; but in psychotherapy, the nature or even existence of specific active ingredients is controversial. One person's placebo, for example, relaxation, is another person's active ingredient. Constructing a psychotherapy placebo cannot be done by fiat because it may include unrecognized ingredients that are beneficial or toxic. Kazdin and Wilcoxon (1976) point out the importance of the credibility of the psychotherapy placebo because placebo effects require a belief in nonplacebo effects. If a treatment has little face validity, it will not arouse positive expectations and may promote demoralization.

External validity deals with the question, to what extent can the results be generalized or extended to people, settings, times, measures, and characteristics other than those in this particular experimental arrangement? This brings us to the major failing of current comparative studies.

Before comparing treatments, it makes sense to establish that each treatment produces specific benefits in addition to the antidemoralizing effects of a caring setting, explanatory framework, etc. For pharmacotherapy, this is relatively simple, given the credible pill placebo case management comparison. (For psychotherapy, as I emphasize, the pill placebo case management comparison in the setting of a pharmacotherapy-psychotherapy comparison offers a useful baseline.) However, assuming that specific benefits have been shown for both treatments, one must recognize that this specificity is sample dependent. For instance, many placebo-controlled trials of imipramine failed to show a specific effect of imipramine despite apparently adequate power, dosage, and sample definition. We now know that patients with one subgroup of major depressions (with atypical features) will have symptoms that respond poorly to imipramine. So retrospectively we can account for imipramine failure (if the correct measures were taken), but prospectively we could not. This raises the problem of sample calibration, as an appropriately treatment-responsive sample is a necessity for comparative trials.

To establish the relative merits of psychotherapy and a standard medication, one might simply compare randomly assigned medication versus psychotherapy. However, this comparison lacks both internal and external validity. If the psychotherapy is superior to medication, it remains unclear whether this is the result of superior psychotherapeutic benefit or invalid medication prescribing practices. Also, despite using diagnostic standards, if one picks a medication-unresponsive sample, the results should not be generalized to a medication-responsive population. However, a pill placebo case management control answers both questions. The internal validity issue is immediately resolved if the medication is superior to pill placebo by the degree of improvement usually found. The external validity question is also resolved because the sample is demonstrated to be medication responsive. Furthermore, medication administration must be valid and not toxic.

One can then contrast psychotherapy with the credible pill placebo case management condition. If a psychotherapy is no better than placebo plus 30 minutes of nondirective, nonspecific support, it does not warrant much practical attention. If the psychotherapy has been shown effective in one group compared with a credible comparison group in a series of clinical trials, then there remains the problem of assessing the causes of this outcome difference, for example, sample variation or treatment variation. However, one might be concerned that, if medication proved superior to psychotherapy, which did not exceed pill placebo, perhaps an atypically psychotherapy-unresponsive sample had been picked, or perhaps psychotherapy-suitable candidates flee potentially receiving medication, or perhaps the psychotherapy was poorly done.

The most important issue is whether—in some substantial series of studies—the pharmacotherapy or psychotherapy has already proven superior to a credible, nonspecific, nontoxic, comparison group. If this has been shown, then, if a particular trial fails this level of efficacy, questions should be raised about the generalizability of this particular study. Unfortunately, many psychotherapies have demonstrated superiority only to waiting list or non–credibly treated control subjects, so a negative trial may indicate a general lack of specific efficacy rather than a sample or technique peculiarity.

Whether the psychotherapy was adequately done requires skilled training and appropriate process analyses. That psychotherapy-responsive patients have an antipathy to medication and therefore will not enter a trial where they may receive medication is, so far, a groundless ad hoc speculation. However, it is not beyond investigation. One might take treatment applicants and randomly select them for assignment to one of two tracks. First-track patients are then randomly selected for comparative treatments, whereas second-track patients get to choose. The key contrast would be if the average outcome of the first-track group differs from that of the second.

The often reported, modest superiority of *combined* pharmacotherapy and psychotherapy, compared with equivalent psychotherapy or pharmacotherapy *alone*, is consistent with results found in samples in which pharmacotherapy is largely ineffective. However, without a pill placebo group, one cannot be sure.

Combined Treatment and the Importance of Pill Placebo

The respective contributions of pharmacotherapy and psychotherapy may be most evident by comparing combined treatment with its components. In a 2×2 factorial design, pharmacotherapy versus pill placebo is crossed with psychotherapy versus no treatment. Because psychotherapy is usually delivered without placebo, this design does not accurately represent psychotherapeutic practice and is therefore a problematic design.

One could extend the 2×2 design to a 2×3 design, that is, psychotherapy versus no psychotherapy crossed with pharmacotherapy, pill placebo, and no treatment (Klerman et al. 1974). A problematic cell is assigned to neither pill nor psychotherapy. As indicated above, using the wait list as a control group leads to positively biased estimates of efficacy. Therefore, it should be deleted, leaving five meaningful cells.

Also, process analyses should compare the psychotherapies delivered unaccompanied with medicine or pill placebo. A pure additive model implies that treatments do not affect each other, but that is unreasonable here. Psychotherapy of a depressed patient carried out in the context of successful antidepressant effect might have quite a different tempo and level of aspiration than psychotherapy carried out alone. Pharmacotherapy might facilitate psychotherapy, just as psychotherapy, by enhancing patient compliance, might facilitate pharmacotherapy.

The importance of a pill placebo control is made clear by Hollon et al.'s (1991) study, which compared cognitive therapy, pharmacotherapy, and the combination in the treatment of depression. The authors conclude that, although the combined modality was not significantly favored, the lack of a pill placebo control group made it impossible to determine whether the sample was pharmacologically responsive. They state, "we have come to share Klein's (1989) view that the tendency to not include pill-placebo controls (maintained in a double-blind fashion) . . . has made it difficult to determine whether pharmacotherapy as operationalized was indeed effective for the samples actually studied."

Power et al. (1990) provide a good example of the importance of a proper placebo contrast in a combined study. In a 10-week study, 101 patients with generalized anxiety disorder were randomly allocated to cognitive-behavior therapy (CBT) alone; CBT combined with diazepam or with placebo; diazepam (5 mg, three times daily); or placebo. CBT did best, and there was no negative effect of diazepam or placebo when combined with CBT. However, both diazepam and placebo as solo treatments did poorly and were indistinguishable.

Without a placebo group, this study could be interpreted as demonstrating CBT superiority to diazepam. Given the placebo group, it becomes much firmer that CBT specifically benefited this group, but diazepam did not. Therefore, whether CBT is superior to diazepam in diazepam-specific responders with generalized anxiety disorder is moot.

Adequate Treatment

A second source of concern is treatment adequacy. Meterissian and Bradwejn (1989) argue that optimal pharmacotherapy should meet certain basic conditions including maintaining adequate doses kept at a maximum for 4–6 weeks, serum monitoring, using adequately trained pharmacotherapists, and switching or augmenting treatment in nonresponders. Walsh et al. (1997) demonstrated the feasibility of the drug-switching design when the first medication was ineffective or poorly tolerated. In the Meterissian and Bradwejn review of the psychotherapy-pharmacotherapy literature for depression, not a single study met all of the criteria and few met more than two, implying inadequate pharmacotherapy. If pharmacotherapy studies do not model good pharmacotherapeutic practice, perhaps psychotherapeutic studies do not model good psychotherapeutic practice. Suspicion falls upon the mandatory use of manuals.

Wilson (1996) vigorously contests this view. He cites Schulte et al. (1992), who compared using manuals for in vivo exposure treatment of specific phobia, with using an individualized therapy in which therapists were free to select whatever technique they saw fit, with a control treatment in which each patient received a yoked therapy tailored to a patient in the individualized condition. The standardized treatment was significantly superior to the other two immediately and at 2-year follow-up. However, the superiority of standardized treatment was the result of individualized therapists failing to use in vivo exposure. The individualized treatments that did use exposure techniques did as well as exposure using manuals. This raises the issue of whether or not manual-guided procedures are necessary, given a general understanding of the superior value of certain interventions, such as exposure techniques for patients with phobias.

Optimum Design

A recent special feature of the *Journal of Consulting and Clinical Psychology* (1996) discusses the optimum experimental design for comparing pharmacotherapy with psychotherapy. I argue that, without a pill placebo case management control group, it is moot whether the sample selected is actually medication responsive or properly treated. By using this control group, a direct comparison is possible between the psychotherapy and a minimum treatment condition that provides the essentials that Jerome Frank (Frank and Frank 1961) claims forms the basis of psychotherapeutic benefit. This tests whether the psychotherapy provides specific benefits. Jacobson and Hollon agree, although for different reasons. Jacobson and Hollon (1996a) say, "It is agreed that the inclusion of such controls would facilitate the interpretation of the findings" and further "that pill placebo controls are optimal but not essential to comparisons between CBT and pharmacotherapy" (Jacobson and Hollon 1996b).

The conclusion that the use of a pill placebo case management control is optimal markedly advances the field. Jacobson and Hollon do not agree that previous comparisons of pharmacotherapy and psychotherapy that lack this control were a waste of time and money, but I conclude that most comparative therapeutic studies and research summaries are so intrinsically flawed by major failings in design, sampling, execution, and lack of replication that they cannot support firm conclusions.

Lack of Essential Independent Replication

An overriding issue is independent replication. Generalizing from a sample is best done when it represents a defined population, ideally by random selection. This is not done; we depend on samples of convenience from our clinics and hope that we define them well enough that the effects found apply to similarly labeled patients elsewhere. We become more confident if our findings are independently confirmed, even if on samples of convenience.

Comparative studies of pharmacotherapy and psychotherapy have lacked properly controlled independent replications. Any current discussion is based upon tenuous evidence and should be conducted tentatively. The statement that the replicated fact/conclusion ratio is vanishingly small will be denied by meta-analysis enthusiasts, so I briefly address this approach.

Meta-Analysis

A number of meta-analyses, starting with Smith et al. (1980), attempted to establish the validity of psychotherapy, as well as its superiority to pharmacotherapy. This claim needs detailed discussion.

R. A. Fisher's distinguished methodological career was crowned by convincing his statistical colleagues of the necessity of randomized treatment comparisons. Randomization ensures that, at baseline, treatment groups differ no more than random processes allow, not only with regard to variables we know about but also with regard to those we do not know exist.

Lambert and Bergin (1994) state,

> A problem in the Smith et al. review is that they had to rely on cross-study comparisons in which behavioral therapy in one study was compared with verbal therapy from another study. In this situation, many variables besides treatment modality also differ across studies. Comparisons like this, of which there are many in the Smith et al. (1980) report, cannot be as conclusive as comparisons in which the compared treatments are offered within a given study.

Furthermore, meta-analysis sweeps aside the validity of treatment provision, the need for blind and independent evaluation, whether control groups were comparable or credible, or even whether waiting lists rather than valid control groups were used. Also, meta-analysis obscures the heterogeneity, reactivity, and differential importance of different measures, by either amalgamating them into an average-effect size or by picking effect sizes according to the meta-analyst's preferences.

More Meta-Analytic Substance

Robinson et al. (1990) clearly compared psychotherapy to placebo control in clinical patients. Their research was based on 58 studies of psychotherapy for depression, restricted to samples of patients identified as primarily suffering from depression. Twenty-nine studies with a wait list control group yielded a significant ($P < .05$) mean effect size of 0.84 (SD = 0.69). However, for nine studies with a placebo control group, the insignificant mean effect size was only 0.28 (SD = 0.52).

Robinson states,

> As our analyses demonstrate, clinical research has firmly established the efficacy of psychological interventions for depression. . . . It remains unclear, though, which aspects of psychotherapeutic treatment were responsible for producing this improvement. When the effects of psychotherapy were compared with those of placebo treatments, no reliable differences emerged. . . . [And] despite their improvement, clients treated with psychotherapy remained distinguishable from healthy controls.

Of enormous import, Robinson et al. demonstrated that the investigator's allegiance may play an overriding role in determining differential treatment outcomes because partialling for allegiance removes any difference in effectiveness between studies. Does the invested investigator conduct treatment better or (unconsciously) bias observations and analyses more effectively? Since this question is moot, studies by enthusiastic or parental investigators require independent replications.

Meta-analysis may be useful when several controlled, low-power studies of well-defined samples have similar results that individually miss significance, but as a group show a signal. This is not a conclusory argument that the treatment works, but rather that proper, high-power studies are warranted. Such a modest meta-analytic role is quite different from its ambitious misuse.

Are All Psychotherapies Equivalent?

Stiles et al. (1986) succinctly state that psychotherapy is more effective than no treatment, but "No such consensus exists concerning the relative effectiveness of diverse therapies." The famous dodo bird verdict (Luborsky et al. 1975) that "all have won and all must have prizes" implies outcome equivalence. How can that be?

The argument that therapist behaviors, in different therapies, are really similar has been discarded since process analyses show marked differences. These procedural distinctions became more concrete with the advent of manual-guided therapies. Alternatively, there may be inherent reparative tendencies. Unfortunately, it remains vague why all psychotherapies should uniformly stimulate these obscure processes rather than hinder or be simply irrelevant.

Most often accepted is Jerome Frank's thesis (Frank and Frank 1961) that all therapies possess common features (prestigious healer, positive expectancies, explanatory framework, special therapeutic setting, affective arousal, prescribed therapeutic activities) that do the job rather than the distinguishing features. But what is the job? Frank's trenchant point is that the common features act on the common demoralization that results from illnesses and life defeats. Common therapeutic features are not "nonspecific," because they specifically attack demoralization, which makes them effective.

Frank asserts that much depressive and anxious symptomatology is the result of demoralization. Therefore, if demoralization is not caused by unchangeable external or internal circumstances, one can expect effective psychotherapy. If demoralization is the result of remediable circumstances, the antidemoralizing effects of psychotherapy might mobilize the patient to improve his or her environment, producing a beneficent cycle. If demoralization prevented learning from experience, one can expect psychotherapy to help eliminate maladaptive avoidances. In specific phobias, demoralization allows anticipatory anxiety to overwhelm the patient, thus preventing exposure to the phobic object and in turn preventing the patient from learning that he or she is capable of stoically containing the anxiety. With continued exposure, the anxiety diminishes and may disappear.

Problems With Power

Being unable to find a statistically reliable difference between treatments does not affirm that they are identical, because the study may be too poorly powered to detect real differences, usually because of too few subjects. Other obscuring problems are a lack of subject uniformity causing outcome spread, a lack of procedural uniformity, unreliable measures, etc. Kazdin and Bass (1989) recommend sample sizes of 71 per group to retain .8 power with $\alpha = .05$, two-tailed. Since this sample size is rarely attained in comparative therapy studies, type II errors (failures to detect real differences) must be frequent.

Maintenance and Follow-Up Trials: Longitudinal Data

An important psychotherapeutic claim is that psychotherapy eliminates the underlying causes of manifest psychopathology, so maintained benefit and prophylaxis occur. This benefit seems superior to medication, whose symptomatic and prophylactic benefits require maintenance treatment. However, definitive studies demonstrating this advantage are few.

Clearly, the most valid maintenance trials are by Ellen Frank et al. (1990, 1991), who studied 128 acutely depressed patients with at least three previous episodes who responded to combined treatment with imipramine and Interpersonal Therapy (IPT) and then entered a 3-year maintenance trial. The patients randomly received placebo or imipramine alone or IPT (given either alone, amplified by placebo, or amplified by imipramine). The results are quite clear for survival time. Imipramine (which was not improved by combination with IPT) had a major effect, compared with the effects found in the poorly performing placebo group. There is a modest superiority for IPT with and without placebo compared with the effects of placebo, but clear inferiority to imipramine. One might argue that IPT, given only monthly, had actually shown a surprisingly good effect as compared with that of placebo. At 1 year, 65% had relapsed on placebo; 46%, on placebo plus IPT; 46%, on IPT alone; 18%, on imipramine; and 8%, on imipramine plus IPT.

The Frank et al. studies are a marked design improvement with regard to most comparative maintenance studies because all the patients had improved initially and then were randomly selected to dismantled components of the combined treatment. This is different from simply following up responders or completers, who are a subsample of a group originally randomly selected to acute treatment.

Simply following up treatment responders, as Blackburn et al. (1986), Simons et al. (1986), and Evans et al. (1992) did, creates another ambiguity. Hollon et al. (1991) state,

> It remains possible that cognitive therapy's apparent preventive effect represents the consequences of differential retention rather than any bona fide treatment effect. The typical follow-up study focuses on patients who both complete and respond to the respective modalities. Given the 20–40% attrition rates and 60–75% response rates associated with the respective interventions, this means that the samples entering follow-up might constitute only 35–60% of the sample initially assigned. If different types of patients are likely to either complete or respond to the respective modalities, the acute treatment period could act like a *differential sieve*, producing systematic differences in the sets of patients entering the follow-up from the different modalities. It is conceivable that the differences observed to date result not from any preventive effect attributable to cognitive therapy but rather from a greater propensity for patients at risk for relapse . . . to successfully complete pharmacotherapy than cognitive therapy.

Furthermore, studies often superficially report longitudinal data. Brown and Barlow (1995) illustrate the difference between simple cross-sectional and longitudinal evaluations of fluctuating conditions. Although cross-sectional data indicate that the subjects improved over the follow-up, the fact that some responders have relapsed and a number of nonresponders have improved during this time interval was obscured until the data were analyzed longitudinally.

Sequential Treatment

Singularly little data exist concerning the utility of pharmacotherapy in those who have done poorly on psychotherapy or vice versa. If patients who did poorly from one modality did well on another, that situation argues for different modes of action.

Conceptual Summary

It has proven difficult in clinical samples (excluding simple phobias and obsessive-compulsive disorder treated by exposure and response-prevention therapies) to show that psychotherapies differ much from each other or exceed credible psychotherapy placebos or pill placebo case management.

Stiles et al. (1986) state,

> . . . dismantling studies of cognitive-behavioral approaches to depression have also tended to go against the specificity-of-effects position. Thus, Kornblith et al. (1983) reported a dismantling study. A full cognitive-behavioral treatment was compared with a didactic condition lacking the instigational push of homework assignments, a condition lacking only the self-reinforcement element, and an active control treatment—problem-oriented, psychodynamic group psychotherapy. All four treatments were equally effective.

Jacobson et al. (1996) recently found identical null dismantling results in a three-group study of 150 patients whose treatment ranged from the full cognitive approach to simple behavioral activation.

Comparative treatment research must be hypothesis-driven, otherwise efforts are completely impractical. It is disappointing that researchers have rarely delivered differential prescriptions that clearly paid off. Enormous allegiance effects heighten skepticism about parentally fostered studies. Demonstrating that a proposed mechanism of psychotherapeutic success is the actual mechanism or even that it antecedes therapeutic benefit has not been shown.

The direct contrast of psychotherapy with pharmacotherapy in clinical populations has often shown psychotherapeutic superiority. This is problematic because in the majority of cases pharmacotherapy was not optimal, and the samples were not shown to be medication responsive. Without a pill placebo control group, it cannot be assumed that specific pharmacotherapy benefit actually occurred in such a trial. The establishment of an acceptable psychological placebo has proven irretrievably difficult because of its theory-dependent nature.

Although presumably the psychotherapies and pharmacotherapies have different modes of action, it has proven difficult to show that they affect either different subsets of patients or different ranges of symptomatology or incapacity. Combined therapy generally shows a modest additive benefit, although many analyses are compromised by lack of appropriate cell-wise statistical comparisons or proper placebo controls.

Within samples, substantial heterogeneity exists, leading to marked outcome variance, particularly with regard to depression severity. Moderate benefits will often be undetectable, given the low power inflicted by small cell size and marked outcome variance. Independent replications are rare, particularly by skeptics.

The single-pharmacotherapy versus single-psychotherapy design fails to model the options of clinical practice, which includes switching drugs or adding an adjunct, if little has happened by 6 weeks. Such switching may not be usual psychotherapeutic practice, because one can see difficulties, having spent the first 6 weeks presenting one framework of understanding and then switching to another. However, a pharmacotherapeutic shift is not ideologically problematic.

A number of proposed remedies amount to a flight from the real difficulties, for example, to give up placebo controls or abandon programmatic comparisons or retreat to process, single-case, or event analyses. I recommend the opposite. To evaluate patient treatments, we must jointly study pharmacotherapies and psychotherapies in large multisite studies, as opposed to studies of small samples, calibrated against waiting lists and conducted by enthusiasts, which rarely produce usable knowledge. (Multiple sites incur their own problems, however).

Comparative studies should not be carried out by single-minded therapeutic enthusiasts, but by collaborations between scientists with opposing views willing to put them to the test. Studies comparing psychotherapy and pharmacotherapy must be internally calibrated for pharmacotherapy benefit by a pill placebo control group and jointly supervised by the respective expert clinicians. We must face the fact that our current comparative research approaches have yielded little. This may give us the resolution to recognize that it is time to stop inflexible persistence in fruitless parochial pursuits.

Toward the Twenty-First Century

In psychiatric comparative clinical trials, the track record of our national science institutes, for example, the National Institute of Mental Health (NIMH), is sparse. The well-designed NIMH-supported depression study was completed by 1984, and there have been no successors. Our Therapeutics Department at the New York State Psychiatric Institute has been at the forefront of generating pill placebo controlled, comparative, collaborative studies of pharmacotherapy and psychotherapy. These studies show the feasibility of joint pharmacotherapy and psychotherapy collaborative studies in which the responsibility for the valid service delivery is under the expert supervision of co-investigators: David Barlow, Jack Gorman, Laszlo Papp, Katherine Shear, Scott Woods (panic disorder with moderate agoraphobia), Edna Foa and Michael Liebowitz (obsessive-compulsive disorder), and Richard Heimberg and Michael Liebowitz (social phobia).

Developing and funding collaborative, cross-disciplinary, therapeutic studies has not been a central NIMH initiative. Clinical trials are not even represented within the NIMH structure. Funds at NIMH are limited, such studies are expensive, and there is competition at the National Institutes of Health in general, NIMH in particular, between basic and clinical (person-oriented) science. Even within clinical science, the comparative evaluation of treatments competes with studies of disease mechanisms, for example, epidemiology, brain imaging, genetics, and molecular biology, that have superior academic appeal. Progress in treatment evaluation is almost entirely the result of the creative tenacity of the principal investigators.

The vast, unmet, sociomedical need for proper, comparative, treatment evaluation can be remedied only by legislative action. During the 1950s, clinical psychopharmacology was dismissed by the NIMH leadership as a fad. Through lobbying by Nathan Kline and Mary Lasker, Congress specifically allocated money for a Clinical Psychopharmacology Service Center at NIMH. A recent, ineffectual, congressional attempt to similarly steer NIMH-supported research toward clinical relevance was their stipulation that 15% of the NIMH budget should go to "services research." However, this is so ill-defined that, despite many explanations, the scientific field remains confused as to what services research is, what will be or has been funded, and what the scientific evaluation standards are.

If Congress wishes to improve care by scientifically evaluating comparative treatments, it must clarify its goals by relevant hearings and appropriate dedicated money to accomplish this. In these cost-cutting, budget-balancing days, this seems utopian, but a salient means of reducing medical costs, without denying useful services, is to divert money from ineffective to better treatments. This must be viewed within the larger context; that is, no government agency is specifically charged with proactively improving the public health. Several proposals, particularly in the area of pharmacology, have been proffered to remedy this lag (Klein 1995; Ray et al. 1993; Vinar et al. 1991).

Patient support groups recognize that current treatments are inadequate, so they see the need for research but do not clearly understand that the current research effort rarely addresses developing a firm scientific basis for the complexities of practice. Joining the current research leadership in defending NIMH budgets is worthwhile but unlikely to foster advances in practice. The huge gap between the remarkable neuroscience and molecular developments and their translation into clinical progress is glossed over by our academic leadership.

Engendering such a public realization entails political debate. All change is risky, but it was congressional micromanipulation that demanded the public health–relevant Clinical Psychopharmacology Service Center at NIMH, in contrast to the NIMH decisions that counterproductively disbanded it. The democratic political process requires an informed public. Therefore, it is our responsibility to call the situation as we see it and foster the necessary public debate as to how to remedy the lack of properly controlled, collaborative, therapeutic evaluation.

References

Antonuccio DO, Danton WG, DeNelsky GY: Psychotherapy versus medication for depression: challenging the conventional wisdom with data. Professional Psychology: Research and Practice 26:574–585, 1995

Blackburn IM, Eunson KM, Bishop S: A two-year naturalistic follow-up of depressed patients treated with cognitive therapy, pharmacotherapy and a combination of both. J Affect Disord 10:67–75, 1986

Brown TA, Barlow DH: Long-term outcome and cognitive-behavioral treatment of panic disorder: clinical predictors and alternative strategies for assessment. J Consult Clin Psychol 63:754–765, 1995

Critelli JW, Neumann KF: The placebo: conceptual analysis of a construct in transition. Am Psychol 39:32–39, 1984

Evans MD, Hollon SD, DeRubeis RJ, et al: Differential relapse following cognitive therapy and pharmacotherapy for depression. Arch Gen Psychiatry 49:802–808, 1992

Eysenck HJ: The effects of psychotherapy: an evaluation. Journal of Consulting Psychology 16:319–324, 1952

Frank E, Kupfer DJ, Perel JM, et al: Three year outcomes for maintenance therapies in recurrent depression. Arch Gen Psychiatry 47:1093–1099, 1990

Frank E, Kupfer DJ, Wagner EF, et al: Efficacy of interpersonal psychotherapy as a maintenance treatment of recurrent depression: contributing factors. Arch Gen Psychiatry 48:1053–1059, 1991

Frank JD, Frank JB: Persuasion and Healing. Baltimore, MD, Johns Hopkins University Press, 1961

Hollon SD, Shelton RC, Loosen PT: Cognitive therapy and pharmacotherapy for depression. J Consult Clin Psychol 59:88–99, 1991

Jacobson NS, Hollon SD: Cognitive-behavior therapy versus pharmacotherapy: now that the jury's returned its verdict, it's time to present the rest of the evidence. J Consult Clin Psychol 64:74–80, 1996a

Jacobson NS, Hollon SD: Prospects for future comparisons between drugs and psychotherapy: lessons from the CBT-versus-pharmacotherapy exchange. J Consult Clin Psychol 64:104–108, 1996b

Jacobson NS, Dobson KS, Truax PA, et al: A component analysis of cognitive-behavioral treatment for depression. J Consult Clin Psychol 64:295–304, 1996

Kazdin AE: Research Designs in Clinical Psychology, 2nd Edition. New York, Macmillan, 1992

Kazdin AE, Bass D: Power to detect differences between alternative treatments in comparative psychotherapy outcome research. J Consult Clin Psychol 57:138–147, 1989

Kazdin AE, Wilcoxon LA: Systematic desensitization and nonspecific treatment effects: a methodological evaluation. Psychol Bull 83:729–758, 1976

Klein DF: Review of *American Psychiatric Press Review of Psychiatry*, Vol. 7. Am J Psychiatry 146:263–264, 1989

Klein DF: Improving medication and legislation by controlled experimentation. Psychiatric Annals 25:67–69, 1995

Klein DF, Rabkin JG: Specificity and strategy in psychotherapy research and practice, in Psychotherapy Research: Where Are We and Where Should We Go? Edited by Williams J, Spitzer R. New York, Guilford, 1984, pp 306–331

Klerman GL, DiMascio A, Weissman M, et al: Treatment of depression by drugs and psychotherapy. Am J Psychiatry 131:186–191, 1974

Kornblith SH, Rehm LP, O'Hara MW, et al: The contribution of self-reinforcement training and behavioral assignments to the efficacy of self-control therapy for depression. Cognitive Therapy and Research 7:499–528, 1983

Lambert MJ, Bergin AE: The effectiveness of psychotherapy, in Handbook of Psychotherapy and Behavior Change. Edited by Bergin AE, Garfield SL. New York, Wiley, 1994, pp 143–189

Laska EM, Klein DF, Lavori PW, et al: Design issues for the clinical evaluation of psychotropic drugs, in Clinical Evaluation of Psychotropic Drugs: Principles and Guidelines. Edited by Prien RF, Robinson DS. New York, Raven, 1994, pp 29–67

Luborsky L, Singer B, Luborsky L: Comparative studies of psychotherapies: is it true that "everyone has won and all must have prizes"? Arch Gen Psychiatry 32:995–1008, 1975

Meterissian GB, Bradwejn J: Comparative studies on the efficacy of psychotherapy, pharmacotherapy, and their combination in depression: was adequate pharmacotherapy provided? J Clin Psychopharmacol 9:334–339, 1989

Power KG, Simpson RJ, Swanson V, et al: A controlled comparison of cognitive-behaviour therapy, diazepam, and placebo, alone and in combination, for the treatment of generalised anxiety disorder. J Anxiety Disord 4:267–292, 1990

Ray WA, Griffin MR, Avorn J: Evaluating drugs after their approval for clinical use. N Engl J Med 329:2029–2032, 1993

Robinson LA, Berman JS, Neimeyer RA: Psychotherapy for the treatment of depression: a comprehensive review of controlled outcome research. Psychol Bull 108:30–49, 1990

Schulte D, Kunzel R, Pepping G, et al: Tailor-made versus standardized therapy of phobic patients. Advances in Behavior Research and Therapy 14:18–23, 1992

Simons AD, Murphy GE, Levine JL, et al: Cognitive therapy and pharmacotherapy for depression; sustained improvement over one year. Arch Gen Psychiatry 43:43–48, 1986

Smith ML, Glass JV, Miller TI: The Benefits of Psychotherapy. Baltimore, MD, Johns Hopkins University Press, 1980

Stiles WB, Shapiro DA, Elliott R: Are all psychotherapies equivalent? Am Psychol 41:165–180, 1986

Vinar O, Klein DF, Potter WZ, et al: A survey of psychotropic medications not available in the United States. Neuropsychopharmacology 5:201–217, 1991

Walsh BT, Wilson GT, Loeb KL, et al: Medication and psychotherapy in the treatment of bulimia nervosa. Am J Psychiatry 154:523–531, 1997

Wilson GT: Manual-based treatments: the clinical application of research findings. Behav Res Ther 34:295–314, 1996

CHAPTER 14

Less Is More

*Financing Mental Health Care
for the New Century*

Steven S. Sharfstein, M.D.

As the millennium approaches and we look back on the turbulent twentieth century, we can appreciate in broad perspective the dramatic changes that have occurred in medicine and psychiatry. The twentieth century has been one of discovery in the psychological and biological bases of mental health and mental illness. Extraordinary progress has taken place in the diagnosis and treatment of mental disorders. We understand human development in much greater depth and precision than ever before. The mysteries of the brain and how it functions are unraveling at a rapid pace. Despite these advances, opportunities for care and treatment are constrained by large social and economic forces.

This chapter reviews these forces, anticipating a continuing struggle in the twenty-first century for adequate support to treat and prevent mental illness. Managed mental health care, a phenomenon of the 1990s, is just the latest chapter in the persistent effort to ration needed care and treatment. It is the effort today to use a market-based approach to allocate society's resources among competing demands for care and treatment.

Managed care is the most recent example of the effort to ration health care resources. Prior eras include the economies of scale of large asylums and the deinstitutionalization of patients from these facilities in the mid-twentieth

century. This chapter places these cycles of reform in context to help anticipate what we might expect in the next century.

The Burden of Mental Illness

Mental illness is a huge economic and social burden on the family and society.
The capacity of the family to bear this burden and work in harmony with available and accessible treatments is particularly taxed in today's managed care environment, which emphasizes care outside of institutions. Managed care has
not cured mental illness nor relieved the economic burden, but it has shifted
this burden on to the family and local communities. Cost shifting is a recur-
ring theme throughout cycles of health care reform in the twentieth century.
Mental illness is expensive for all concerned. For the individual, it represents a direct and severe economic threat, decreasing productivity and income, and if chronic in relapsing, inevitably leading to economic dependency
and poverty. For many families, the expense in dollars and time is overwhelming, and families must reach out to the larger community for help and support. For the community, the economic burden, whether supported by health
insurance premiums or tax dollars, is large, and if such resources are inadequate, the quality of community life is compromised. Homeless people with
obvious chronic psychosis are one example of the inadequacy of economic
support for this vulnerable population. That a schizophrenic population wan-
ders in late-twentieth-century America is a disgrace. The lack of willingness
of the body politic to tax itself sufficiently to support adequate care and treatment for this vulnerable population or legislate parity, that is, nondiscriminatory health insurance coverage for treatment of the mentally ill, is a sad
commentary on American civilization.
So as the twentieth century comes to a close, we continue to wrestle with
the shortfalls in resources that can be characterized by the phrase "less is
more." The disparity between treatments that are effective and the need for
care and the access to that care is growing.

Cycles of Reform: Less Is More

The second half of the nineteenth century provided for the first broad reform
that took place throughout the republic, initiated with idealism and purpose,

but rapidly deteriorating into a clinical and economic model emphasizing economies of scale and long-term institutionalization.

The citizen reform movement, led by Dorothea Dix, emerged in the 1850s in reaction to the plight of "the insane" in many local communities. People were confined in attics and basements. Some led degrading lives in almshouses. Others wandered homeless throughout America. Moral indignation, compassion, and idealistic notions of treatment and cure combined to lead to the asylum movement in the United States. Dix's efforts over three decades led to the founding of some 32 state facilities in 18 states. These large facilities became even larger as local communities discovered the opportunity to cost-shift the care of many dependents to state dollars by transferring their care to these institutions. In New York, the disembarkation port for America's immigrants, smaller facilities rapidly became huge communities of the dependent and mentally ill. Pessimistic clinical notions on the incurability of mental illness as a brain disease combined with the economies of scale of large institutions. This led to a growing number of individuals confined for months, years, even lifetimes in these facilities.

By the mid-1950s, the peak of public asylum psychiatry was reached with 550,000 Americans confined to mental hospitals. The average length of stay was 9 months, but many patients spent a lifetime in these facilities. One of two hospital beds was occupied by a psychiatric patient. Exposés and investigative journalism revealed many of the excesses of these hospitals. Reform accelerated with the federal formation of the Joint Commission on Mental Health and Illness and the publication of *Action for Mental Health* in the early 1960s. The availability of potent tranquilizing medications in the mid-1950s led to renewed hope and the sense that these large, now expensive facilities could be depopulated. The Federal Community Mental Health Centers Program, passed by Congress in 1963, federally legislated the idealistic goals of putting treatment sites back in local communities and closing state facilities (Foley and Sharfstein 1983).

The era of deinstitutionalization, the second major era of less is more, like the era of asylum psychiatry, began with optimism and hope. The rapidity of change and the scale of activity led, however, to a process of wholesale dumping on unprepared local communities and the beginning of the public health crisis of the homeless person with schizophrenia.

This era could not have been accomplished except for new opportunities for states to shift care of the chronically mentally ill to the federal government, which would fund services for patients with chronic illness in the community—not only through the Community Mental Health Centers Program, but especially through funding of Medicare and the Social Security disability programs. The impact of these programs led to a decline from a high of 550,000 individuals in the mid-1950s in state asylums to only approximately 125,000 remaining in state facilities by the mid-1970s.

The development of community programs began in earnest throughout the 1970s and 1980s with expanded outpatient day treatment and residential alternatives for patients. In the 1980s, once again, concern regarding costs of care led to the concept of managed care, which, in turn, has produced the third era of reform of less is more.

Cost Shifting: The Recurring Theme

In the search for efficiency and effectiveness, the financing of care has been a shell game with its objective being to get someone else to pay the bill, whether the shift has been from local communities to state hospitals in the late nineteenth century and into the twentieth, representing a shift from local tax base to state level, or from the state to federal level in the process of deinstitutionalization, or the more broadly conceptualized privatization of care that has taken place as a result of managed care. The cost of cost shifting is a predominant theme in the search for accountability. Clinical realities, however, must be kept in mind.

Most major mental illness is chronic or relapsing. The economics of chronic or relapsing illness requires a longitudinal perspective, the initial investment of resources to try to prevent disability later. Most health insurance has emphasized an acute care model of illness and cure. The need for ongoing treatment is poorly addressed in such models. Large asylums took care of the problem through a policy of chronic institutionalization, which led to excess morbidity and scandal. Deinstitutionalization deteriorated into a policy of neglect for the chronically ill and relapsing patient in the community. Managed care neglects the needs of the chronically ill by defining medical necessity narrowly and in the context of a care episode.

The other reality is the phenomenon of clinical uncertainty. Much of psychiatric care is extremely individualized despite our improving effort to categorize, diagnose, and develop treatment protocols and clinical pathways. The response of a patient to treatment is more than a statistical phenomenon. There are now many options for treatment. The art of care is as important as the science of treatment for many patients. Asylums and deinstitutionalization ignore the problem of clinical uncertainty with their brutal sledgehammer approaches. Managed care attempts to reduce the role of clinical uncertainty through the development of gatekeeping, utilization review criteria, and outcome management. This, combined with the use of markets to allocate services, is the current circumstance for psychiatric care into the twenty-first century. How psychiatric care will fare depends on a number of variables relating to both the public and private sectors.

Psychiatric Care in the Marketplace: Priorities, Incentives, and the Public Health

In the private marketplace, psychiatric care has been handled differently than the rest of medical care by health insurance. Insurance benefits have been more limited because of several factors. The fear that liberal benefits would disproportionately increase demand for services and the stigma attached to mental illness are the main reasons for limited insurance coverage. Further, for over 100 years it has been the state's responsibility to provide mental health services to those without insurance and to the insured whose benefits have run out.

Although nearly all private insurance policies have some coverage for treatment of mental illness, most have so-called inside limits in which psychiatric care is treated in a more restricted fashion compared with general medical care. These limits include higher cost sharing, visit limits on outpatient care, and limits on number of hospital days. Lifetime limits of $25,000 or $50,000 for psychiatric care as contrasted with $1 million lifetime limits for general medical care are common.

For psychiatric care, therefore, especially for catastrophic illness, the patient and the family are at risk to a greater extent than for the treatment of cancer or heart disease. These patients have more out-of-pocket expense, forgo care, or must turn to the public sector for their care. Private insurance coverage has not been a source of support for catastrophic economic loss as the result of mental illness.

In addition to inside limits, employers who pay for most of private health insurance in this country have implemented other strategies to reduce costs. Managed care has introduced the concept of *carve-outs* in which mental illness and substance abuse are handled differently from the rest of the situations covered in the health insurance contract. Carve-outs include subcontracting benefits to an independent company or subsidiary of a large insurance company to manage the treatment of mental illness through case managers or other gatekeepers, utilization review criteria, and high-cost case management. These carve-outs may affect the choice of health care providers, as health insurance companies may have an exclusive relationship with a network of preferred providers, and in order to receive insurance benefits, individuals must turn to this particular network for care.

Although managed care has been primarily an effort to manage costs, paradoxically it has led to the expansion of insurance benefits through parity legislation that has been passed in several states, notably Maryland and Wisconsin. Minimum mandated benefits have been legislated in more than 30 states, providing a basic minimum of care under private health insurance for mental disorders and/or substance abuse. The parity legislation as well as minimum mandated benefits are efforts to overcome adverse selection and market failure to provide health insurance coverage for mental disorders and substance abuse. By spreading the risk over a larger population, the economic feasibility, that is, insurability, of mental illness is increased and, when combined with managed care, costs are very much under control.

As increasingly more Americans enroll in health maintenance organizations (HMOs), that is, prepaid capitated care, perspectives for coverage of mental illness and substance abuse change, depending on the policy within an individual HMO and the capacity to take care of individuals with severe mental illness. Staff model HMOs have been parsimonious in providing psychiatric treatment. Independent practice association HMO models have provided more opportunities for necessary care through a managed approach. HMOs also turn to the carve-outs for their care management and sometimes to referrals when the basic mental health care within an HMO is inadequate to provide the needed treatment.

Because private health insurance inadequately covers psychiatric care and the market for such insurance is limited, the public sector remains the mainstay for care and treatment. Increasingly, patients with public insurance are directed into managed care, and this has varied from state to state. As more Medicare beneficiaries enroll in HMOs, mental health care is provided through the private sector, albeit in a managed care context. Medicaid programs, which are important sources of support for the psychosocial rehabilitative care and treatment of the severely and persistently mentally ill, are increasingly coming under the private managed care industry. This process of privatizing the public programs, Medicare/Medicaid and the state categorical programs, will continue into the twenty-first century and may equalize the opportunities for care and treatment. On the other hand, the rationing of care that occurs in the public sector could become worse under such scenarios of privatization. Longer-term treatment and rehabilitation may be cut with privatization.

A critical issue for financing of care into the twenty-first century is where the safety net is. The catastrophic care safety net for the underinsured and uninsured and the severely and persistently ill is tattered today. The need for such a backup system for these patients is underscored by the numerous homeless as well as severely mentally ill individuals being cared for by families who make great sacrifices to protect these vulnerable people. Some patients never get well and suffer progressive deterioration despite good access to treatment. The treatment of individuals with severe and persistent conditions is a major public health crisis in the United States today. This is especially true in psychiatry.

Notwithstanding the need for such a backup system, managed care has underscored the appropriateness of lower-cost alternatives to the hospital and a continuum of care for most patients. Just as diabetes or chronic cardiac disease can be managed with frequent outpatient visits and intensified medication management, much of psychiatric care with patients who have acute exacerbations of chronic illness can be treated with outpatient treatment, day hospitalization, domiciliary care, and other alternatives. Traditionally, the market for health insurance recognized only inpatient treatment as the legitimate site for care for mental illness. For years, hospital stays were longer than necessary and alternatives were underfunded. Alternative economic incentives, such as capitation, can promote care in other settings and can work as long as we are able to provide continuity of care, easy access without barriers, and the introduction of both consumer and provider options for flexibility and treatment decisions.

Numerous studies have shown the cost-effectiveness of alternatives to hospitalization. These studies often compare traditional inpatient treatment to halfway houses, day treatment, or intensive outpatient care. Almost all show decreases in costs as well as outcomes that are equal to and sometimes better than inpatient care. This more efficient resource use can expand opportunities for individuals who are not receiving care but who might benefit from it.

What About Psychiatry?

Psychiatrists are faced with major changes in their expected roles within the new delivery system and in their identity as physicians. It is important to emphasize that psychiatry has a strong and growing medical and scientific basis. It is a branch of medicine and relies on the medical model of illness, on a biopsychosocial model of behavior, and, from an ethical perspective, on the Hippocratic doctor-patient relationship.

The discoveries of biological psychiatry have led to a renaissance of the medical model in psychiatry. The emergence of the *Diagnostic and Statistical Manual* (American Psychiatric Association 1952), the pathophysiological approach to understanding symptoms and syndromes, and treatment planning that emphasizes reduction in symptoms and return to function all underscore the important physician identity of psychiatrists. A prime example of the psychiatrist as physician is seen in the case of treating major mental illness, in which it is becoming increasingly clear that the brain, its structure and function, lie at the basis of psychotic disorders. The problem with the medical model is its potential for reductionistic thinking.

To combat reductionism, psychiatry emphasizes the biopsychosocial model, which is based on the attempt to connect the brain and its pathology with the psychology of the mind and social systems for an overall understanding of disturbed behavior. As psychiatrists move beyond the biology of neurochemicals and genetics, they consider the meaning of mental phenomena and the interplay of the brain, consciousness, and social environment. One of the great threats to the field under managed care scenarios is to confine psychiatry to the medical model and the biology of mental illness. This limitation must be resisted.

A third pillar of a psychiatrist's identity is the ethical demands of the Hippocratic doctor-patient model. The commitment to the individual patient is at the heart of this model. In the face of the pressures to provide population-based treatment through a public health model or prepaid capitation such as in HMOs, the psychiatrist is pulled away from this ethical commitment to the individual patient. Population-based care requires physicians to be just as concerned about the many who may need treatment but are not accessing such treatment as they are about the patients who are in their offices.

In the managed care era, psychiatrists are challenged to deal with market-based language and concepts in modifying their primary role as physicians. Care provided is often called *products*, and patients and families are called *customers*. In this new model, psychiatrists are extremely expensive labor whose utilization must be carefully rationed and rationalized. Such market-based thinking does not care about the medical, biopsychosocial, or Hippocratic models, and the questions posed focus on managing patients more cheaply by less expensive labor. The managed care perspective leads to a fragmentation of a psychiatrist's identity as well as the core values that motivate and inform the profession.

The psychiatrist brings unique and important values to the treatment team caring for psychiatric patients. The differential diagnosis may be the singular skill for which the psychiatrist is best suited. Medication management, including the decision not to medicate, is uniquely within the domain of psychiatric care. The psychiatrist also is ideally suited to perform the role of consultant, not only on the biomedical questions but also on the overall psychosocial treatment planning, questions of safety and social control, and the all-important issue of prognosis. The psychiatrist is well suited for team leadership in this regard and certainly is uniquely qualified to be such a leader in the complicated business of integrated treatment of complex cases that demand specialized expertise. These include unstable psychotic patients, patients with organic brain diseases, severely characterologically ill patients, seriously suicidal patients, substance-abusing patients, forensic cases with high levels of dangerousness, seriously medically ill patients with psychiatric problems, and cases where there are litigious and manipulative patients or families.

It is also true that psychiatrists can perform a variety of other roles, such as psychotherapists, a time-honored profession and part of the core training experience. Psychotherapy is still a residency review committee (RRC)–required imperative although the quality of its teaching varies. Many psychiatrists are recruited from medical students who have a special interest in psychotherapy.

Another important role for psychiatrists will be as *principal physicians*, especially for chronically mentally ill patients, highly somatizing patients, and disturbed patients who act out around the medical illnesses. This role requires primary care skills by psychiatrists, with a willingness to manage medical problems even as they are dealing with the psychiatric symptomatology.

Psychiatry must proactively assert what it is it can do in the new overall system of managed care in the United States. Despite the market-based pressures to downsize specialties, the logic around the psychiatric task is such that the value of psychiatry will emerge and assert itself well into the twenty-first century.

Mental Health Care and Its Financing in the Twenty-First Century

At some point early in the twenty-first century, universal health insurance will become part of the American experience. What will happen to mental health care broadly defined in that context?

The remedicalization of psychiatry and the increasing effectiveness of treatment will underscore the basic similarities between psychiatric and general medical care. Mental health care will become integrated into the overall health care system, and this will lead to the end of discrimination against the mentally ill as we know it today. Universal health insurance will be nondiscriminatory with regard to mental health benefits.

What this means is a basic and enduring commitment to mental health care as a part of general health care. This encompasses hospital-level treatment of acute illness and exacerbation of persistent illness, outpatient visits, both psychosocial and biological treatments, as well as the provision of more intensive alternative care. Prospective budgets and payment on the fee-for-service retrospective basis will be on the basis of services and not psychiatric or other diagnostic categorization.

All health insurance contains policies related to cost containment. These policies should and will be identical for mental health and general health in the twenty-first century. Differential day and visit limitations between general and mental health, as well as other dollar limits, will be a historical footnote. An equitable universal system will encourage access without sacrificing catastrophic coverage. Universal health insurance will apply cost containment principles identically in a nondiscriminatory fashion to mental health and other general health care.

Despite the above, there will be the need to retain a smaller, publicly funded backup system for high-cost, long-term, institutional-level care. In Canada and other countries, such a system has persisted despite the provision of universal health. This safety net is necessary because, despite even the most dramatic advances in treatment, the aging of the population and other factors will lead to the need for such approaches. The vast majority of Americans, however, will be treated in the integrated health and mental health care continuum, which will emphasize outpatient, day hospital, and residential alternatives to inpatient care.

Such approaches require a better understanding than we have today of the optimal level of care for certain patient subgroups, such as patients with chronic psychosis. Information from outcome studies is needed now more than ever. This information requires cost-effectiveness and cost-benefit analyses, ongoing collection of epidemiological data, and cost-offset studies that look at the total picture of health and mental health. In this information age, it is critical to provide this type of information in order to expand opportunities for effective treatment for psychiatric patients.

Is Less Ever More?

Even with the optimistic scenario outlined above and its premise that psychiatry will truly become a legitimate and full partner in the delivery of medical care in the United States, pressures regarding cost containment will continue to emphasize that less is more. But is less ever more in the provision of psychiatric care? When psychotherapy is provided by masters-level clinicians at lower cost, is this truly equivalent to the same care provided by well-trained doctors? When intensive day treatment is substituted for inpatient care at lower cost, does this provide superior outcome to the stay in a hospital? Does brief, solution-focused therapy provide superior outcomes to longer, more intensive psychodynamic psychotherapy?

These are issues that will be resolved by better health services research and outcome studies as well as the political and social battles that will continue well into the twenty-first century. With increasing evidence that treatment is indeed effective and necessary and a less stigmatized understanding of the robust epidemiology of mental illness and substance abuse, the issue of resource limitations becomes less of an arbitrary discrimination against providing mental and substance abuse benefits and more a question of a careful triage and use of flexible practice guidelines, which will provide the most effective and efficient care for the individual patient.

Can markets and the competitive model truly do this? Managed care, as we know it today, makes its profits by risk selection, denial of care, and the dumping of the most seriously ill. It needs the regulatory oversight of government to deal with the excesses of this mentality. Universal health care, with a more energetic and active role of government, is not a popular solution in the United States and promises bureaucratic rigidity, paperwork, and inefficiency. Obviously, we need to work toward a balance between the extremes of the free market and excessive government regulations. To afford necessary and effective treatment, we require the pooling of resources and the spreading of risk in order to deal with the continuing phenomena of mental illness and substance abuse. Strong advocacy is ever necessary to make these promises into realities. In the search for the appropriate balance of access, cost, and quality, this advocacy must be informed by good data and humane values.

The American Psychiatric Association and Its Advocacy for Economic Justice for the Mentally Ill

Over the past quarter-century, the American Psychiatric Association under the leadership of its medical director, Dr. Melvin Sabshin, has been an enlightened and steadfast advocate on behalf of economic opportunities for the mentally ill that parallel the scientific advances and create great hope for families across the nation. The American Psychiatric Association (APA), through its Office of Economic Affairs, has been able to put together critical information that has been helpful across the country, state by state, in the fight for parity, that is, nondiscriminatory coverage. At the federal level, under the leadership of Jay Cutler, advocacy has been enlightened and informed on such critical programs as Medicare and Medicaid, the Community Mental Health Centers, and research. The advocacy of the APA, although always focused on the profession of psychiatry, has emphasized a broad view of the field and the needs of the mentally ill and their families in the context of changing treatment opportunities. By working closely with coalitions of organizations representing other professions as well as families and patients, the APA has been a leader in the fight for better funding for treatment and support for individuals with mental illness. These individuals have especially benefited by having Dr. Sabshin as the psychiatrist leading the way for the past quarter-century and continuing to do so as the new century approaches.

Reference

American Psychiatric Association: Diagnostic and Statistical Manual: Mental Disorders. Washington, DC, American Psychiatric Association, 1952

Foley HA, Sharfstein SS: Madness and Government: Who Cares for the Mentally Ill? Washington, DC, American Psychiatric Association, 1983

CHAPTER 15

Ethical Conduct of the Psychiatrist

Jeremy A. Lazarus, M.D.

To frame the subject of the ethical conduct of the twenty-first century psychiatrist, it is necessary to review how medical ethics have evolved, where they currently are, and where they may or will be headed. Although some issues in psychiatric ethics will remain immutable, others will be open to interpretation and difference of opinion. The preamble to the Code of Medical Ethics of the American Medical Association states, "The following Principles, adopted by the American Medical Association, are not laws but standards of conduct, which define the essentials of honorable behavior for the physician" (AMA CEJA 1996). These standards of conduct are changeable, and indeed this century has seen major changes in the way physicians interpret medical ethics. These changes have been the result of alterations in the practice of medicine and psychiatry, societal changes in values, and world events. Although this chapter is not able to cover in detail all of these influences on the ethics of the next century, it provides some guidance and context for a discussion of what ethical standards might be like for psychiatrists in the twenty-first century.

Foundations of Psychiatric Ethics

The first ethical code for physicians was included in the Code of Hammurabi in 2000 B.C.E. Subsequently, in the fifth century B.C.E., the Greek Oath of Hippocrates came to serve as a statement of ethical ideals for the physician. With the Middle Ages came the code of Maimonides, which contained further elaboration on ethics. Thomas Percival's 1803 Code of Medical Ethics was the most significant contribution to the refinement of ethical guidelines for physicians since the Oath of Hippocrates. The American Medical Association (AMA) published its first ethical code in 1847. The American Psychiatric Association (APA) relied on the code of the AMA and the Hippocratic Oath until 1973, when it first published *The Principles of Medical Ethics With Annotations Especially Applicable to Psychiatry* (APA 1973). The history of ethics in the APA is detailed in several books (Barton 1987; J. A. Lazarus, "A History of Ethics in the APA after World War II," publication pending). The period between the first annotated code in 1973 and the present has been extremely active for ethics elucidation within psychiatry and the APA. The APA not only developed its own elaboration on the AMA code, but also enforced that code through its Ethics Committee.

Social value changes played a major role in a movement away from doctor-oriented paternalism to patient autonomy and informed consent. This was related in part to the influence of bioethical thinking in medical ethics (Beauchamp and Childress 1994). The civil rights movement, the women's movement, the Holocaust, and technologic advances in medicine paved the way for new formulations and positions in medical and psychiatric ethics. Today, we are experiencing massive changes in health care delivery, changes in resource allocation and funding of health care, and new roles for psychiatrists. All of these will affect the future ethical positions of the field.

Yet with all these changes, the principles upon which organized psychiatry has stood are relatively simply contained in the current version of *The Principles of Medical Ethics With Annotations Especially Applicable to Psychiatry* (APA 1995) and the *Code of Medical Ethics: Current Opinions With Annotations* of the AMA Council on Ethical and Judicial Affairs (AMA CEJA 1996). The Constitution of the APA requires the APA to abide by the ethical code of the AMA. When there have been disagreements with ethical positions of the AMA, the APA has attempted to resolve those differences and thereby not come into constitutional conflict. There may come a time in the next century when the APA may not be able to support an ethical position of the AMA, thereby creating an exception of some sort to the constitutional mandate of the APA.

Forces for New Ethical Challenges in the Twenty-First Century

The primary factors influencing ethical challenges into the twenty-first century include rising health care costs, new technologies, new research into mental illness, shifts in psychiatric education and workforce, and the locus of health care treatment.

As health care costs in the 1990s are now using up to 15% of the gross national product, there has been increasing pressure to moderate or reduce this growth. The pressures have come from employers who pay workers' health insurance premiums, the states that partially fund rising Medicaid costs, and *the White House and Congress, which are attempting to reduce or contain Medicaid and Medicare expenditures into the early twenty-first century.* Although there has been some moderation in health care costs for employer groups in 1996, there is no evidence to date that market forces on managed care will effectively constrain rising health care expenditures *in the future.* This may in part be the result of the lack of universal access to health care, the aging population, and ever-improving technologies and treatments of illnesses. These forces and their resultant effect on medical ethics have been described in detail (Lazarus and Sharfstein 1994; Morreim 1991). Since the failure of President Bill Clinton's Health Security Act in 1994, Congress and market forces have attempted to restrain rising health care costs by incremental health care reform and shifts of patients into managed care. Although the General Accounting Office estimated that savings in some health maintenance organizations (HMOs) ranged from 3% to 15% in health care expenditures, there remained an uncertain conclusion about the extension of these savings to the population at large (Office of Technology Assessment 1994).

These pressures to moderate health care costs while maintaining quality of medical treatment and increasing access to health care services have placed medical systems and professionals into increasingly complicated ethical dilemmas. Medical ethicists, recognizing these pressures, have attempted to craft solutions to this health care crisis (Daniels 1985; Eddy 1994; Engelhardt and Rie 1988). The conclusions of these authors and the actual experience articulated by the Congressional Budget Office leads to the inevitable conclusion that, if United States society does not increase its commitment to health care expenditures, some form of allocation of health care resources is inevitable. This allocation, or rationing, creates unprecedented ethical challenges for health care professionals and systems (Daniels 1987). Some direction is provided by the AMA (AMA 1995) and others (Sabin and Daniels 1994; Wolf 1994).

The principal ethical question is how health care professionals either balance or integrate their responsibilities as patient advocates and members of society. If a professional is working in a system with a fixed budget, be it public or private, there inevitably occur situations where not all optimal health care services can be provided to the covered population. Ways the physician or system deals with these dilemmas vary. They can range from the professional always considering the needs of a population of patients first while treating the individual patient to having no input into how allocation decisions are made. Strong arguments exist along this continuum (Mechanic 1990; Pellegrino 1986, 1995). A debate at the APA Annual Meeting in 1996 regarding the restriction of care because of costs captured both sides of this dilemma (APA 1996). Both sides did agree that for-profit systems without adequate disclosure and concurrence by patients, professionals, and payers created the greatest tendency toward potentially unethical treatment. Attempts at societal, patient, and professional concurrence in any allocation system are under way in Oregon. The APA has addressed these issues in its principles of health care reform (APA 1993).

Problems for psychiatrists and other professionals when financial incentives may influence choice or extent of care has also been the subject of much heated debate (Lazarus 1997; Rodwin 1993). It is the opinion of this author that financial incentives primarily applied to the improvement of quality of care are ethically sound. Incentives provided for other purposes are ethically suspect and place physicians in a conflict of interest, balancing their own benefit with that of the patients (Thompson 1993).

The influence of new technologies has had much less influence on ethics in psychiatry than in other branches of medicine. Although psychiatry uses its fair share of laboratory tests, it is not a technologically laden specialty. New uses of positron-emission tomography (PET) scans and other innovations that will permit us to more accurately map the brain and its chemical functioning may begin to present ethical dilemmas. If, for example, tests are developed to more accurately diagnose, treat, or prevent mental illness, the costs associated will need to be incorporated into health care budgets. The potential for resistance to the use of high cost tests, especially if there are only a few who will benefit, will place psychiatry into similar dilemmas as other specialties. A careful ethical analysis in these situations will assist psychiatrists in finding the right course and effectively advocating for patients. Ongoing stigma against the mentally ill will undoubtedly influence these decisions, and the profession needs to be vigilant so that our patients are treated fairly.

New research into psychiatric illness will provide answers and treatments for the mentally ill. Along the steps of progress, however, will be questions, as genetics, neurobiology, and societal effects play a role in psychiatric disorders. As the possibility of genetic engineering of personality traits becomes a reality, psychiatry and society must face the inevitable pressures to mold and accentuate certain desirable or perhaps competitively improved individuals. If research finds educational or treatment approaches to violent disorders, society will need to find a way to fund these initiatives. Societal reengineering for better mental health will present new challenges to psychiatric ethics. Just as the psychiatric profession's high hopes in the twentieth century about its ability to influence world behavior faded, the twenty-first century may indeed have the tools to bring that about. The real possibilities of a person being genetically engineered for certain mental and physical characteristics will present new battlegrounds of controversy in medical and psychiatric ethics. Societal fears of mind control by genetic engineering may have more merit in the next century. There will undoubtedly be some who will be excited by such possibilities and others who will abhor it. Psychiatrists will need to address these questions carefully.

While psychiatric workforce issues are covered elsewhere in this book, it is important to recognize that in areas heavily populated with psychiatrists there is increasing competition for the patient population. This competition can influence professional relationships, educational opportunities, and patient care. Although some areas of the United States are underserved in terms of numbers of psychiatrists, other areas may be overserved, leading to potential intraprofessional problems. Psychiatrists may either resolve these problems through market forces or through their professional organizations. The splitting off or fragmentation of groups of psychiatrists away from professional organizations will influence how these potential ethical dilemmas will develop and be resolved. For example, if psychiatrists working in organized systems of care, for example, HMOs or the public sector, do not maintain their professional organization input or join competing and unaffiliated professional organizations, fragmentation may develop. There is a deep concern among many of us that, without an umbrella organization for psychiatry providing an ethical focus, new standards of practice unfettered by traditional medical ethics might emerge to the potential detriment of patient care and the integrity of the profession. These themes have been widely discussed (English 1993; Fink 1989; Rothman 1991).

As the psychiatric workforce stabilizes into the next century, these ethical dilemmas will eventually sort themselves out. In the interim, however, the powerful market forces that are shaping health care will create deep points of controversy for the psychiatric workforce.

The first half of the twentieth century had three predominant loci of psychiatric treatment: the psychiatric hospital, the public system, and the private practitioner's office. The second half of the twentieth century has witnessed the emergence of other health care delivery systems such as HMOs, group practices, clinics without walls, partial hospitals, intensive outpatient or crisis treatment centers, in-home services, and residential care. Team or collaborative approaches to treatment have expanded from the public sector to managed systems of care in the private sector. These alterations in locus of treatment and shared professional responsibility will continue to present new dilemmas to psychiatrists (J. A. Lazarus, "Ethical Issues in Divided Treatment," publication pending). As some patients feel more connected to a system of care versus an individual doctor, new problems may emerge. The covenant of trust exemplified by the Hippocratic Oath continues to be the central value of the medical profession (Glass 1996). Treating professionals, who value the doctor-patient relationship, may be surprised by the willingness of patients to switch to other systems or providers because of insurance changes. On the other hand, private systems may encourage reliance on a system rather than on a doctor to maintain loyalty to the system. Other systems may continue to stress the importance of continuity of the doctor-patient relationship. If there is a reduction in financial barriers to patients continuing with their treating doctors, even if there are insurance changes, for example, through affordable point-of-service plans or portability, this issue may vanish.

In summary, the forces of change into the next century will create new dilemmas for psychiatrists. The remainder of this chapter focuses on potential ethical problems for the psychiatrist, as a result of these forces, which will influence ethical conduct in the next century.

New Roles Bring New Problems

The rapid changes in health care have presented psychiatrists with new roles and opportunities. Jobs have been created as utilization reviewers, managed care medical directors, group practice administrators, chief executive officers of corporations, and outcome researchers. Each of these new roles brings challenges, not only in role, but in ethics. Physicians are rapidly becoming employees as opposed to owners of practices (Kletke et al. 1996). These new roles are covered in detail elsewhere (Lazarus and Sharfstein 1997). The ethical question arises as to whether the ethical principles of the individual psychiatrist apply to the psychiatrist in a new role. There is a limited literature on these issues other than the publications of the AMA, APA, and other medical organizations (American College of Physicians 1992; AMA 1993; APA 1989,

1991). The APA has been relatively silent in articulating ethical principles for administrative psychiatrists as distinct from clinical psychiatrists. The work of an APA task force to develop guidelines for psychiatrists in organized systems of care may help in this process. In addition, inadequate attention is paid to the bioethical principle of justice in the AMA and APA principles of medical ethics. Dissatisfaction with the APA code has also been articulated by some (Sabin 1994). Ethical dilemmas may especially be apparent when psychiatrists in nonclinical roles receive financial incentives for utilization targets. In addition, working in for-profit systems may create significant ethical challenges, as an employed psychiatrist may need to weigh clinical care delivery with system profits. The degree to which there is an absolute firewall between the administrative psychiatrist and demand for profit or productivity will undoubtedly influence the extent of the conflict. These conflicts take the shape of conflicting standards between business and medical ethics (Mariner 1995).

Many psychiatrists in administrative positions in organized systems of care indicate that their ethical belief is an obligation to the population of patients their organization serves. They would then balance individual patient needs with the needs of the population and the money available to treat that population. This ethical belief has operated for decades in public systems of care with limited budgets where psychiatrists do not receive any potential gain for their actions. In private for-profit systems, there is the additional factor of an outside investor or stockholder benefiting by care being limited. Ethical guidelines need to be developed to inform this practitioner. New philosophies of treatment relating to short-term, crisis intervention, or solution-focused therapy have evolved to respond to the market demands for less costly and more effective forms of treatment. The question arises are these new treatment philosophies derived from our expanded knowledge or from arguments to enhance profit. The scientific basis for time-limited types of treatment versus clinically determined treatment has come under attack (Miller 1996). Miller concludes that the scientific basis for supporting time-limited interventions as equal or superior to clinically determined length of treatment is flawed. Unfortunately there is limited available outcome research to help us. What is available gives mixed results on the question of outcomes in varying systems of delivering psychiatric care (McFarland 1994; McFarland et al. 1996; Wells et al. 1992). Those psychiatrists in administrative positions may choose those studies as the basis for their decisions or some other set of data from their own systems.

These new roles will continue to present formidable challenges to psychiatrists trained as clinicians to do what is in the best interest of the patient. In organized systems of care, interests compete for allocated money across groups of patients, professionals, and often stockholders. These competing interests may lead some down a slippery slope of limiting care for a given patient, arguing that the care is a medically unnecessary treatment, whereas, in fact, the intent is to enhance profit. Some administrative psychiatrists have confided to this author the pressure toward utilization targets and varied interpretation of medical necessity criteria based on available funds for an insurance group. Another psychiatrist recently informed the author of the need to bargain with a utilization review psychiatrist for needed care. This bargaining took the form of allowing a certain number of partial hospital days if the psychiatrist would guarantee discharge from inpatient care on a certain day. This mongrelization of medical judgment inevitably would lead to a type of situational ethic and away from a principled medical ethic relying on scientific guidelines and medical judgment. One solution to this dilemma would be that those in administrative positions would clearly articulate to patients and practitioners the underlying ethical philosophy that governs their actions if different from that of the practitioner. Another alternative would be for the administrative psychiatrist to shed the M.D. mantle and become a businessperson working through business ethics. This might help to alleviate the psychiatrist's confusion in roles and clarify to the public where the psychiatrist takes his or her direction.

The medical profession must also take a proactive position of discussing in ethical terms these new dilemmas for physicians. This could be done by increased attention to these subjects by inclusion in ethics curricula in medical schools, residencies, and in postgraduate training. Although some medical schools have increased their medical ethics curricula, medical students have voiced concern about spotty approaches to ethics teaching (Durso 1996). The APA has attempted to deal with these issues by conducting training workshops at the American Association of Psychiatric Residency Training Directors meetings and by developing a Model Ethics Curriculum (APA 1996). Perhaps as these dilemmas are exposed and discussed, solutions based on a firm sense of medical ethics will ensue. In the interim, administrative psychiatrists in the next century may be left to follow a limited set of guidelines for ethical direction.

Psychiatric Ethics and the Marketplace

Current market forces are demanding high-quality health care with improved access and at the lowest possible cost. In addition, there is a new emphasis on accountability both to the payers for insurance and to the public. There is no difficulty in setting the traditional and published ethical positions of the AMA and APA up against these demands. Patient advocacy is primary, no matter what the health care system. However, the medical profession does indicate an obligation to society. The AMA Council on Ethical and Judicial Affairs (AMA CEJA 1996) has stated that

> Physicians are not ethically obligated to deliver care that, in their best professional judgment, will not have a reasonable chance of benefiting their patients. Patients should not be given treatments simply because they demand them. (CEJA 2.035)

The AMA has also clarified its opinion on the allocation of health care resources (AMA CEJA 1996). This important section of the CEJA document clarifies that

> A physician has a duty to do all that he or she can for the benefit of the individual patient. Physicians have a responsibility to participate and to contribute their professional expertise in order to safeguard the interests of patients in decisions made at the societal level regarding the allocation or rationing of health resources. (CEJA 2.03)

This important distinction between the ethical value system of the AMA/APA and other discussions of physician behavior in systems of care is an important one. Some would argue that the treating physician should also consider the health care needs of a population served. This argument is in contradistinction to the position of the AMA, which assigns the societal obligation away from the treatment setting. It appears unlikely that those positions of the AMA/APA will change, unless there is a systemwide overhaul of the health care system allowing physicians to believe that their patient advocacy role is administered fairly and not compromised. Perhaps this could occur if universal access to insurance benefits through either private systems or through some governmental single payer system could be ensured.

With regard to the issue of providing quality care at the lowest possible cost, there are considerable pitfalls in the marketplace. The current competitive nature of psychiatric care is driving down the amount of funds that payers are providing for psychiatric and substance abuse treatment. This is especially true in mature managed care markets using capitation as a form of payment. Unfortunately, capitation rates continue to fall while comprehensive psychiatric services are being promised. This leaves many to wonder if there is honest disclosure of what really will be provided and the real limitations once capitation rates have fallen significantly. Some ethicists see no more peril in managed systems of care as opposed to fee-for-service systems (Boyle and Callahan 1995).

Psychiatrists in these systems need to decide whether competent psychiatric treatment can be provided at very low capitation rates. If the answer is no, psychiatrists might opt out of these systems or remain in them if they believe they can influence better care in the future. When competent care can be provided at lower cost, it is entirely ethical for psychiatrists to be involved. This continues to be the area of greatest controversy and least fact as we all await accurate outcome data. If scientifically valid outcome data supports what is happening in the marketplace, psychiatric ethics has already supported providing equal quality treatment at the lower cost. If outcome data indicate that more expensive treatments have materially better outcomes, then they should be provided. If a system does not provide those treatments, then they should disclose those facts to enrollees in a straightforward and clearly understandable manner.

In the area of accountability, physicians have always supported continuing education and peer review. They have always been accountable to the public by way of medical licensing boards. The APA has had an extremely active ethics process that enforces the code of ethics. The APA has devoted considerable resources to these efforts (Lazarus and Sharfstein 1992). Newer forms of accountability to patients or systems of care, if done sensitively and for the purpose of improving the quality of care patients receive while minimizing intrusions into the doctor-patient relationship, should be fully supported by the ethics of the profession. When certain forms of accountability do not result in those improvements and are a detriment to patient care, they should be resisted or modified to conform with psychiatric ethics.

Statements of ethical principles that are consistent with some of the current market forces already exist. They will be better accepted by psychiatrists if they are seen as truly helpful to patient care and clinical outcome and not primarily for marketing purposes. In addition, the amount of resources going into accountability measures, while funds for clinical treatment fall, raises concerns for the proper balance. Psychiatric patients continue to be discriminated against with regard to health care benefits and therefore are already unjustly treated. Further erosions or limitations in funding place even more strain on psychiatrists attempting to behave ethically with their patients. When there is universal access to benefits—parity of benefits for the mentally ill and all involved in the treatment of the mentally ill, following scientific guidelines and outcomes data—psychiatric ethics will have no difficulty in adapting to market forces.

New Treatments and
the Ethical Psychiatrist

As noted in other chapters in this book, the advances in psychiatric treatment into the next century should be remarkable. As our nosology, research, and available treatments continue to expand, psychiatrists will have a broader array of approaches to the psychiatrically ill. Psychiatrists will need to leave less effective forms of treatment and embrace newer forms and interventions that yield superior patient outcome. When research does not indicate superiority of one form of treatment over another, it will still be appropriate for the psychiatrist to use his or her medical judgment in determining treatment. It has and will continue to be important to question new treatments and to recognize when they are experimental and need to be disclosed appropriately to patients. The formation of the Practice Research Network of the APA should be an important proving ground for various forms of treatment. As this century closes, the first complete set of the APA practice guidelines should be complete. Yet, even now there are demands for *standards* of practice that go beyond the guidelines. Demand for evidence-based medicine increases (Clancy and Kamerow 1996). Psychiatric disorders affect quality of life and functional capacity (Glass 1996), and the presence of these disorders in primary care practice is well documented (Spitzer et al. 1995). It is likely that the psychiatrist in the next century will have even more of an interface with colleagues in primary care and other specialties. This will emerge from larger integrated systems of care recognizing the need for adequate prevention and treatment of mental illness within their systems. As stigma against mental illness diminishes and treatments continue to improve, demand for psychiatric treatment will undoubtedly increase. It will be imperative from an ethical point of view that psychiatrists use new treatments appropriately and interact with medical colleagues to improve the overall health of patients treated.

Concerns will continue to be raised about research using patients with psychiatric illness. This issue has been discussed in detail (Lazarus 1994), relating especially to the issue of informed consent. Recently the Maryland Attorney General's Office has begun an effort to clarify and reform state law concerning research involving cognitively impaired subjects (Schwartz 1996). New types of treatment for psychiatric illness may well emerge presenting new ethical challenges for the psychiatric researcher. The fundamental ethical principles regarding research should not be altered, and psychiatrists must guard the safety of their patients and obtain appropriate informed consent.

As noted earlier in this chapter, the possibilities for genetic manipulation of personality or personality traits may pose a new ethical dilemma for psychiatry. To date, psychiatry has been spared the ethical dilemmas surrounding genetic or fetal manipulation. Yet we must recognize that these same issues may face us. Psychiatry has yet to make any opinions on genetic or fetal research but must be prepared to engage in those discussions.

The ethical question of physician-assisted suicide will undoubtedly carry into the next century. While the AMA and APA are firmly opposed to physician-assisted suicide, there are groups of physicians who strongly support it. Even if it is ruled legal in some states or federally, the AMA and APA may well not support its members engaging in this form of end-of-life intervention. Many concerns have been raised about inexact standards for determining those patients truly terminally ill and at the end of life. In addition, questions have been raised about whether physician-assisted suicide requests are truly those of the patient or those caretakers who may understandably wish to be relieved of their caretaking burdens. Although laws may allow physician-assisted suicide in the future, the place of psychiatrists (if willing to be involved) would most likely be in assessing competence and presence or absence of a psychiatric illness influencing decision making.

In the twenty-first century, psychiatrists may be asked to operationalize certain societal imperatives. These might be related to rationing limited health care resources. Psychiatrists and other physicians may be called upon to themselves ration health care. The response of organized medicine will be crucial in that most certain debate. Psychiatrists may be called upon to influence societal goals, a situation that may resulting in ethical conflict, as in the physician-assisted suicide debate. A similar situation recently occurred in regard to whether psychiatrists could ethically treat prisoners on death row, if by so doing the prisoners could be competent to be executed. After long discussion with the AMA, the APA took the position that psychiatrists could ethically treat the incompetent prisoner on death row only if the death sentence was commuted. Another example illustrative of potential problems is the Kansas Sexually Violent Predator Act. The Kansas Act, similar to statutes in several other states, provides for a form of commitment for certain "sexually violent predators" who would not qualify for the usual civil commitment for those with a mental illness. The Kansas Act raises the specter of the use of psychiatric commitment for political purposes as occurred in the Soviet Union and elsewhere. Thus, psychiatrists will need to be vigilant about being used as an agent of society against the interests of the individual and will need to strongly advocate against the abuse or misuse of psychiatry.

Stigma and Patient Advocacy

The APA has taken a leadership position along with patient advocacy groups in attempting to erase stigma against the mentally ill. These efforts appear to be paying off. Yet the APA Ethics Committee has tended to discourage psychiatrists from actively involving their own patients in these efforts. This has derived from the principle of not influencing the patient in a manner that is not consistent with treatment goals. This author has, however, spoken with numerous psychiatrists who do not fully agree with this position. For example, they consider it appropriate to provide various patient information booklets related to patient advocacy or attempt to involve patients in political actions that have ramifications for the treatment of the mentally ill. It is conceivable that there will be a gradual shift toward more involvement of the treating psychiatrist in these areas. This may occur because of more acceptance on the part of patients of psychiatrists advocating for them politically, changing patterns of psychiatric practice limiting the negative consequences of such psychiatrist involvement, and an increase in materials provided by the APA that can be given to patients as education. Overall, however, psychiatrists will need to decide how the value of providing such information to patients outweighs whatever negative consequences might occur in the treatment. These issues will undoubtedly continue to affect psychiatrists in the next century as we attempt to find ways to advocate for our patients' needs with ever-diminishing resources. It is hoped that the relationship between the APA and patient advocacy groups will remain strong and help to mitigate the dilemma for many psychiatrists who may direct their patients to these groups.

Boundaries in the Next Century

There has been no single ethical issue that has galvanized the efforts of the APA Ethics Committee more than sexual misconduct and boundary violations. These ethical transgressions are discussed in detail in numerous publications (Frick 1994; Gabbard 1994; Gabbard and Nadelson 1995). The APA has been a leader in educating psychiatrists and other physicians about the tragedies as a result of sexual misconduct (AMA CEJA 1991). The APA has also enforced its ethical code by suspending or expelling over 120 psychiatrists over the last decade, most often for sexual misconduct. The frequency of other types of boundary violations or nonsexual misconduct preceding sexual misconduct has also been a major point in ethics education and risk prevention for psychiatrists and other health care professionals. Questions continue to be raised about the ethics of the APA annotation relating to sexual misconduct with former patients. These questions relate to the changing nature of psychiatric practice with new models of treatment not using dynamic psychotherapy or providing primarily medication management. Though not all agree with the strict dictum "once a patient, always a patient" (Gabbard 1992; Lazarus 1992), there has yet to be a group of psychiatrists who were involved with former patients to come forward to demonstrate no harm to those patients. Unless that were to occur, the ethical position of the APA should remain unaltered.

As psychiatrists' practices change over the next century, is it likely that the ethical conduct regarding boundaries or sexual misconduct should change? Actually, as other medical specialties, primary care physicians, and state medical licensing boards become more familiar with patient harm from sexual misconduct and boundary violations (those boundary transgressions in treatment which cause patient harm), the ethical or licensing sanctions have begun to approximate the enforcement work and opinions of the APA. Even those psychiatrists who do no psychotherapy may be subject to the same boundary concerns as those providing psychotherapy (Epstein and Simon 1990). The unfortunate tendency of nonsexual boundary violations as a precursor of sexual misconduct should serve as a sentinel signal to psychiatrists in any form of practice.

Some treatment interventions in modern psychiatric practice do place the psychiatrist in situations with patients outside of the consulting room. This includes treatment in intensive outpatient treatment situations, in-home family therapy, and residential or nursing home care. In these situations, blurring of psychiatrist-patient boundaries, if carried out as an explicit part of treatment, may be quite helpful. If not for therapeutic purposes, however, these boundary blurrings may create problems for patient and psychiatrist. It is also important to note that psychiatrists may more likely be serving patients in rural settings and small towns. There psychiatrists have no choice but to act like a country doctor by treating multiple family members, seeing patients frequently in social settings, and engaging in business relationships outside of the therapeutic situation. This probable increase in psychiatrists in underserved areas may create pressure to modify in a more direct way the principles related to boundaries and to make explicit what has been a general understanding of these differences in rural settings. To prevent harm to patients and to maintain the integrity of the profession, it will still be incumbent on the twenty-first century psychiatrist to maintain a professional relationship with patients.

Will Psychiatric Ethics Survive?

Just as some medical ethicists have questioned whether medical ethics will survive (Pellegrino 1993; Relman 1992), so must psychiatry ask the question about psychiatric ethics. Probably the greatest challenge as we move into the next century will continue to be the changing economic influences in psychiatric care. This has created unprecedented changes in type and place of psychiatric treatment as well as a business focus to patient care. This business focus has often created a dilemma for the psychiatrist as both clinician and administrator or clinician and stockholder. If psychiatric ethics moves to more of a business ethic, then the traditional covenant of trust between doctor and patient may be irrevocably shattered. It would mean moving from that covenant (Crawshaw et al. 1995; Webb 1986) to a corporate ethic of doing the least for your customers without dissatisfying them. If that metamorphosis occurs, there truly would be the gradual elimination of psychiatric ethics, which depends so much on the doctor-patient relationship as a distinct and principally nonbusiness relationship. To guard against this occurring, efforts are under way with the formation of an Ethics Institute within AMA to study among other things professionalism in medicine. Psychiatry will be a part of the dialogue by its involvement with the Council on Medical Specialty Societies, which has a similar process under way. These new initiatives represent the core value that the profession of medicine holds in professionalism in the practice of medicine. So when we address whether psychiatric ethics will survive, the principal question relates to the fundamental elements of the doctor-patient relationship and the corollaries that follow. It appears certain that psychiatrists will need to be more businesslike and incorporate some business principles in administering their practices and their systems. But this can be accomplished without a radical transformation of psychiatric ethics by appropriate delegation of business duties and attention to the clinical situation.

Conclusion

It is likely that the twenty-first century psychiatrist will occupy new roles but continue in the clinical treatment of the mentally ill. Economic forces along with health care policy reform may influence where, when, and how psychiatrists are able to treat patients. Society will have a greater influence than ever before in deciding how health care resources will be allocated. All of these factors will influence how psychiatrists will conduct themselves.

Some suggested ethical guidelines to consider (both for psychiatrists and the systems in which they work) into the next century include the following:

1. Psychiatrists have an ethical obligation to rise above any profit motive and serve as patient advocates.
2. Psychiatrists should provide treatments that are potentially beneficial and chosen by informed patients.
3. Beneficial psychiatric treatments should include those empirically demonstrated to provide benefit that is valued by patients, regarded as part of a standard of care, and recommended by established practice guidelines.
4. If allocation decisions are made, the manner in which these decisions are made and the influence of the treatment philosophy on patient care should be disclosed to patients in a clear manner in advance.
5. Treatment decisions should, to as great an extent possible, continue to be a joint enterprise between psychiatrist and patient.
6. Psychiatrists serving in administrative roles have the same professional ethics as clinicians. If they choose to follow a different set of ethics, they are ethically obliged to disclose their ethical standards to other physicians and patients.
7. Organized systems of care should foster a spirit of patient advocacy by professionals who are treating patients.
8. If there is an obligation assumed by a system of care to conserve society's resources, then all involved (patients, professionals, administrators, and stockholders) should benefit, profit, or be adversely affected by making proportionate gains or sacrifices.
9. Psychiatrists must continue to behave in a manner that will maintain trust in the doctor-patient relationship and not engage in behavior that will harm the patient.
10. Psychiatrists should be actively involved in any social policy debates that affect psychiatric patients.
11. Psychiatrists must advocate for fair treatment of psychiatric patients in all health care systems.

New research and new treatments will bring new ethical challenges. Societal forces may play additional roles in forcing psychiatrists to examine traditionally held values. With all of these forces for change, however, the profession can remain fundamentally secure in a body of knowledge and tradition of ethics that will not easily be shaken. Medicine, for most physicians, will continue to be seen as a moral enterprise and not as a business. When the time comes for the text to be written on twenty-second century psychiatry, it is this author's hope that professionalism and the primary importance of the doctor-patient relationship will remain as core values for psychiatry.

References

American College of Physicians: Ethics Manual, 3rd Edition. Ann Intern Med 117:947–960, 1992

American Medical Association: Guidelines for the Conduct of Managed Care. Chicago, IL, American Medical Association, 1993

American Medical Association: Ethical issues in managed care. JAMA 273:330–335, 1995

American Medical Association Council on Ethical and Judicial Affairs: Sexual misconduct in the practice of medicine. JAMA 266:2741–2745, 1991

American Medical Association Council on Ethical and Judicial Affairs: Code of Medical Ethics: Current Opinions With Annotations. Chicago, IL, American Medical Association, 1996

American Psychiatric Association: The Principles of Medical Ethics: With Annotations Especially Applicable to Psychiatry. Washington, DC, American Psychiatric Press, 1973

American Psychiatric Association: Conflicts of interest. American Psychiatric Association Ethics Newsletter 5(2), 1989

American Psychiatric Association: Principles of Health Care Reform. Washington, DC, American Psychiatric Press, 1993

American Psychiatric Association: The Principles of Medical Ethics: With Annotations Especially Applicable to Psychiatry. Washington, DC, American Psychiatric Press, 1995

American Psychiatric Association: A Basic Model Ethics Curriculum for Psychiatric Residents. Washington, DC, American Psychiatric Press, 1996

American Psychiatric Association Annual Meeting Debate: Is Restriction of Benefits Because of Costs Unethical? New York, NY, May 1996

American Psychiatric Association: Ethics in Managed Care Conference, Baltimore, MD, 1991

Barton WE: The History and Influence of the American Psychiatric Association. Washington, DC, American Psychiatric Press, 1987

Beauchamp TL, Childress JF: Principles of Biomedical Ethics. New York, Oxford University Press, 1994

Boyle PJ, Callahan D: Managed care in mental health: issues. Health Aff Fall, 1995, pp 6–22

Clancy CM, Kamerow DB: Evidence-based medicine meets cost-effectiveness analysis. JAMA 276:329–330, 1996

Crawshaw R, Rogers DE, Pellegrino ED, et al: Patient-physician covenant. JAMA 273:1553, 1995

Daniels N: Just Health Care. Cambridge, MA, Cambridge University Press, 1985

Daniels N: The ideal advocate and limited resources. Theoretical Medicine 8:69–80, 1987

Durso C: Hunting for hidden ethics. The New Physician May/June, 1996, pp 17–23

Eddy DM: Rationing resources while improving quality: how to get more for less. JAMA 272:817–824, 1994

Engelhardt HT, Rie MA: Morality for the medical-industrial complex. N Engl J Med 319:1086–1089, 1988

English JT: Presidential address: patient care for the twenty-first century: asserting professional values within economic restraints. Am J Psychiatry 150:1293–1301, 1993

Epstein RS, Simon RI: The exploitation index: an early warning indicator of boundary violations in psychotherapy. Bull Menninger Clin 54:450–465, 1990

Fink PJ: Presidential address: on being ethical in an unethical world. Am J Psychiatry 146:1097–1104, 1989

Frick DE: Nonsexual boundary violations in psychiatric treatment, in American Psychiatric Press Review of Psychiatry, Vol 13. Edited by Oldham JM, Riba MB. Washington, DC, American Psychiatric Press, 1994, pp 415–432

Gabbard GO: Once a patient, always a patient: therapist-patient sex after termination. The American Psychoanalyst 26:6–7, 1992

Gabbard GO: Sexual misconduct, in American Psychiatric Press Review of Psychiatry, Vol 13. Edited by Oldham JM, Riba MB. Washington, DC, American Psychiatric Press, 1994, pp 433–456

Gabbard GO, Nadelson C: Professional boundaries in the physician-patient relationship. JAMA 273:1445–1449, 1995

Kletke PR, Emmons DW, Gillis KD: Current trends in physicians' practice arrangements from owners to employees. JAMA 276:555–560, 1996

Glass RM: The patient-physician relationship: JAMA focuses on the center of medicine. JAMA 275:147–148, 1996

Lazarus JA: Sex with former patients almost always unethical. Am J Psychiatry 149:855–857, 1992

Lazarus JA: Critical ethical issues and conflicts. The Journal of the California Alliance for the Mentally Ill 5:1, 1994

Lazarus JA: New Financial Incentives and Disincentives for Psychiatrists. Washington, DC, American Psychiatric Press, 1997

Lazarus JA, Sharfstein SS: APA acts against ethics violators. Psychiatric News XXVII(20):14, October 16, 1992

Lazarus JA, Sharfstein SS: Changes in the economics and ethics of health and mental health care, in American Psychiatric Press Review of Psychiatry, Vol 13. Edited by Oldham JM, Riba MB. Washington, DC, American Psychiatric Press, 1994, pp 389–413

Lazarus JA, Sharfstein SS (eds): New Roles for Psychiatrists in Organized Systems of Care. Washington, DC, American Psychiatric Press, 1997

McFarland B: Health Maintenance Organizations and persons with severe mental illness. Community Ment Health J 30:221–242, 1994

McFarland BH, Johnson RE, Hornbrook MC: Enrollment duration, service use, and costs of care for severely mentally ill members of a Health Maintenance Organization. Arch Gen Psychiatry 53:938–944, 1996

Mariner WK: Business vs. medical ethics: conflicting standards for managed care. Journal of Law, Medicine and Ethics 23:236–246, 1995

Mechanic D, Ettel T, Davis D, et al: Choosing among health insurance options: a study of new employees. Inquiry 27:14–23, 1990

Miller I: Time-limited brief therapy has gone too far: the result is invisible rationing. Professional Psychology: Research and Practice 27:567–576, 1996

Morreim EH: Balancing Act: The New Medical Ethics of Medicine's New Economics. Dordrecht, The Netherlands, Kluwer, 1991

Office of Technology Assessment, Congressional Budget Office: Understanding estimates of national health expenditures under health reform (Publ No OTA-H-594, GPO stock 052–003–01374–6). Washington, DC, U.S. Government Printing Office, May 1994

Pellegrino ED: Rationing health care: the ethics of medical gatekeeping. J Contemp Health Law Policy 2:23–45, 1986

Pellegrino ED: The metamorphosis of medical ethics: a 30-year retrospective. JAMA 269:1158–1162, 1993

Pellegrino ED: Guarding the integrity of medical ethics: some lessons from Soviet Russia. JAMA 273:1622–1623, 1995

Relman AS: What market values are doing to medicine. The Atlantic Monthly, March 1992, pp 99–106

Rodwin MA: Medicine, Money, and Morals Physicians' Conflicts of Interest. New York, Oxford University Press, 1993

Rothman DJ: Strangers at the Bedside: A History of How Law and Bioethics Transformed Medical Decision Making. New York, Basic Books, 1991

Sabin JE: Caring about patients and caring about money: the American Psychiatric Association Code of Ethics meets managed care. Behav Sci Law 12:317–330, 1994

Sabin J, Daniels N: Determining "medical necessity" in mental health practice. Hastings Cent Rep 24:5–14, 1994

Schwartz J: Initial Report of the Attorney General's Research Working Group. Annapolis, MD, Office of the Maryland Attorney General, October 8, 1996

Spitzer RL, Kroenke K, Linzer M, et al: Health-related quality of life in primary care patients with mental disorders. JAMA 274:1511–1517, 1995

Thompson DF: Understanding financial conflicts of interest. N Engl J Med 329:573–576, 1993

Webb WL: The doctor-patient covenant and the threat of exploitation. Am J Psychiatry 143:1126–1131, 1986

Wells KB, Burnam MA, Rogers WH, et al: The course of depression in adult outpatients: results from the medical outcomes study. Arch Gen Psychiatry 49:788–794, 1992

Wolf SM: Health care reform and the future of physician ethics. Hastings Cent Rep (March–April):28–41, 1994

SECTION III

The Psychiatric Workforce and Its Education

INTRODUCTION

Having explored the evolving knowledge base of our discipline as we struggled with models of practice, and sobered by new economic realities as well as the difficulties in assessing joint psychological and pharmacological treatment, we now move to the issue of how many psychiatrists do we need and, in the United States, where will they have gone to medical school.

In Chapter 16, The Psychiatric Workforce, James Scully reviews both the forces and the varied opinions that will shape United States physician workforce needs and policy. Scully traces for us the thrust to increase United States physician supply in the 1960s after the passage of Medicare legislation. In slightly more than a decade, the United States doubled the number of medical graduates. The dust had hardly settled on policies and actions to increase physician supply when federal policy planners began to argue that we had a surplus of physicians. Initially, however, the planners proposed that psychiatry was one of the few specialties with a shortage. Today in the United States, federal policy, Scully points out, addresses a desire to reduce the number of first-year residents in all specialties other than primary care (family practice, general pediatrics, and general internal medicine). Attempts to implement this federal policy will be by reducing federal financial support for graduate medical education (residency training). This, it is anticipated, will result in a reduction of residency positions. This reduction, in turn, would reduce the need for international medical graduates (IMGs) in the United States. This reduced need would occur at a time when IMGs fill nearly one-half of United States psychiatric residencies. The loss of residency positions, if severe, could cause serious issues for health care delivery in sectors of the United States.

Scully also reviews and compares United States psychiatrist workforce numbers with their numbers in other industrialized countries. He concludes that the number of psychiatrists a country needs is significantly determined by how the country defines psychiatric practice (we might also add, in light of Sharfstein's chapter, how they fund psychiatric care).

In Chapter 17, The International Medical Graduate in American Psychiatry, Richard Balon, Rodrigo A. Muñoz, and Nyapati R. Rao explore the major impact on American psychiatry of non–United States-trained physicians (IMGs). After World War II, IMGs established the power of psychoanalysis and helped spread knowledge of the major pharmacological advances initiated in Europe. IMGs have played major roles in the elective offices and councils of the American Psychiatric Association. We are left to ponder a less clear role for new IMGs. It is not clear to us at this time, as previously noted, how reductions in federal (central government) support for residency education will affect both United States psychiatry in the long term and the opportunity for IMGs to come to the United States.

In Chapter 18, Psychiatric Education for the New Millennium, Carolyn B. Robinowitz addresses how to both educate a new generation of psychiatrists and concurrently develop approaches to maintain the competencies of those in practice. Her current position as a medical school dean of students and before that as founding director of the American Psychiatric Association's Office of Education equip her well to address this topic.

Robinowitz reviews the advances in our science, the shifting economics of health care, and shifts in practice patterns. Whereas earlier in this volume we discuss these issues, now we are asked to look at how we will educate and train residents to respond to the new realities of the practice of our discipline. We learn that we will be required to educate and train with decreased resources. Our clinical services in academic medical centers are currently being reorganized to respond to these changes—changes that make obsolete the training paradigms of the past generation. Current models of clinical training acceptable to residents' accrediting organizations will, Robinowitz argues, need to be changed to respond to these new realities. In spite of these changes, she argues, new technologies and curriculum organization will enable us to fulfill our educational mission, both for residents in training and practitioners. Although she devotes much of this chapter to what will change, Robinowitz reminds us not to forget that the core of our work will not. As psychiatrists, we must always remember our critical role in relating to and communicating with our patients.

CHAPTER 16

The Psychiatric Workforce

James H. Scully Jr., M.D.

As we approach the twenty-first century, symbolic issues of transition and change might be expected. Nevertheless, proposed changes in the size and composition of the United States medical workforce seem to be quite real. These potential changes could have profound effects on the profession of psychiatry in America.

As economists tried to explain the rise of health care costs in the United States in the past 30 years, a general consensus began to develop that there was an oversupply of physicians. The oversupply of physicians, rather than producing increased competition and subsequent lower costs, it was argued, actually increased costs. The oversupply coupled with the third-party insurance, fee-for-service model of paying for health care encouraged increased health care utilization and increased societal health care costs. More doctors provided more or excess care, and increases in costly technology compounded the problem from the point of view of health economists. Data that purported to show that United States citizens were not healthier as a result of the nation's high health care expenditures gave added credence to the view that health care spending was out of control.

Highlighting recent public concern over health care expenditures are concerns of the financial integrity of the United States Medicare program. Begun over 30 years ago, Medicare not only guaranteed affordable care for the elderly and disabled people, but it funded a significant portion of the cost of graduate (residency) medical education. The program was set up in a way that economically encouraged increased numbers of hospital-based residents. When the decision was made for Medicare to fund graduate medical education, no one thought this was a problem. At the time, there was a general consensus that a shortage of physicians existed. Any program to provide medical services to the elderly without necessary physicians would have failed. At that time, psychiatry was thought to be a specialty in even more shortage than most.

In response to the physician shortage, in the late 1960s and early 1970s a doubling of the number of graduates from United States schools of medicine occurred. Most schools increased their class size, and more than 40 new medical schools opened. Rather than producing approximately 8,000 new physicians each year, nearly 16,000 new physicians were graduated by 1975 within a decade of the passage of the Medicare legislation. Concurrent with the increase in graduates, was a shift in career choice away from what is today called primary care. Specialty practice became the dominant career choice.

Recruitment of Unites States medical graduates into psychiatry was relatively good in the sixties. The best recruiting schools were the private schools of the northeast and public schools based in large cities. Psychoanalytic theory predominated in the departments of psychiatry, and psychoanalytic training was considered by many as the most prestigious and elite subspecialty in psychiatry.

At the same time, psychiatry was becoming more estranged from the rest of medicine. In 1972, the requirement of the internship prior to a psychiatric residency was dropped. Ostensibly, this was because graduate medical education was being reorganized and free-standing internships were dropped. Psychiatry, however, not only eliminated the internship, but eliminated the requirement for a core clinical experience working with the medically ill. Working with medically ill patients as a physician, not just as a student, was no longer essential in becoming a psychiatrist.

Declining United States medical graduate interest in psychiatry in the 1970s was seen by some as a result of the estrangement of psychiatry from medicine as exemplified by the elimination of the internship (Table 16–1). By 1977, The American Board of Psychiatry and Neurology, under pressure from the field, reinstituted a requirement for at least 4 months of medicine or pediatrics and a month of clinical neurology for all psychiatrists in residency training and increased training from 3 years to 4. The restored medical training requirements for psychiatry and attention to recruitment may have contributed to the increased numbers of medical students choosing psychiatry (Table 16–2) in the 1980s.

At about the same time that psychiatry recruitment increased in the early

Table 16–1. Total residents by census year

Census year	No. of residents	Difference from prior year
1994–1995[a]	6,089	+30
1993–1994[a]	6,059	−36
1992–1993	6,095	−64
1991–1992	6,159	+143
1990–1991	6,016	−56
1989–1990	6,072	+24
1988–1989	6,048	+219
1987–1988	5,829	+321
1986–1987	5,508	+20
1985–1986	5,488	+176
1984–1985	5,312	+203
1983–1984	5,109	+223
1982–1983	4,886	+205
1981–1982	4,681	+163
1980–1981	4,518	+111
1979–1980	4,407	−258
1978–1979	4,665	−243
1977–1978	4,908	+64
1976–1977	4,844	+79
1975–1976	4,765	−49
1974–1975	4,814	+76
1973–1974	4,738	+39
1972–1973	4,699	+483
1971–1972[b]	NA	NA
1970–1971	4,216	+251
1969–1970	3,965	+156
1968–1969	3,809	

Note. Data are based on a 100% survey of all programs approved for general and/or child psychiatry training. All percentages are computed by excluding unreported data from totals. NA = not available.
[a]Census includes American Osteopathic Association (1993)–approved programs, which accounted for 35 residents in 1993–1994 and 38 in 1994–1995. [b]Census was not conducted in 1971–1972.

Table 16–2.   Recruitment of U.S. medical school graduates into psychiatry: comparison of National Residency Matching Plan (NRMP) results for 1988 through 1998

Year	U.S. students registered in match	PGY-1 residency selections— U.S. senior students only Psychiatry
1988	14,499	745
1989	14,117	722
1990	13,908	664
1991	13,943	641
1992	14,032	526
1993	14,094	476
1994	14,207	438
1995	14,621	476
1996	14,539	448
1997	14,614	462
1998	14,610	428
% change 1997–1998	–0.03%	–7.36%
% change 1988–1998	0.077%	–42.55%

Note.   PGY-1 = postgraduate year 1.

1980s, the Graduate Medical Education Medical Advisory Council (GMENAC) was organized by the federal government to study both current physician supply and future requirements. GMENAC produced a needs-based study of physician requirements. This study looked at the available epidemiological data on mental illnesses in the United States population and estimated the percentage of individuals who might need treatment from psychiatrists. GMENAC then factored in the workload of an average psychiatrist at that point in time in their algorithm to determine needs. This model predicted an estimated need for 50,000 adult and over 30,000 child psychiatrists. Because, at the time, there were fewer than 4,000 child psychiatrists, this led to the statements that child psychiatry was the greatest shortage specialty in the country. GMENAC also predicted a significant oversupply of physicians by the end of the century.

GMENAC was followed in the 1980s by the Council on Graduate Medical Education (COGME), which also has argued that we are producing a physi-

Table 16–3. Source of medical training of U.S. psychiatric residents by year: 1991–1992 through 1996–1997

	Year					
	1991–1992	1992–1993	1993–1994	1994–1995	1995–1996	1996–1997
Non-IMG, no. (%)	4,665 (77.4)	4,431 (73.8)	4,140 (69.0)	3,909 (64.6)	3,705 (61.4)	3,468 (59.0)
IMG, no. (%)	1,364 (22.6)	1,570 (26.2)	1,858 (31.0)	2,140 (35.4)	2,325 (38.6)	2,408 (41.0)
Unreported, no.	130	94	61	40	57	76
Total, no. (%)	6,159 (100.0)	6,095 (100.0)	6,059 (100.0)	6,089 (100.0)	6,087 (100.0)	5,952 (100.0)

Note. IMG = international medical graduate.

cian surplus. In the meantime, recruitment of United States graduates into psychiatry in the late 1980s through the National Residency Matching Plan (NRMP) peaked in 1988 (see Table 16–2) with a corresponding increase in the total resident population through 1991. This has been followed by a decline in recruitment of current United States medical graduates through the NRMP (Table 16–2) of nearly 40% by 1996. At the same time, the total number of psychiatric residents has remained stable at approximately 6,000 for the past 8 years. This has occurred because of a dramatic increase in the number of international medical graduates (IMGs) recruited into psychiatry residencies (Table 16–3).

The stabilization of the number of psychiatry residents has occurred at a time when, as noted, there is a general consensus that an oversupply of physicians, especially specialists, exists. The potential oversupply, it is argued, affects the cost of health care. The Institute of Medicine (IOM) report *Primary Care: America's Health in a New Era* (Donaldson et al. 1996) strongly supports the transformation of the United States health care workforce to one of primary care clinicians. *Clinicians* are defined to include nurses and physician assistants as well as primary care physicians, and the IOM further recommended that state governments review the restrictions on the scope of practice of primary care nurse practitioners and physician assistants and eliminate or modify those restrictions that impede collaborative practice and reduce access to quality primary care (Donaldson et al. 1996, p. 174).

The IOM also opposed the concept of mental health *carve-outs*, the separate and unique behavioral health care plans that have arisen in the managed care era. The proponents of primary care recognize that "a major portion of mental health care is rendered in the primary care setting and always will be, sometimes despite strong disincentives; . . . a sensible vision of primary care must have mental health woven into its fabric . . . " (Donaldson et al. 1996, p. 135) The report recognizes the common failure of primary care providers to recognize psychiatric disorders and calls for collaborative models to integrate primary care and mental health services more effectively. No special role for psychiatry was discussed in the report. Indeed, the tone of the IOM report was one that discounted any special role for physicians in general and promoted the role of nonphysician providers. The inevitable consequences for psychiatry, if the IOM recommendations or similar ones were implemented without modification, would be a drastic reduction in the need for psychiatrists. The psychiatrists needed would probably function as consultants, perhaps such as those in the system in Great Britain, where psychiatrists are primarily consultants to other physicians and where the general practitioners treat the majority of those patients who seek treatment for nonpsychotic psychiatric disorders. It should be noted that the workforce requirements for psychiatrists in Great Britain under this model is only about 4 psychiatrists per 100,000 population.

A similar model has been proposed for the United States by others as well. Weiner forecasted a demand for psychiatrists by using a model of health maintenance organization (HMO) staffing patterns, including the care of the chronic mentally ill, extrapolated on a national level (Weiner 1994). Current HMO staffing ratios of 3.8–4.8 psychiatrists per 100,000 population would actually need to decline to provide for psychiatrists to treat the more seriously mentally ill and maintain the 4 per 100,000 population. Using these models, because data from the American Medical Association (AMA) indicates that we now have about 16 psychiatrists per 100,000 population (AMA 1996), we have an oversupply of psychiatrists and need only 25%–30% of the current numbers.

Workforce numbers in other countries that have single payer systems of national health insurance rather than managed care may be useful for comparison. Those countries all have more central control over health care expenditures than does the United States. As noted above, Great Britain has about 4 psychiatrists per 100,000 population. New Zealand has about the same, whereas Australia has 8.8 psychiatrists per 100,000 population. Interestingly, in Australia, psychiatrists provide all forms of psychotherapy, including long-term individual psychotherapy. In New Zealand, they do not, and there is minimal coverage for private fees. Nonetheless, the cost per person is about the same in each system (Andrews 1989).

Canada has a psychiatrist/population ratio of about 10/100,000. Perhaps the highest ratio in Europe is in Holland, where there are approximately 12 psychiatrists per 100,000 population. In all these countries with more than 4/100,000, psychiatrists provide psychotherapy along with inpatient and consultative services. The clear critical issue in determining psychiatrist need in a country is the breadth of the psychiatrist's clinical responsibilities.

As noted above, the COGME was authorized by the United States Congress to assess the physician workforce trends and recommend both federal and private efforts to address physician workforce needs. In the past 10 years, they have produced eight reports. Their most recent report affirms earlier findings that they have made regarding an excess in the number of specialist physicians and a call to reduce those numbers (COGME 1996).

COGME concludes that the only scenario that will accomplish the task of reducing the supply of specialist while maintaining the generalist supply is a combination of both reducing the number of first-year residents from 140% of United States medical graduates (USMGs) to 110% of USMGs while increasing the proportion of generalists to at least 50% annually. This plan is referred in shorthand discussions as the "110/50:50" proposal. Reductions in any future physician supply can come only from either the IMG or USMG component, or a combination of both (Kindig and Libby 1996).

Restated, the size of United States medical school graduating classes can be reduced, individual schools can close, or the number of IMGs entering the United States can be reduced. Other less palatable options are also possible to implement COGME proposals. These options include either not all graduates of United States medical schools being able to enter postgraduate training positions in the United States or USMGs leaving the country to practice abroad or leaving medicine altogether and seeking employment in other field. This last phenomenon, while unknown in America, has been described in other countries. Stories of physicians in other countries driving taxicabs because of physician oversupply and government restrictions are well known. One of the vice-presidents of the Association of American Medical Colleges has predicted a large oversupply of physicians that could lead to physicians in the United States being unemployed. The oversupply that he indicated in the growth in graduate education numbers will be the result of increases in the number of IMGs. He declared (Dickler 1995) that the quandary posed by IMGs "is the single biggest issue in graduate medical education, and no one can seem to get their arms around it."

If the Eighth COGME Report (1996) was implemented as written, we would see a cut in the total number of trainees by nearly 25%. If these recommendations are carried out and no special exemption is granted to psychiatry, we can expect cuts of 44% in the number of first-year psychiatric residents to approximately 600. If one combines the 1994 United States allopathic and osteopathic graduates plus 10%, the number is 19,600 positions. Because there are currently nearly 25,000 physicians in postgraduate year 1 (PGY1) positions, this would require a cut of more than 5,000, or 22%. If then there is a requirement of 50% in primary care, then all the cuts would be from the specialties, including psychiatry. Our share of the cut without any special exemptions would be 44%.

It must be noted that not everyone agrees that the United States is heading toward a massive oversupply of physicians. Serious questions are raised regarding the methodology of studies that argue for oversupply (Cooper 1994, 1995). Cooper proposes that the number of specialists needed will continue to rise slowly, depending on technological advances in the coming decade. Psychiatry may not fit this pattern but will not be in great oversupply either, he argues.

Discussion of oversupply and changes in the availability of specialty practice opportunities has already affected medical student residency choice. Residency numbers in several specialties, such as family medicine, have risen, whereas numbers in anesthesiology have declined. The changes lead some planners to advising that the *market* will work to set the relative numbers of specialists. They do not believe that it will be necessary for the government to directly intervene by establishing explicit guidelines for hospitals to produce 50% of all physicians in primary care. Others dispute this and believe that the market-driven change will take too long to limit massive physician oversupply. In response to this issue, the Veterans Administration (VA) has proposed several classifications of specialists (Petersdorf 1992). Proposed cuts in specialty training positions would be distinct for each specialty. Reductions would be directed at non–primary care areas. Specialties such as psychiatry would be considered more like primary care than like the technical and surgical subspecialties, thus facing fewer reductions in positions in the VA proposal.

Independent of the number of training positions allocated in the United States is the United States dependence on IMGs in psychiatry to either maintain or expand the number of psychiatrists. Any restrictions in the number of IMGs allowed to train will have a profound impact on psychiatry. The proposal to limit the number of IMGs to 10% of all United States medical graduates in training would be uniquely negative on psychiatry if all specialties showed equally the reductions. Such a profound reduction would require a major recruiting effort among United States students just to obtain the 800 new psychiatric residents each year needed to maintain our current number of practitioners. This is far fewer than the 1,200 we have had training per year for the last decade.

Severe restrictions in IMG numbers from the current near 30% of all medical trainees to 10% would cause major disruption in academic health centers and disrupt care for many in the underserved areas currently served by IMG-dependent hospitals. New York is especially vulnerable to this proposal. Over half the psychiatric residents in New York are IMGs, and nearly a third of all of the IMGs in psychiatry residency training in the United States are in New York (American Psychiatric Association 1995). We in American psychiatry have asked these physicians to join us, and they have helped care for a large number of the poor that United States physicians have chosen to avoid. Now they are perceived by some not as part of the solution to our health care problems, but as part of the problem (Mullan et al. 1995). It is important, in coming years, to attend to the issue of how we treat those doctors who are here versus those physicians who have graduated from the nearly 1,400 medical schools around the world who may wish to come here. Does the United

States have the same obligations to both groups? Do all physicians, wherever they are from, have equal rights to seek training in the United States? Do all physicians trained in the United States have the same right to practice in the United States?

How we in psychiatry deal with this issue will be critical to the future of our profession. In the early twenty-first century, United States psychiatry will be forced to address the major shift in resources available for residency training and health care. We may not, under current proposals, be able to maintain our current numbers or wish to do so. We will need to develop strategies to argue for adequate numbers of psychiatrists and agree on the practice responsibilities of psychiatrists. Although psychiatry is practiced uniquely in each country, all will face issues of resource utilization.

References

American Medical Association: Physician Characteristics and Distribution in the US. Chicago, IL, American Medical Association, 1996

American Psychiatric Association: Census of Residents. Washington, DC, American Psychiatric Association, 1995

American Osteopathic Association: Osteopathic Physician Distribution. Chicago, IL, American Osteopathic Association, 1993

Andrews G: Private and public psychiatry: a comparison of two health care systems. Am J Psychiatry 146:881–856, 1989

Cooper RA: Seeking a balanced physician workforce for the 21st century. JAMA 272:680–687, 1994

Cooper RA: Perspectives on the physician workforce to the year 2020. JAMA 274:1534–1543, 1995

Council on Graduate Medical Education: Eighth Report: Patient Care Physician Supply and Requirements: Testing COGME Recommendations (1996). Rockville, MD, U.S. Department of Health and Human Services, July 1996

Dickler R: The AAMC Reporter 4(8), April 1995

Donaldson MS, Yordy KD, Lohr KN, et al. (eds): Primary Care: America's Health in a New Era. Washington, DC, National Academy Press, 1996

Kindig DA, Libby DL: Domestic production vs. international immigration. JAMA 276:978–982, 1996

Mullan F, Politzer RM, Davis CH: Medical migration and the physician workforce: international medical graduates and American medicine. JAMA 273:1521–1527, 1995

Petersdorf RG: Response to Title VII Reauthorization Need-Based Financial Aid Provisions (Action AAMC #92-95), December 21, 1992

Weiner JP: Forecasting the effects of health care reform on US physician workforce requirements. JAMA 272:222–230, 1994

CHAPTER 17

The International Medical Graduate in American Psychiatry

Richard Balon, M.D.
Rodrigo A. Muñoz, M.D.
Nyapati R. Rao, M.D.

International medical graduates (IMGs), those physicians trained in medical schools outside the United States, have been a major presence in American psychiatry since its beginning. From more than 140 countries, they are a heterogeneous group from various linguistic, ethnic, cultural, and medical education backgrounds. At present, approximately 25% of the general membership in the American Psychiatric Association (APA) are IMGs. Similarly, nearly 50% of first-year residents in psychiatry during 1995–1996 were IMGs.

International medical graduates have been the subject of various misconceptions, discriminations, and biases. Their role in American psychiatry has not been fully appreciated. This chapter reviews the history and the problems IMGs face and focuses on important contributions IMGs have made. The future role of IMGs in American psychiatry is also discussed.

Brief History of International Medical Graduates in the United States

From time immemorial, physicians have traveled to foreign countries in search of higher learning to improve their skills. Ancient civilizations such as China, India, and Japan have examples of such sojourns by their medical leaders. In more recent Western civilization, centers of medical academic excellence existed in Edinburgh and London in the eighteenth century, Paris in the early nineteenth century, and Germany in the late nineteenth and early twentieth centuries. (Adolf Meyer, founder of psychobiology, migrated to the United States in 1892.) Until the 1930s, it was common for Americans to travel abroad to centers of medical academic excellence for their medical education rather than study in the United States. Benjamin Rush, who is best known as a signer of the Declaration of Independence and whose face appears on the APA insignia, was an American who obtained his medical education in Edinburgh, Scotland.

The migration of international physicians to the United States significantly increased after World War II as the United States, with its enhanced prestige, wealth of resources, and excellence in medical education began to attract more IMGs. An important difference in physician migration occurred in the twentieth century, as physicians who came to the United States chose to stay in the United States, unlike the physicians of earlier times who traveled to Europe from various parts of the world only to return to their home countries. The migration of foreign physicians to the United States was hastened by political persecution in Europe around and after World War II. Some of the most prominent IMG psychiatrists of European origin who came to the United States during this period include Franz Alexander, Nathan Ackerman, Frieda Fromm-Reichman, Heinz Kohut, Lothar Kalinowsky, and George Tarjan.

Migration was further aided when Congress passed the Exchange Visitor Law in 1950, permitting foreign nationals in various professions to enter the United States for limited periods of time for advanced training in their respective areas.

Until the late 1950s, foreign physicians did not have to pass a qualifying examination. As the number of IMGs grew, some voiced concerns about the competence and readiness of the IMGs to seek postgraduate training in the United States. As a result of these concerns, Congress created the Educational Commission for Foreign Medical Graduates (ECFMG) to verify credentials as well as test the readiness of foreign physicians to enter medical training in the United States. The first standardized examination, a 1-day multiple-choice test in basic and clinical sciences and a test to evaluate the candidate's proficiency of the English language, was administered in 1958. Different versions of the qualifying examination have been used in subsequent years. The Visa Qualifying Examination (VQE), a 2-day test that IMGs were required to pass to obtain an exchange visitor's visa as well as to become eligible for training in the United States, was created in 1975. Subsequently, in 1984 the Foreign Medical Graduate Examination in Medical Sciences (FMGEMS) replaced the VQE. There had been a strong movement to create a common examination for both United States medical graduates (USMGs) and IMGs, and in the early 1990s, the unified United States Medical Licensing Examination (USMLE) was introduced.

The number of IMGs in American medicine has been steadily increasing. At the present time, more than 23% of all physicians in the United States are IMGs.

Changes of Ethnic and National Representation Among International Medical Graduates in the United States

Immigration laws have changed periodically to adapt to social, economic, and political realities. As mentioned earlier, as large numbers of IMGs entered the country as refugees and later as exchange visitors consequent to the creation of exchange visitor visa status by the Congress in 1950, many physicians converted to permanent resident status and continued to live in the United States. Criticism arose that the conversion of IMGs from exchange visitors to permanent resident status was depriving foreign nations of their trained professionals. Consequently, in 1955 a requirement was added to the exchange visitor visa that the physician return to his or her home country for 2 years before seeking permanent resident status.

In 1965, the Immigration Act was amended to give professions in short supply, such as medicine, preference in granting permanent visa status. This act also removed quotas based on national origins. As a result of this law, more physicians from non-European countries were allowed to enter the United States as permanent residents. Although Europe had been the major source of IMGs prior to 1965, Asia and Latin America took the lead after 1965. Graduates of foreign medical schools represent about 23% of actively practicing physicians in the United States at the present time (Iglehart 1996). In 1994, the ECFMG granted the largest number of certificates to physicians from India (25.9%), the Philippines (8.1%), Pakistan (5.9%), countries of the former Soviet Union (4.2%), China (3.7%), and Egypt (2.6%) (Iglehart 1996). United States citizens, principally from medical schools in the Dominican Republic, Grenada, Mexico, and Montserrat, were granted 4.9% of all certifications in 1994 (Iglehart 1996). The exact numbers for psychiatrists are not available, but it is clear that among IMGs there has been an overall shift toward physicians from non-European countries. It is plausible that psychiatry has followed a similar pattern. Some of the prominent IMG psychiatrists from Asia and Latin America include Hagop Akiskal, Otto and Paulina Kernberg, Rodrigo Muñoz, Henry Nasrallah, Pedro Ruiz, Ming Tsuang, and Elizabeth Weller.

Major Issues and Obstacles Encountered by International Medical Graduates Who Are Entering American Psychiatry

As with other immigrants moving to the United States, IMGs born outside of the United States face problems of acculturation and adjustment to the new country. Davidson (1982) described five stages of "cross-cultural transition." In stage one, cultural shock and frank paranoid feelings about the new culture are common. In stage two, one mourns the "lost culture." In stage three, vertical thinking becomes prominent with a consolidation of the old cultural and personal identity in response to a feeling of not being claimed, of being different and rejected. In stage four, cultural structuralism and assimilation take place, cultural distances for an IMG become smaller, and American customs and values are more readily sought and accepted. Finally, in stage five, there are finally creative contributions to the new country and culture, and one strives to become a full participant and a good citizen. These stages may vary in their length, depending on one's "original culture" and individual characteristics.

The process of acculturation may overlap or be complicated by various issues and obstacles, such as passing the ECFMG examination, getting a residency position, obtaining licensure and board certification, getting a permanent job, becoming a member of a hospital staff and, more recently, becoming a member of a health maintenance organization (HMO) panel. These problems are faced by all IMGs, United States and non–United States alike. In addition, starting in 1998, IMGs are required to take a Clinical Skills Assessment (CSA) examination.

A foreign medical school graduate who wants to enter postgraduate training in the United States must earn ECFMG certification, which is achieved by taking an examination that tests clinical competence and English language proficiency. Until the early 1990s, the ECFMG administered its own examination that was different from the National Board Examination. The existence of two different examinations has been the basis of complaints of discrimination against IMGs. Finally, a new examination, the USMLE, was created. This examination is administered in three steps and can be taken by United States and non–United States medical students or physicians. At present, to obtain ECFMG certification an IMG must 1) pass steps 1 and 2 of the USMLE, 2) demonstrate competency in oral and written English, and 3) satisfy other ECFMG credentialing requirements.

Obtaining a residency position is another obstacle. The permanent rumor that the majority of programs prefer USMGs and that some programs reject IMGs outright has been confirmed by many anecdotes. The most recent example was a University of Michigan memorandum regarding the house staff that stated, "no international medical graduates (except Canadian) may be appointed" (Mitka 1996). However, this issue requires more rigorous study. A recent study (Balon et al. 1997) highlighted the possibility of discrimination against IMGs in the selection process of psychiatry residents. Some of the residency programs in psychiatry limited the influx of IMG applicants at the first level—request for an application. The reasons for this practice are not known, but discrimination could be a possible explanation.

Licensure to practice medicine in the United States is controlled by 54 different licensing jurisdictions, mostly states, each with its own policies and regulations. Some states require that physicians pass a licensing examination and complete a certain number of years of postgraduate training. However, many states have different rules for acceptable examination scores. For instance, in the case of the Federation Licensing Examination (FLEX), some states accept a weighted average score and others require a minimum score on separate parts of the examination. Also, some states require that all scores are passed at a single sitting while others accept scores from different sittings. That has created a difficult problem for many IMGs who attempt to move from one state to another.

American medical graduates have not encountered these difficulties. According to the U.S. General Accounting Office (1990), in the past, "Most states require[d] that foreign medical school graduates pass a different licensure examination and complete more years of postgraduate (residency) medical training than their U.S. counterparts." The introduction of the USMLE examination removed one of the differences, as the rules apply. The introduction of CSA in 1998 brings back different requirements for IMGs. Because this examination is given only in Philadelphia and is expensive, it will probably limit the number of IMGs entering the United States. In addition, IMGs have to complete more years of postgraduate training in most of the states, and approval of foreign medical schools varies from state to state. Questions about the applicant's medical school could be absurdly detailed; for example, one IMG was asked about the number of books in his medical school library. In addition, some states have also limited the time in which licensing examination scores will be accepted (5–40 years). This ruling creates difficult situations, even for some American graduates of foreign schools. An example is the case of a distinguished residency training director, a professor of psychiatry in his late fifties, who decided to move to Florida before his retirement. He wanted to obtain a Florida license but found that as a United States–born IMG, he had to take the FLEX examination because he had graduated from a Swiss medical school. He had attended medical school in Geneva, Switzerland, on the GI Bill after World War II and had practiced psychiatry for years in the United States. He passed the examination, which he characterized as the "least substantiated and most difficult in my life."

The process of obtaining licensure might be complicated by other requirements, such as passing Special Purpose Examinations and completing personal interviews. The recent Council on Graduate Medical Education (COGME) study (unpublished data) showed that several states had higher average processing times for IMG applicants and greater endorsement processing times for IMGs.

Another obstacle for IMGs has been the certification by the American Board of Psychiatry and Neurology, Inc. (ABPN). IMG performance on this examination has been historically worse than that of USMGs. For instance, in 1989, 65% of IMG candidates failed and only 31% of USMGs failed the ABPN examination. (For various reasons, the ABPN and APA stopped publishing the passing rate for IMGs after 1989.) Even though discrimination has been the most frequently discussed explanation for the poor performance of IMGs, there are other important factors. Part I of the examination is multiple choice, a format unfamiliar to many IMGs. Part II is an oral examination format, familiar to many IMGs. However, they are taking the examination in a "foreign" language. Linguistic regression brought on by performance anxiety affects the capacity to communicate in an acquired language more than it does in one's native tongue (Weintraub 1997). Another factor may be poorer residency training. It has been alleged that many top programs in the country avoid accepting IMGs and that IMGs are therefore concentrated in residency programs that provide poor training.

Discrimination against IMGs during the oral examination has been a frequent complaint. It is well known that IMGs have been underrepresented among the ABPN examiners and directors. Val and Quick (1983) reported that the percentage of IMGs who reported being associated with the ABPN as either a consultant, a director, or an examiner fell considerably below the percentage of IMGs in a general sample of psychiatrists, even when corrected for the lower proportion of IMGs holding board certification. The ABPN along with the APA have tried to rectify this discrepancy. The APA established the Task Force to Facilitate Communication Between APA and ABPN under the leadership of Rodrigo Muñoz, M.D. In 1995, Pedro Ruiz, M.D., was appointed as the first IMG director of the ABPN, and in 1997, Elizabeth Weller was elected as the first female IMG director of the ABPN. However, IMG representation, especially among senior examiners, remains low.

No studies exist on the difficulties of obtaining hospital privileges and memberships on HMO panels. However, it is plausible that some HMO panels do not approve many IMGs because of the applicant's lack of ABPN certification.

Unique Contributions of International Medical Graduates to Clinical Care, Education, and Research in American Psychiatry

Despite the lack of definite statistics about IMG contributions to American psychiatry, there are many examples of their significant contributions.

Historically, IMGs played a vital role in caring for the most severely mentally ill. The percentage of IMGs practicing in public mental hospitals during the 1970s ranged from a low of 5.3% of the total physician staff in Arkansas to a high of 87.2% in Rhode Island, with a national average of 50.4% (Jenkins and Witkin 1976). This trend has continued throughout the 1990s. Results of the 1994 APA membership survey revealed that IMGs were clearly overrepresented in city, county, and state hospitals when compared with representation of graduates from United States medical schools (10.7% versus 5.2%) (Balon and Muñoz 1996). However, the same survey demonstrated that IMGs were underrepresented in solo office practice, group office practices, and medical schools.

Several prominent IMGs have had a profound impact on various areas of clinical care. George Tarjan, the first IMG president of the APA, was instrumental in the development of the field of mental retardation. Leo Kanner coined the term *infantile autism* and provided a comprehensive account of this syndrome.

American psychoanalysis has benefited from contributions of many IMGs, either recently or in the past. Heinz Kohut and his followers (e.g., Anna and Paul Ornstein) postulated some of the dominant paradigms of self psychology that are used in the treatment of narcissistic personality disorder. Another important paradigm in the psychoanalytical treatment of narcissistic personality disorder associated with ego psychology–object relations was postulated by Otto Kernberg. The work of Kohut and Kernberg profoundly changed our view and treatment of narcissistic personality disorder. The *American Journal of Psychotherapy* is edited by Toksoz B. Karasu. Other prominent psychoanalysts—IMGs of the past—include Sandor Rado (director of the first psychoanalytic institute established within a university medical school), Alfred Adler, Erich Fromm, and Frieda Fromm-Reichman. Kurt Goldstein, who came to the United States from Germany, was a leader of the holistic or organismic theoreticians and was also involved with Gestalt psychology and existentialism.

Recently, Hagop Akiskal, M.D., brought attention back to the careful clinical observations of mood disorders, chronic low depression, dysthymia, and the relationship between mood disturbance and personality pathology. The work of Juan Mezzich, M.D., and others contributed ethnic and cultural considerations in the *Diagnostic and Statistical Manual of Mental Disorders*, 4th Edition, including the Appendix, Outline for Cultural Formulation and Glossary of Culture-Bound Syndromes (American Psychiatric Association 1994).

One of the most prominent figures of twentieth-century American psychiatry and psychiatric education is Adolf Meyer, who emigrated to the United States from Switzerland. His numerous contributions to psychiatry include a biographical-historical approach to the study of personality, his advocacy of social action for mental health, and the conceptualization of psychobiology.

Many prominent researchers in American psychiatry have been IMGs, including Henry Nasrallah, M.D., who specializes in the area of schizophrenia; Ming Tsuang and Javier Escobar in the area of psychiatric epidemiology; Hagop Akiskal, Bernard Carroll (dexamethasone suppression test [DST]), and Natraj Sitaram (cholinergic system and mood disorders) in the area of mood disorders; Elizabeth Weller and S. Arshad Husain in the field of child psychiatry; and Samuel Gershon in the area of psychopharmacology.

Despite the many unique contributions to American psychiatry, only a few IMGs have been appointed as chairs in the department of psychiatry. Currently, five IMGs serve as chairs—Javier Escobar at the UMDNJ–Robert Wood Johnson Medical School in New Jersey; Angelos Halaris at the University of Mississippi in Jackson; Toksoz B. Karasu at the Albert Einstein College of Medicine in New York; Henry Nasrallah at Ohio State University in Columbus; and Ole Thienhaus at the University of Nevada in Reno.

The Critical Role of International Medical Graduates in the Problems of the Psychiatric Workforce in the United States

The percentage of IMGs among the physician workforce in the United States has been steadily increasing from about 10% in 1963 to almost 25% in 1995 (Mullan et al. 1995). This growth has been stimulated by two public policies. The first was an

> . . . immigration policy that has recognized the advantage of allowing foreign-national physicians to enter the United States to participate in graduate medical education as exchange visitors. These physicians would receive advanced medical education, provide services to the hospitals in which they trained, and return to their countries carrying the latest and best in U.S. medical training, benefiting all concerned. (Mullan et al. 1995)

The second policy was based on the perceived physician shortage in the United States in the 1960s and 1970s. Many IMG physicians who came to the United States in the 1960s and 1970s describe urgent phone calls from United States hospitals and being offered one-way plane tickets to the United States. However, at the same time, the annual number of USMGs was steadily on the rise and actually doubled. Immigration policies relaxed, and many IMGs never returned to their countries of origin.

The number of physicians in the United States has been escalating, and no clear agreement exists about the physician staffing needs in the United States. Since the 1980s, many health care analysts have warned of a physicians' glut, which has frequently been blamed on IMGs. This led to suggestions to limit the number of residency slots to 110% of the number of graduates of United States medical schools (Ritvo and Kindig 1996). This proposed policy would drastically limit the number of IMGs entering graduate medical education (GME), as the number of available residency positions is roughly 140% of the number of USMGs. Other suggestions included the call by the Pew Health Professions Commission (1995) to slash the number of medical school slots by 20%–25%. On the other hand, some experts believe that the existing surplus is small and that it is likely to be of modest size during the next 15 years, after which it will recede, and also that major surpluses are local and regional (Cooper 1995; Dalen 1996). Finally, as the country struggles with the ongoing need for physicians, suggestions to limit the number of residency slots to the "magic number" of 110% of graduates of United States medical schools may be irrelevant.

Even the staunchest proponents for limiting the number of IMGs entering GME have appreciated the important contributions to the provision of health care in this country by the IMG community (Mullan et al. 1995). They also point out that after filling residency positions that remain unfilled by USMGs, IMGs relocate to office-based practices in similar patterns to their USMG counterparts.

The situation in American psychiatry has mirrored the situation in American medicine in general. The number of USMGs interested in psychiatry has steadily declined during the last decade. For instance, the number of USMGs choosing psychiatry through the National Residency Matching Program dropped 5.9% (from 476 to 448) from 1995 to 1996. This was slightly higher than the 1994 number (438), but almost 40% lower than the 1988 number (745). Nevertheless, the number of residency slots in psychiatry has remained relatively stable over the last decade, with IMGs filling the remaining slots. In July 1996, more than one-half of first-year residents in psychiatry were IMGs. However, here the similarity ends. After graduating from residency programs, IMGs do not always move to practices similar to their USMG counterparts. They often care for the poorest patients in the public sector, where they are clearly overrepresented (Balon and Muñoz 1996). They have been critical providers of health care for the poor in a number of states, especially in the Northeast (S. Weissman, as quoted in "Match Results Show Numbers Continue to Slip in Psychiatry," 1996). The crucial role of IMGs in the inner city and remote rural hospitals has been recognized by the APA, the American Academy of Child and Adolescent Psychiatry, and the American Association for Geriatric Psychiatry. In a joint statement presented to the House Ways and Means Subcommittee on Health on April 16, 1996, these three organizations strongly opposed targeting IMGs for the elimination of or disproportionate reductions in federal support.

Some experts suggest that the number of recruits into psychiatry should be about 800 to 850 per year to maintain the current number of psychiatrists. Others (J. Scully, as quoted in "IMGs Boost Psychiatry Match Rate Once Again," 1996) would like to see about 5% of all USMGs (about 670) choose psychiatry and then add IMGs to reach a minimum of 850 residents. Even this unrealistic proposal (in 1996, only 3.3% USMGs chose psychiatry) expects IMGs to fill at least 20% of the residency slots.

Psychiatry may be heading for an even bigger shortage, assuming that 1) surpluses are local and regional; 2) the surplus will recede in about 15 years; 3) the number of IMGs will be limited to 110% or whatever number of USMGs; and 4) the number of USMGs interested in psychiatry will remain low as a result of economic considerations, effects of managed care, and the uncertainties about the future of the profession. The first to suffer from this shortage will be severely mentally ill patients and the poor, with research, education, and administration following. IMGs will have to play a critical role in maintaining the levels of psychiatric services in the United States.

Other factors are rarely addressed in the discussions of psychiatric staffing and the role of IMGs. It is estimated that by the year 2050, almost half of the United States population will be minorities. By the end of the twenty-first century, no single racial or ethnic group will be in the majority in the United States. In fact, for major cities such as Los Angeles, New York, and Miami, the future is already here; non-Hispanic whites make up less than half of city residents (Updata 1996). Most minority patients are treated by minority physicians. Black and Hispanic physicians play a unique and important role in caring for poor, black, and Hispanic patients in California (Komaromy et al. 1996). However, a shortage of minority physicians will continue, at least in the near future.

Minorities continue to be underrepresented among United States medical students. For instance, Hispanics compose at least 9% of the United States population; however, less than 5% of all United States physicians and medical students are Hispanics. Asian American medical students are less interested in psychiatry. However, most IMGs are minority physicians with some degree of cultural competence who expect to devote their professional activities to the care of minorities. We may have to take into consideration some kind of cultural competence for physicians taking care of these growing minorities. American psychiatry cannot afford to limit the number of IMGs entering psychiatry, as the need for IMGs may be increasing in the near future as they continue to play a crucial role in the care of patients with severe mental illness and minorities.

International Medical Graduates and Organized Medicine in the United States

The involvement of IMGs in organized medicine in the United States has been traditionally low for various reasons. Organized medicine has not *widely* opened the doors to minorities and IMGs in the past. Some IMGs have been mistrustful of organized medicine, as they felt it did not represent their interests and wanted only their membership dues. However, during the last two decades there has been definite progress in the relationship between IMGs and organized medicine.

The American Medical Association (AMA) appointed its first Ad Hoc Committee on Foreign Medical Graduates in 1978, and a second Ad Hoc Committee in 1985. In 1989, the Board of Trustees of the AMA created the IMG Advisory Committee. This committee was replaced by the IMG Caucus in 1996. IMG leaders within the AMA are working to establish an IMG Section. The IMG Advisory Committee and the IMG Caucus served in an advocacy role in IMG issues, such as unfair practices that exclude IMGs from licensing, credentialing, obtaining residency positions, or practicing medicine. They also review existing AMA policies in support of IMGs; revise or develop new policies, as needed, that support IMGs; identify emerging workforce policies and legislation that may impact IMGs; and increase communication with state medical societies and state licensing boards on IMG issues. The AMA has adopted a number of policies on IMG issues, such as licensure, speech tests, unfair discrimination, participation in medical societies, and residency training. The AMA also created an International Medical Graduates Section during its House of Delegates meeting in December 1996. The new IMG Section will focus on a variety of issues facing IMGs, including residency training, managed care problems, and the alleged physician surplus.

The APA's record on IMG involvement is actually better than that of the AMA's. In 1979, the Committee on Foreign Medical Graduates (renamed in 1990 the Committee on International Medical Graduates) was restructured from the existing Task Force on Manpower and Foreign Medical Graduates and has been active in advocating issues of IMG members of the APA. The committee's newsletter, the *International Psychiatrist Newsletter*, published continuously since 1991, is distributed free to all IMG members of the APA. The committee has organized numerous presentations, seminars, and workshops during APA meetings, as well as a series of workshops for IMG residents, and it was instrumental in establishing The George Tarjan Award. This award is bestowed annually on an individual who has made significant contributions to the enhancement of the integration of IMGs into American psychiatry.

Another achievement was the establishment of the IMG Caucus in the APA Assembly. In 1977, the Assembly Executive Committee passed a resolution that provided representation of minority and underrepresented groups in the APA Assembly. These groups include American Indian/Alaskan Natives, Asian Americans, blacks, Hispanics, gay men and lesbians, IMGs, and women. The IMG Caucus was established in 1993 and its representative and deputy representative were seated in the Assembly.

However, IMGs remain significantly underrepresented among the APA leadership. IMGs composed about 9.2% of the APA leadership in 1993, whereas they actually represented 24% of the general membership. Until recently, only one IMG, George Tarjan, had been president of the APA (Rodrigo Muñoz became president-elect of the APA in 1997), and usually no more than one IMG is on the Board of Trustees. The collaboration of organized medicine and IMGs has been only slowly improving, and much remains to be accomplished.

Possible Future Trends of Immigration and Practices of International Medical Graduates in the United States

The issue of IMG immigration into the United States has become a political one. However, politicians are not enthusiastic about addressing the overall question of the supply of physicians, including the number of residents (Iglehart 1996). The immigration of IMGs into the United States will continue and probably not taper in the near future. This might be actually good news for psychiatry as a profession as well as for patients with severe mental illness.

The majority of the incoming physicians will most likely immigrate from countries in Asia and Latin America, as these countries have been producing surpluses of physicians. The United States continues to be economically attractive for medical school graduates from developing countries. As minority populations will increase, especially in California, New York, New Jersey,

Florida, Illinois, and some of the Southwestern states, IMGs will probably continue to gravitate to those places. We can also assume that IMGs will continue to play a critical role in the care of severely mentally ill, minority, and poor populations, as well as an increasing role in academic psychiatry and in organized medicine.

Conclusion

IMGs have played an important role in and have made significant positive contributions to American psychiatry. American psychiatry has been able to maintain the current level of practicing psychiatrists because of the continuous influx of IMGs. Poor, severely mentally ill, and minority patients have been and will continue to be treated predominantly by IMGs—who have been an intellectually stimulating force in American psychiatry as well. At present, the United States cannot afford to reduce the number of IMGs in psychiatry. As we enter the twenty-first century, IMGs are a constant presence and will continue to be a major positive force in American medicine and psychiatry. We need to reevaluate workforce issues and the participation of IMGs in United States medicine and psychiatry. It is crucial to integrate IMGs into American psychiatry and organized medicine without discrimination.

References

American Psychiatric Association: Diagnostic and Statistical Manual of Mental Disorders, 4th Edition. Washington, DC, American Psychiatric Association, 1994

Balon R, Muñoz RA: International medical graduates in psychiatric manpower calculations. Am J Psychiatry 153:296, 1996

Balon R, Mufti R, Williams M, et al: Possible discrimination in recruitment of psychiatry residents? Am J Psychiatry 154:1608–1609, 1997

Cooper RA: Perspectives on the physician workforce to the year 2020. JAMA 274:1534–1543, 1995

Dalen JE: US physician manpower needs. Arch Intern Med 156:21–24, 1996

Davidson L: Foreign medical graduates: transcultural psychoanalytic perspectives. J Am Acad Psychoanal 10:211–224, 1982

IMGs boost psychiatry match rate once again. Clinical Psychiatry News 24:1–2, 1996

Iglehart JK: The quandary over graduates of foreign medical schools in the United States. N Engl J Med 334:1679–1683, 1996

Jenkins J, Witkin MJ: Foreign Medical Graduates Employed in State and County Medical Hospitals (Statistical Note 131). Rockville, MD, National Institute of Mental Health, July 1976

Komaromy M, Grumbach K, Drake M, et al: The role of Black and Hispanic physicians in providing health care for underserved populations. N Engl J Med 334:1305–1310, 1996

Match results show numbers continue to slip in psychiatry. Psychiatric News XXXI(8):1, 60, April 19, 1996

Mitka M: Michigan IMGs blast residency rule as discrimination. American Medical News 39:5, 1996

Mullan F, Politzer RM, Davis CH: Medical migration and the physician workforce. International medical graduates and American medicine. JAMA 273:1521–1527, 1995

Pew Health Professions Commission: Critical Challenges: Revitalizing the Health Professions for the Twenty-First Century. The Third Report of the Pew Health Professions Commission. Center for the Health Professions, University of California San Francisco, San Francisco, CA, November 1995

Ritvo ML, Kindig DA: A report card on the physician workforce in the United States. N Engl J Med 334:892–896, 1996

Updata (A bi-monthly publication from the Robert Wood Johnson Foundation's Office of Health Statistics and Analysis) 3(3), 1996

U.S. General Accounting Office: Medical Licensing by Endorsement—U.S. GAO Report to Congressional Committees (Publ No AD/HRD90–120). Washington, DC, U.S. General Accounting Office, May 1990

Val E, Quick S: Foreign medical graduated and board certification: myths and realities. Am J Psychiatry 140:184–188, 1983

Weintraub W: The international medical graduate as a psychiatric resident: one training director's experience, in International Medical Graduates in Psychiatry in the United States: Challenges and Opportunities. Edited by Husain SA, Muñoz RA, Balon R. Washington, DC, American Psychiatric Press, 1997, pp 53–64

CHAPTER 18

Psychiatric Education for the New Millennium

Carolyn B. Robinowitz, M.D.

Medical educators are always interested in the future. Psychiatrists in particular are interested in the interrelationships of past, present, and future. Understanding this interrelationship in our patients is one of the basic tenets of our clinical practice. Some of this interest may come from curiosity—wanting to know what caused and what will be, as well as desiring to influence it. Educators have special concerns and responsibilities for the future. They prepare their students not only for today and tomorrow, but for a long career. This effort involves the connection of training for the present with education for a more uncertain and distant future. As such, residency training and education must expand beyond the historical maxim of "see one, do one, teach one." Unfortunately, many teachers teach as they were taught. They frequently employ the model of the charismatic teacher and use precepts they learned a quarter of a century earlier. Thus, while medical education tends to promote the awareness of new information and its integration into practice, in another sense, medical educators (as other educators) often tend to recapitulate what they most valued in the past.

The twenty-first century conjures up many images. The Stanley Kubrick movie *2001: A Space Odyssey* is one. With its lush Strauss music, it creates richly evocative pictures of Darwinian apes and movement—into the unlimited boundaries of space and the immense possibilities of the computer (in-

301

cluding that of its malevolence). The mystery of the twenty-first century depicted in the movie has diminished somewhat as we approach the new millennium. Many of what were once fantasies of artificial intelligence and informatics are real and, once known and experienced, are not so powerfully overwhelming. Yet, we still base our predictions for education in the future on uncertainties—ongoing changes in the science of our field, as well as the way health care will be delivered. Indeed, although molecular biology is seen by many as the critical science of today and the future, 25 years ago it did not exist as we now know it.

As other authors note in this volume, the rapid and wide-reaching, wide-ranging developments in biomedical research and technology have led to increasingly sophisticated approaches to diagnosis and treatment. Advances in psychopharmacology have revolutionized psychiatric practice. An extensive array of psychopharmacological products designed to address neurotransmission at specific receptors have augmented or replaced the limited agents available only a few decades ago. The psychopharmacological research approaches that created new agents for the treatment of mood disorders and schizophrenia are beginning to yield agents for treating personality disorders and alcohol and cocaine craving and withdrawal, and even for retarding the progression of dementias of the Alzheimer's type. It is reasonable to expect additional great strides in the next decades. We will be able to provide more to our patients; but the new approaches and understandings, while expanding the core knowledge expected of trainees and practitioners, make more difficult the task of residency and postresidency education and training.

Psychiatry, perhaps more than any other medical specialty, has changed in ways related only in part to the expansion of its scientific base and the rapid growth of new knowledge. As empirically derived knowledge has replaced ideology, we have reconsidered the paradigms that have guided our treatments. Paradigms, which only a quarter of a century ago were based primarily on psychodynamic concepts of development and behavior, and in which the use of biological therapies were viewed as evidence of "treatment failure," have undergone transformation to include psychobiological and sociocultural facets as well. This "sea change" in understanding and approaches represents a major, and for some, painful, transformation and, in turn, has been accompanied by another set of changes fueled by major shifts in the economics of health care. These economic changes have revolutionized the delivery of care. These latter changes have been seen by some as attempts to control the escalating costs of high-technology health care. Others have defined the changes as a way to use resources more effectively to provide service to all citizens. Still others have viewed them as siphoning off funds from health care by providing financial rewards for entrepreneurs and stockholders in for-profit health care systems. Finally, others see them as a way of rationing care. All of these reasons may be true in some circumstances. Whatever the rationale, however, economic or science, there is, today, a different manner of conceptualizing care as compared with that a quarter-century ago—a way that is particularly uncomfortable for the middle-aged psychiatrists who make up the bulk of psychiatric educators (Goodman et al. 1992).

In psychiatry, the merger of scientific advances with new economics of practice has had a marked impact on hospital care. Lengths of stay formerly measured in weeks are measured in days; 23-hour admissions are not uncommon. This decrease has changed the locus of care for many individuals with severe and/or acute mental disorders from the inpatient to the ambulatory setting. The nature of hospital care, especially in academic medical centers, has changed even further. Academic centers (which have had higher costs because of educational and research demands) have attempted to compete with community nonteaching hospitals for patient referrals and are now facing restructuring to become more competitive in the marketplace. This transformation has occurred as the dollars available to support education and training have decreased. In this environment, many hospitals have downsized considerably. Opportunities to use revenue from patient care to subsidize teaching and research have diminished or disappeared. Teaching and research (unless supported by protected funding) could become a nonaffordable luxury in the twenty-first century (Blackwell and Schmidt 1992).

Meetings of the psychiatric educational establishment (the chairs of departments of psychiatry and the residency training directors in psychiatry) have frequently focused on the heightened impact of economics on academic psychiatry's clinical and educational functions, as well as the financial well-being of academic departments of psychiatry. These discussions highlight a concern for the viability of what was once academic psychiatry. Concerns for the scientific productivity of the field as well as the quality and quantity of the future workforce are real in the current economic climate. Unfortunately, much energy has been devoted to cursing the darkness or complaining about the quality of the candles. There has been less success in finding ways to cope or thrive in the new environment or to develop models to both fund and educate psychiatric residents and current practitioners for the future. Academic departments have been markedly lax in addressing the educational needs of current practitioners.

The task ahead for psychiatric education is not easy, but it is clear that no matter what the near-term obstacles, psychiatrists will always be needed. Other physicians, such as neurologists, internists, or family physicians, are neither sufficiently skilled in the diagnosis or therapeutics of caring for patients with chronic mental disorders nor interested in learning. Furthermore, the increasing complexity of medical management of some patients, used in combination with psychotherapies, requires medical knowledge and skills only the psychiatrist can provide. These evolving complexities begin to redefine the roles of psychiatrists in the new millennium and, therefore, the new psychiatric residency's requisite curriculum.

Twenty-First-Century Residency Education Goals and Requirements

What will the goals of the psychiatric residency be in the twenty-first century? Because we cannot be sure of the future, what should we teach? How will we link training and education? What basic skills and approaches will be essential for the long term? How will psychiatrists' practices be defined? Will psychiatrists be generalists who care for all sorts of psychiatric maladies of varied degrees of severity? Will psychiatrists mainly serve as specialists and consultants for secondary referrals of patients who are more severely mentally ill? Patients whose disorders do not respond to standard treatment will, of course, always be referred to psychiatrists. Will psychiatrists need to rely mainly on primary care physicians for referrals, or will patients continue to access them directly? Whatever the outcome for these varied questions, the likely scenario requires the development of new residency experiences with potentially far fewer residents.

Psychiatric residents need to develop, attain, and maintain the capacity for scientific thinking. This includes the capacity to critically review the psychiatric literature. The resident must be able to perform a problem-oriented assessment and management plan for each patient. Treatment planning will be based on anticipated outcomes and cost-effectiveness. Of all mental health professionals, only the psychiatrist has the skills for such comprehensive approaches to patient problems and treatment planning along the biopsychosocial continuum.

The psychiatric resident will need to master the new neuroscience knowledge base, while retaining an ability for compassionate care. As we have developed better science, the field has been seen by some as losing its soul. Reflecting these new priorities is the nature of departments of psychiatry. While the expansion of knowledge is important and the research advances have changed patients' lives as well as the image of the field, it still is essential for residents to communicate with patients, to understand the role of illness on functioning and behavior, and to assist in modifying destructive behavior. These communication skills, critical in treating our patients, also enable the psychiatrist to be a member as well as leader of the treatment teams that will care for patients. These teams of physicians and other health care and mental health providers will work in a range of traditional and new health care settings.

In addition to having strong interpersonal skills and neuroscience knowledge, psychiatrists must be knowledgeable of the indications (and contraindications) for, and skilled in (some of) the increasing numbers of, treatment approaches and options. Skills in assessment and management, approaches to treatment resistance (with patients often referred from other health care and mental health providers), and rehabilitation of patients with chronic mental illness will be needed. The ability to use the ever-increasing and therapeutically more specific pharmacological agents will be essential. With the increased attention to primary care medicine in the psychiatric setting (particularly in the care of those with chronic mental illness), overlapping areas (e.g., human immunodeficiency virus [HIV] disorders, sleep disorders, pain management, neuropsychiatry) will need to be addressed. Residents will need to understand the scientific basis of treatment, as well as be sufficiently educated to assess and monitor treatment effectiveness, and be able to evaluate new treatments as they become available (Accreditation Council for Graduate Medical Education 1997; Yager et al. 1988).

Curricular expansion and elaboration of goals are further complicated by the growth in psychotherapies. The mid-twentieth-century reliance on long-term psychodynamic treatment alone has been superseded by development of a plethora of short-term, brief, focused, individual and group interventions using behavioral as well as psychodynamic paradigms. To learn and teach these approaches, resources—that is, patients and supervisors—must be available. Not every program has a faculty member highly familiar with each technique. Indeed, not all residencies can teach each approach. Ways must be developed first to distinguish core concepts and tactics of varied psychotherapies and then to educate residents in them. Next, each residency will, after examining its resources, develop ways to teach and educate residents in them. Differing residencies will highlight differing approaches. Current thinking suggests identifying one or two that emphasize psychodynamic-interpersonal approaches, another for cognitive-behavioral approaches (and these may be both individual and/or group), and one for couples-family approaches (Verhulst and Tucker 1990).

Manual-based short-term psychotherapies constitute a specific new form of psychotherapy. These can be taught through treatment manuals (which provide discussions of theory, indications, and contraindications), videotaped and videodisk material, and supervised practice. As the number of psychotherapies expands, as previously noted, training, not education, must focus on residents practicing a few psychotherapies (e.g., interpersonal psychotherapy, brief focal psychotherapy, and cognitive-behavioral approaches are ones that have been demonstrated to benefit specific conditions). In addition to understanding and assimilating the basic skills of these approaches, residents must also develop a sense of how to apply them flexibly in diverse clinical situations. It should be noted that even new or manual-based psychotherapies can be taught through live audiotaped or videotaped observation, and skills can be taught through tapes and videodisks. Such materials also can be the basis for a focus on critical incident approaches (e.g., assessment and initial management of suicidal and assaultive patients). Trainees should be expected to use and practice these techniques in relation to their patients as well as discuss experiences in problem-based seminars, using active learning approaches. The clinical effectiveness and professional satisfactions of future psychiatrists who do psychotherapy may depend in good measure on how well they employ these brief psychotherapies.

Residents should also be stimulated to think both creatively and critically by participating in seminars and journal clubs devoted to advances in fundamental and clinical neurosciences, cognitive sciences, and social sciences and by being prompted to draw out potential current and future implications for practice and public policy. More formal training in economics and epidemiology might need to be provided by graduate courses, as well as by specific residency sessions. Residents also should have more formal instruction in education and how to teach, focusing on other health care providers as well as patients and community leaders (e.g., clergy and teachers).

There are many unique educational challenges related to providing residents with the perspectives and proficiencies they will require to survive and thrive in the twenty-first-century environment. These include their experiencing different attitudes and values than those of twentieth-century psychiatric residents. Epidemiology and principles of public health, only shadows in the twentieth century, will now take on a major role. Description and documentation of observations and interventions will become key requirements as residents learn to practice evidence-based medicine. Economics will include knowing and mastering both the organization and administration of different practice models. Residents will learn the use of information management systems for data collection, retrieval, and storage. Other business aspects of practice, legal issues, and ethical advocacy for patients and populations will be new core experiences and require new bases of knowledge. Residents will further need to know the forces that have fueled the development of managed care and how they will shape future practice (Blackwell and Schmidt 1992; Lazarus 1995; Meyer 1993).

Elsewhere, Robinowitz and Yager (1996) have expanded on the proficiencies and skills demanded for successful managed care psychiatric practice. These include skills for what we might more appropriately describe as cost-effective medical care. Many of these skills are necessary for all varieties of competent psychiatric practice in the twenty-first century. They include the ability to establish an empathic relationship with patients; conduct comprehensive assessments; formulate appropriate diagnoses and treatment plans; construct and negotiate a focused treatment plan (e.g., considering and using techniques of crisis intervention and stabilization, determining indications for inpatient and partial hospitalization); provide appropriate and effective therapies, including pharmacotherapy or a specific psychotherapy; be aware of and deal with countertransference problems; and act ethically and with integrity. They also include the ability to work in a cost- and time-effective manner, using principles of critical decision making and evidence-based medicine to decide about the kinds of treatment (including intensity, length of treatment, proposed outcome), and the ability to conduct (or delegate and/or supervise) such focused treatment by using appropriate family, community, and systemic resources. These actions will frequently need to take place in the context of providing care for an entire caseload of patients (Sabin 1991).

Curriculum design, including both classroom and clinical experiences, must address all the new issues noted. Since time for residency is fixed as an independent variable (with quality or outcome the dependent variable), new priorities must be set and met. Each residency program will emphasize distinct areas, but all must address an agreed-on range of training experiences with the teaching of today's expanded core knowledge base. A final goal of each residency will be to teach residents how to be self-directed learners who remain current in the science and skills of our profession after residency graduation.

Where and How Training Will Occur

Psychiatric clinical training will continue a trend toward a decreased use of hospital settings. Learning in the hospital about continuity of care through patient observation and contact will be replaced by learning about patient stabilization, crisis intervention, and responses to brief therapy, medical management, case management, and collaborative care in the twenty-first century. The skills described above will be honed in ambulatory care settings where residents can appreciate the natural history of patients with severe psychiatric disorders. The inpatient hospital will still provide residents the best experience in the fundamentals of initial assessment and treatment planning for patients with severe or acute disorders.

As academic psychiatry departments' service burdens expand, the relationship between residents and faculty will shift. Resident education experiences will need to be protected. Staffing patterns with responsibility for a caseload of patients will frequently pair residents with faculty. This new team will provide experience in the longitudinal care of shifting numbers of patients. Faculty, not residents, may frequently conduct initial patient interviews, so that the decisions regarding problem focus and requisite treatments can be made immediately in a more cost-effective fashion. This faculty-trainee pairing must not be a return to the pre-Flexner system of apprenticeship, but a way to have more protected clinical learning. This is especially important as third-party payers will increasingly demand more faculty presence with a demonstration of faculty involvement with their patients (Robinowitz and Nadelson 1985).

Although faculty will need to be involved with managed care patients, many training programs whose patient population is based nearly totally upon managed care contracts for patient flow and revenue will need to develop models of care where residents under supervision provide direct care to managed care patients. Such approaches will probably demand stringent on-site, hands-on forms of supervision by attending psychiatrists. *Attendings*, previously referred to in psychiatry as *supervisors*, may see all patients face to face for at least some time during the initial evaluation and during each or most subsequent visit(s) in both outpatient and inpatient settings. This model of collaborative care, jointly provided by residents and attendings, is more familiar to primary care residencies than to psychiatric training. This method represents a major shift in the approach to supervision and the importance of the dyad in psychiatric practice. It also requires more labor-intensive participation by faculty psychiatrists in residency activities at a time when faculty are increasingly pressed to generate their own clinical income. These new approaches will also require new methods of resident evaluation to ensure that the resident has acquired core competence.

As the hospital ceases to be the locus of training in the treatment of patients with mental disorders, continuity of care in the new service models becomes a problem. Residents will have difficulty seeing the effects of their interventions on the course of patients unless they are adequately linked to community clinics and varied partial hospital programs where their patients are located.

These new integrated rotations will allow residents to follow patients initially seen in the hospital into other settings, giving residents a new model as part of a longitudinal experience with a larger team. They will also demand that residents spend their time in new ways. Part of each day will be spent on an inpatient unit, part in the outpatient clinic, part in a partial program, and some time during the week at community sites.

In ambulatory or outpatient settings, residents will generate income for their departments by providing services that will include triage, consulting and interacting with primary care physicians, serving as consultation-liaison psychiatrists, following their own patients outside of the hospital, as well as treating patients never hospitalized. Some of these psychiatric services will be provided in a small primary care setting or in large multispecialty group practices. In some instances, psychiatrists could serve additionally as primary health care or principal health care providers. In all instances, emphasis will be on psychiatric diagnosis and treatment (both treatment planning and implementation) in the medical context. Additionally, psychiatrists will work with other mental health (as well as education and social service) professionals to develop an approach to longer-range treatment and rehabilitation. The propensity of managed care to use patient education and self-help will define still another role for psychiatry residents. Many of these areas will be fiscally self-sustaining. Steps will need to be taken such that the new outpatient experience will not adversely affect the resident learning about and experiencing with patients over time the disorders that have always been managed in outpatient settings.

Because of these changes, the traditional block rotations, where residents are assigned full-time to one service, will be modified. A more flexible longitudinal system will evolve in which a team of caregivers (faculty and residents) follows patients throughout the course of their illness (as currently occurs in private practice). The patient's caregiver remains the same although the site may vary from inpatient hospitalization to partial day hospital and/or after-work evening programs, and into a nonhospital ambulatory rehabilitation setting. Such an approach will demand much of those who schedule residents, both to allow elasticity of time and to maintain an understanding of the role of inpatient care. These models will be particularly difficult to implement in residencies that rotate residents through a number of sites, many distant from the main medical center campus.

Learning Materials, Resources, and the New Curriculum in an Era of Reduced Financial Support

Reduced funding for education will require hospitals to share resources, including faculty and facilities. In metropolitan areas, or locales in which there is more than one residency program, shared seminars and other teaching activities may become the norm. Nationally developed standards, curricula, and learning materials that can be adopted and adapted for a particular setting will be used to reduce costs. The American Psychiatric Association and/or the American Association of Directors of Psychiatric Residency Training will need to serve as a resource in developing core curricular materials that can be accessed through the Internet, courses through interactive video or teleconferencing, and other shared learning experiences. Decreased numbers of faculty, combined with increased demands for faculty involvement in clinical services, may diminish the amount of time available for seminars and separate supervision. Part-time or clinical faculty will be increasingly called upon as clinical teachers and supervisors, as they are used in other medical specialties.

An essential new skill for residents will be learning to use tools in clinical informatics—information retrieval and information assessment. As medical students are required to become more computer literate and to use informatics as part of medical reasoning, they will, as residents, be better prepared than many of the faculty. Using computer technology, instruction will focus on how to evaluate and review all mechanisms that screen for, appraise, and distill new clinically important information in a timely manner. Educators must develop ways to teach these skills to clinicians in time-efficient, cost-effective, and user-friendly forms. Trainees should learn how to conduct computer-based literature searches, critically read the literature, and access and use psychiatric information from databases, journals, books, newsletters, and consultants anywhere.

The instant accessibility of information available via the Internet and CD-ROM interactive training materials will move the learning of some concepts away from centralized learning rituals (the core seminars) to distributed, "just-in-time" learning, that is, identifying what you need to know and how to obtain it in a timely fashion. This will lead to increased flexibility, better retention, and more efficient use of time. This approach is frequently used in adult education, providing information on an as-needed basis. It is also programmed to address each individual student's unique learning needs. Students will be expected to learn principles, but the details—ranging from drug dosages and interactions, to differential diagnostic possibilities given a cluster of symptoms, to evidence-based algorithms for treatment—will be easily accessed through computers. These new models address experiential learning based on specific problems, deemphasize the role of the teacher as the pace-setter and repository of all knowledge, and provide reinforcement and new directions based on students' learning and needs. Simulations of real-life environments, virtual patients, and sophisticated interactive capabilities can be used in patient care situations as well as in "libraries" and at home after hours.

Even with new educational forms, content will still be somewhat traditional in that residents must learn diagnosis and treatment. But with the limited availability of inpatients to communicate a broad array of symptoms for which the student might have the opportunity to make diagnoses, a patient "library" available on videodisk will be essential, as will the personal data organizer/handheld computer for maintaining logs of patients seen and their presenting symptoms and histories. Educators will rely on the "virtual" patient, viewed and heard on computer through CD-ROM and other technology. This patient will eventually, with growth in technology, become an "intelligent" patient, who can be programmed to respond verbally to questions and interventions, giving simulations a realistic approach. Computers will also be helpful in pursuing diagnostic and treatment algorithms and giving feedback and follow-up to decisions. Access to the Internet already permits instantaneous access to journal abstracts and full text and will permit access to experts via bulletin boards and via Internet-based consultation services (Fidler and Robinowitz 1987; Robinowitz and Yager 1996).

Paradoxically, in some ways, observations through videotape, one-way screens, and computers may be less necessary in learning as the attending works face to face with the resident. But in a new use, videotapes of interviews as well as computer-based simulations can form a record of resident skills and behaviors over time, as well as provide a record of patient progress (leading to the possibility of reviewers reviewing the videotapes).

Resident Competency Assessment

It is anticipated that there will be more frequent formative assessments, in which trainees will be expected to document their abilities and skills. In the United States, the Psychiatric Resident In Training Examination (PRITE) can be expanded to a series of computer-based examinations that may be taken in modules year round. Each module would be programmed to respond to the level demonstrated by the student, with easier to progressively more difficult questions either with or without feedback. This will provide a more nationally standardized way of determining knowledge and its application that can be tailored to an individual residency's curriculum and rotations.

Accreditation and Certification

With the changes in residency structure and content must come changes in program accreditation requirements. No longer can a series of block rotations measured in weeks or months with traditional core seminars measured in hours or weeks be required to fulfill standards. Program planners and evaluators will need to consider programmatic objectives and outcomes with new forms of measurement. They must be willing to observe, monitor, and assess more flexible and creative approaches that define core competencies and the settings in which they are taught. With more emphasis on individual self-guided learning, resident performance on external assessments becomes an important aspect of program evaluation. Board certification will continue to assess core knowledge but will use a computer-generated examination. The current clinical examination will give way to computer-simulated patients or objective-simulated clinical examination (OSCE), which can be standardized for assessment of candidates.

Workforce Issues and Recruitment

Medical students, by their career choices, demonstrate their awareness of contemporary practice issues. They are concerned about being able to survive economically in the managed care climate in the United States. They are aware of discussions and disagreements as to how psychiatry will be practiced in the twenty-first century. Their actions demonstrate concern as to what model of practice will survive into the millennium. They are further concerned as to whether there is a shortage or surplus of psychiatrists. In this context, medical schools that have been successful in recruiting their graduates into psychiatry are ones in which psychiatry is taught as an important aspect of all of medicine and is seen as valuable by faculty in other departments. Clinical experiences by medical students in psychiatry in medical school must be perceived as relevant to the practice of medicine. Schools recruiting the highest percent of graduates into psychiatry in general are not schools with major research departments of psychiatry but schools engaging students as healers. Contrary to theories suggesting that psychiatry competes with primary care specialties in recruitment, high-recruiting schools tend to have a high recruitment of students into primary care specialties.

In discussing the recruitment of United States medical graduates into psychiatry, we must address the general dissatisfaction of so many psychiatrists, particularly middle-aged and older teachers, in their current work. Communication of their malaise is a powerful disincentive, and their dissatisfaction is both contagious and insidious.

As fewer U.S. students choose psychiatry and residencies are filled with increasing numbers of trainees whose comfort with United States cultural practices and fluency in the English language are frequently initially limited, we run the risk that United States medical students may view these residents, and their residencies, with disdain and eschew them further. Moreover, as the medical student's debt level rises, students increasingly voice their concern about repayment and choose either designated primary care specialties with debt forgiveness or surgical specialties, which still provide considerably higher income than psychiatry (De Titta et al. 1991).

The long-term vitality of the field depends on science and the translation and relationships of science to clinical care. To achieve this requires considerable support and attention to our recruitment of future researchers and teachers. We need to recruit more students and trainees through the medical scientist training programs, ease or forgive debt burden for researchers, and develop special residency programs or tracks to interrelate research and clinical training.

Similarly, attention must be paid at the faculty level to facilitate faculty development and retention as well as recruitment in academic medical centers. Faculty must adapt to survive, but all too often, they are left on their own. Organized psychiatry can help with education and resources. Not only should we not eat our seed corn, but once it is planted, we have an obligation to water, fertilize, and weed to ensure growth. A faculty that feels ignored or not valued will implicitly, if not explicitly by their affect, discourage students from pursuing psychiatry and academic careers.

The Continuing Education of the Practitioner

The rapid growth of knowledge coupled with major shifts in resources for health care quickly date some of the knowledge and skills learned in residency. New methods will need to be developed and applied to sustain the competencies of the practicing psychiatrist. All of the approaches used for residency training and education will be used for a new method of sustained education for the practitioner. Practitioners will be able to use the techniques already described on learning modules tailored to their individual practices with our new computer technologies.

New methods of continuing certification using virtual reality techniques will appear. With rapid knowledge expansion and change in optimal therapeutics, recertification of competence will be critical. Procedures will be developed that address issues that relate to each psychiatrist's practice. The practitioner's clinical acumen will be assessed, just as is the resident's, using the previously described new technologies. Professional meetings will need to develop Internet capabilities to communicate to all members of the profession, not just those in attendance. Planners will need to distinguish what learning and information is best exchanged at meetings versus that best developed through other techniques. In this context, scientific journals will need to be reinvented, and they will need to be available on CD-ROM or the Internet. Journals will also need to reduce the time from when a paper is submitted until publication, as "Internet journals" will offer rapid peer-reviewed routes to disseminate information.

This is both the best and worst of times for academic medicine as well as for psychiatric education. The scientific advances and improvements in the treatment of mental illnesses have been extraordinary and have been accompanied by a decrease in stigma and an increased public understanding of mental illness as *no-fault illness;* yet the economic climate for health care has become volatile, and the impact of managed care systems has often hurt patient care, research, and training programs. Although the role of psychiatry in the promised health care reform of the next decade, century, and millennium remains uncertain, whatever happens, the need will continue for well-trained psychiatrists who can assist patients with their struggles with mental disorders and who can provide patients with the best scientifically based treatment. It remains the role of the psychiatric educator to ensure psychiatrists' growth and development.

References

Accreditation Council for Graduate Medical Education: Accredited Residencies in Psychiatry. Chicago, IL, Accreditation Council for Graduate Medical Education, 1997

Blackwell B, Schmidt GL: The educational implications of managed mental health care. Hospital and Community Psychiatry 43:962–964, 1992

De Titta M, Robinowitz CB, More WW: The future of psychiatry: psychiatrists of the future. Am J Psychiatry 148:853–858, 1991

Fenton WS, Leaf PJ, Robinowitz CB: Male and female psychiatrists and their patients. Am J Psychiatry 144:358–361, 1987

Fidler D, Robinowitz CB: Educational materials and technology for the future, in Training Psychiatrist for the '90s. Edited by Nadelson CC, Robinowitz CB. Washington, DC, American Psychiatric Press, pp 115–122, 1987

Goodman M, Brown J, Deitz P: Managing Managed Care: A Mental Health Practitioner's Survival Guide. Washington, DC, American Psychiatric Press, 1992

Gunzburger LK: U.S. medical school's valuing of curricular time: self-directed learning vs. lectures. Acad Med 68:700–702, 1993

Lazarus A: An annotated bibliography in managed care for psychiatric residents and faculty. Academic Psychiatry 19:65–73, 1995

Meyer RE: The economics of survival for academic psychiatry. Academic Psychiatry 17:141–160, 1993

Nadelson CC, Robinowitz CB: Medical academics and economics: continued conflict or resolution?, in Training Psychiatrist for the '90s. Edited by Nadelson CC, Robinowitz CB. Washington, DC, American Psychiatric Press, 1987, pp 11–22

Robinowitz CB, Nadelson CC: The impact of the new economics on psychiatric training programs and academic departments of psychiatry, in The New Economics and Psychiatric Care. Edited by Beigel A, Sharfstein S. Washington, DC, American Psychiatric Press, 1985, pp 85–95

Robinowitz CB, Yager J: Future of psychiatric education, in American Psychiatric Press Review of Psychiatry, Vol 15. Edited by Dickstein L, Riba MB, Oldham JM. Washington, DC, American Psychiatric Press, 1996, pp 581–604

Sabin JE: Clinical skills for the 1990s: six lessons from HMO practice. Hospital and Community Psychiatry 42:605–608, 1991

Verhulst J, Tucker GJ: Issues for psychiatric education. Psychiatric Annals 20:278–282, 1990

Yager J, Borus JF, Robinowitz CB, et al: Developing minimal national standards for clinical experience in psychiatric training. Am J Psychiatry 145:1409–1413, 1988

SECTION IV

The Future

INTRODUCTION

For this section, we asked the current and former medical directors of the American Psychiatric Association to speculate on how they saw psychiatry in the next century. Their contributions were written without their review of the other contributions. It is striking how their chapters resonate with the contributions of our varied experts.

In Chapter 19, Predictions About the Financing and Delivery of Care, Steven Mirin addresses issues of the provision of care to the mentally ill from a distinctly North American, or, more precisely, United States, perspective. Yet, although the forms that he describes, health maintenance organizations (HMOs) and managed care organizations (MCOs), are particularly American, the perceived problem that they address is universal. The British reader can simply substitute *National Health Service* (NHS) for *HMO* or *MCO*. In the United States, MCOs have reduced the important power and authority of specialists in clinical care. In Britain, this (MCO) function has been undertaken by the general practitioner, who has been given authority to contract and limit the role of specialists. Both models are attempts in different environments to contain health care costs. Mirin walks us through the reasons for the immediate focus on cost containment and then discusses the immediate impact of various cost-containment strategies on practitioners, hospitals, and, most significantly, patients. Then he examines potential future responses of each group to the current realities. He presents a challenge to psychiatry to respond in a way that maintains its role in dealing with the mentally ill.

We conclude with Chapter 20, Psychiatry in the Twenty-First Century: New Beginnings, by Melvin Sabshin. As one of the intellectual leaders and synthesizers of American and world psychiatry for over a quarter-century, he provides a perspective of psychiatry's future from a position inside the rapidly evolving intellectual life of our discipline. Indeed, it is striking that Sabshin's enumeration of new beginnings reads almost like this volume's contents. But Sabshin goes further. He explores the problems that we, the world's psychiatrists, face in the application of our expanded knowledge to varied countries with unique health care systems and varied resources. He addresses the twentieth century's long battle against the stigma associated with mental disorders. In sum, he contends that, although we have not resolved or removed stigma, we have made advances; and he reminds us, as did Mirin, not to forget our patients.

It is significant that Sabshin reminds us not to forget our patients. Indeed, of all of the elements that define our discipline, without an informed empathic appreciation of our patients' needs, and, we might add, of our patients' experience of us, we do not exist as a discipline.

CHAPTER 19

Predictions About the Financing and Delivery of Care

Steven M. Mirin, M.D.

A s we prepare to enter the next millennium, knowledge developed through clinical experience, augmented by exciting new findings from basic and clinical research, has greatly enhanced our ability to treat, and ultimately prevent, mental illness. At the same time, this enormous progress is taking place against a backdrop of shifting economic forces that are reshaping how mental health care is financed and delivered. This chapter focuses on these forces and their implications for the mentally ill and those who care for them.

How Did We Get Here? The Rising Costs of Care

Much has been written about the dramatic rise in health care costs that has characterized the last two decades. With the nation's aggregate health care bill now exceeding $1 trillion, or about 14% of the gross national product, health

The author wishes to thank Claire Ryan and Audrey Nicol for their assistance in the preparation of this manuscript.

care is an important, and growing, segment of our national economy (Levit et al. 1996b). It is also a segment of our economy whose products and services are consumed almost entirely within our borders and whose costs, therefore, are borne essentially by citizens who purchase health insurance, taxpayers who fund state and federal entitlement programs, and patients and their families who bear the cost of copayments, deductibles, and myriad other health-related costs.

The escalating cost of general health care has been paralleled by a substantial increase in the cost of mental health care. Between 1985 and 1995, mental health and substance abuse costs rose at a rate of about 15% annually (Rice et al. 1992). This rise was fueled primarily by the increased availability of insurance coverage for mental health and substance abuse care and a corresponding expansion in the number of institutional and individual caregivers, particularly in the private sector. Thus, in the decade of the 1980s, the number of beds in both freestanding psychiatric hospitals and general hospitals doubled (Dorwart et al. 1991).

Another factor contributing to the increased use of mental health and substance abuse services was the effort of professional trade organizations, such as the American Psychiatric Association (APA), along with federal agencies, such as the National Institute of Mental Health, and a growing number of patient advocacy groups to educate patients, their families, and the general public about the causes of mental illness and the availability of treatment for these disorders. Such efforts, coupled with advances in our knowledge about the interplay of genetic, biological, and psychosocial factors in the etiology of mental disorders and the emergence of new, and often more effective, treatments for illnesses such as schizophrenia, panic disorder, major depression, bipolar disorder, and obsessive-compulsive disorder, helped destigmatize mental illness and encouraged many to seek care who might otherwise have remained outside the treatment system.

Payer Response to Rising Costs: Managed Care

As expanded coverage, destigmatization, and greater access to new, more effective treatments fueled an increase in the use of mental health and substance abuse services, employers, insurers, federal and state governments, and other purchasers of health care began to identify the rising costs of such care as a problem requiring active intervention. Though the costs of these services never amounted to more than 10% of overall health care expenditures (Levit et al. 1991), there was a pervasive feeling on the part of some that mental health and substance abuse care was too costly and, moreover, that such care was either unnecessary, ineffective, or both.

The initial response of employers and insurers to the rising costs of mental health and substance abuse treatment was to effectively reduce both benefits and service utilization by imposing annual and/or lifetime caps on insurance coverage and by introducing higher patient copayments and deductibles. These efforts, however, were marginally effective in controlling costs. As a result, payers turned to "carve-out" strategies in which mental health and substance abuse benefits were segregated from general health care benefits and managed separately. Responding to this market opportunity, a number of fourth-party managed care organizations (MCOs) sprang up whose impressive growth over the last decade was fueled by their demonstrated ability to reduce costs.

The MCOs have employed a variety of strategies to reduce the costs of mental health and substance abuse care. These have generally focused on controlling patients' utilization of services by imposing increasingly stringent "medical necessity" criteria to justify both access to care and continued care. Precertification, concurrent review, and retrospective review of medical necessity characterized the early phases of managed care. More recently, carefully selected provider networks, while discounting fees paid to individual and institutional caregivers, have become an important part of the cost-containment armamentarium for MCOs.

The growth of managed mental health care, though relatively modest in the 1980s, accelerated dramatically in the early 1990s. The success of carve-out arrangements in reducing mental health and substance abuse treatment costs, particularly those related to inpatient care, caught the attention of employers looking for ways to reduce their health insurance premium costs. State governments, concerned about the rising costs of public sector programs that serve the mentally ill, also began carving out mental health and substance abuse care for those insured under the Medicaid program and contracted with for-profit MCOs to manage the care for this population of patients (Rowland and Hanson 1996).

Though clinicians and hospitals began to protest what they saw as a growing balkanization of patients' health care, widely publicized scandals involving kickbacks for patient referrals and billing for unnecessary care by some for-profit, private psychiatric hospitals (Karel 1994) undermined the credibility of all providers and contributed to the perception, on the part of payers and the general public, that more "fat" could be rendered from the mental health care delivery system without compromising the care of those who really needed it. In this atmosphere, complaints that the cost-containment activities of payers and managed care organizations were compromising the quality of patient care generally went unheard.

In the decade of the 1990s, the trend toward managed mental health care accelerated as employers and insurers began to provide economic incentives such as stable (or even declining) health care premiums and the promise of fewer out-of-pocket expenses in order to encourage insured individuals to transfer out of unmanaged, traditional, fee-for-service plans into managed systems of care. For example, point-of-service options in indemnity plans are designed to reward—with lower copayments and more inclusive coverage—those patients who obtain care through selected in-network hospitals, clinics, and clinicians. As a result of these and other incentives, more than 60 million people now receive their care through health maintenance organizations (HMOs) (Interstudy 1996), and more than 60% of all insured individuals, approximately 120 million people, are in plans where their mental health and substance abuse care is managed separately from their general health benefits (National Advisory Mental Health Council 1993).

Impact of Managed Care on Providers and Patients

Impact on Clinicians

Because a chapter of this nature cannot fully explore the subject, suffice to say that, for many clinicians, the impact of managed care has been dramatic and unwelcome. As actual and potential patients have migrated into managed systems of care, many clinicians have had little choice but to follow, accepting the tightly managed benefits, discounted fees, and external review of clinical decision making that characterize managed care systems. Within such systems, clinicians are characteristically required to conform their philosophy of care and their practice patterns to emphasize symptom-focused, short-term treatment models. The type and frequency of treatments delivered are carefully monitored by external reviewers who routinely make judgments about the medical necessity of such treatment, often in the absence of direct contact with the patient. At the same time, *provider profiling* is used to identify clinicians whose practice patterns run counter to the desired mode and those whose clinical decision making and utilization patterns suggest a preference for longer-term care. These providers, along with those who frequently appeal the benefit decisions of managed care reviewers, are at increased risk of being *deselected* from managed care networks.

The growth of managed care has also affected the market for mental health services. As more patients enroll in HMOs or obtain care through managed mental health networks, the clinical and economic imperative to be included in such networks and the competition for patients who are still free to choose any willing provider have intensified. In both these arenas, psychiatrists in particular have found themselves at a competitive disadvantage because, on a per-unit-of-service basis, their fees are generally higher than those of other mental health professionals and, as a group, they are viewed as more reluctant to embrace managed care principles. In addition, there has been a tendency within managed care systems to compartmentalize the roles of various mental health professionals. Thus, psychiatrists are often restricted to providing medical management and/or pharmacotherapy for patients, whereas social workers, psychologists, and other caregivers who are perceived as less expensive are used to provide verbal therapies and case management, if and when these are deemed "medically necessary." The impact of these policies on the quality or cost-effectiveness of patient care has not been well studied, but many clinicians believe that the *split treatment* model is inefficient and often less effective than the more traditional dyadic model, in which clinicians' roles and responsibilities are less ambiguous.

Finally, it is not surprising that increased competition among caregivers has also led to disputes over therapeutic territory. Thus, some psychologists and nurse clinicians have argued that the knowledge and experience base needed to provide competent pharmacological treatment can be obtained without a medical school education or psychiatric residency training. Staunch opposition to this perceived intrusion on medical practice has been offered by the American Psychiatric Association, the American Medical Association, and other professional organizations (Karel 1995; "Hawaii Psychiatrists Again Victorious Over Psychologists," 1996). Thus far, such opposition has prevented psychologists from obtaining prescribing privileges in any state. A number of states, however, do permit prescribing by nurse clinicians, albeit within a limited formulary and with medical oversight.

Impact on Hospitals

The rapid spread of managed care and its dominance within the mental health marketplace have also had a profound effect on institutions that provide mental health and substance abuse care. Indeed, much of the cost-containment focus of MCOs has, thus far, been on hospital-based care, and specifically on restricting the use of inpatient care. As a result of MCO pressure, changing philosophies of care and the expansion of alternatives to inpatient care, hospital admissions for psychiatric care, which occurred at an annual rate of 10 per 1,000 insured people a decade ago, have dropped to a rate of 4 per 1,000. During the same time period, overall inpatient utilization in managed care systems has declined from an annual rate of 150 days per 1,000 insured individuals to approximately 30 days per 1,000 (Goldsmith et al. 1993).

Faced with declining lengths of stay and falling occupancy rates, both free-standing psychiatric hospitals and psychiatric units in general hospitals have been forced to compete for a dwindling number of inpatients by joining managed care networks and expanding their referral streams while also developing alternatives to traditional inpatient care (e.g., partial hospital, residential, outpatient, and home care) (Cooper 1993). Yet, despite these and other survival strategies, hospitals have found themselves with relatively little countervailing power in the marketplace. As a result, most have had to succumb to the demands of payers and MCOs for deep discounts in the reimbursement for their services, while, at the same time, patient acuity and the actual costs of care have increased.

Impact on Patients

Lost in the rush to contain mental health care costs are findings from credible epidemiological surveys (Kessler et al. 1994; Regier et al. 1993) demonstrating that mental health and substance abuse problems are widespread within the general population and that, untreated, they exact an enormous medical, economic, and social toll on individuals, families, and society (Rice et al. 1990). Also not considered thus far is that timely and appropriate treatment is effective, not only in relieving patients' symptoms, but in reducing the adverse impact of mental disorders on patients' social and vocational functioning and on their general health status and future use of all health services (Frank 1981; Strain et al. 1991).

The most immediate concerns about managed care practices center around patients' access to care and the adequacy of that care. Growing constraints on the utilization of services, interference with clinical decision making, and the perceived threat to patients' confidentiality are the most frequently cited concerns (Iglehart 1992). As clinical decisions are increasingly influenced by constraints on benefits, caregivers have had to make difficult choices between advocating for patients and conforming to the expectations of those who control the flow of dollars that support care. In some instances, gag rules in the contractual agreements between MCOs and providers have compromised clinicians' ability to fully inform patients about the limitations of their health care coverage or the policies of their health plan that may limit access to certain kinds of care (Mechanic and Schlesinger 1996). Finally, as pressure to reduce inpatient lengths of stay have increased, some (or many) patients have been discharged prematurely, to the detriment of themselves and their families. These practical and ethical dilemmas are just now being addressed by professional organizations, consumer groups, and legislators (American Medical Association Council on Ethical and Judicial Affairs 1990; Pellegrino 1986).

What Does the Future Hold?

As we anticipate the next millennium, it is clear that some of the trends described above will continue, or even accelerate, whereas others will change direction—it is hoped, to the benefit of patients. The following are some speculations about what we can expect.

Continued Pressure to Reduce Costs in the Private and Public Sectors

Little doubt exists that the cost-containment efforts of managed care systems have been effective. For example, a decade ago the average cost, to employers and HMOs, of providing mental health benefits was about $9 per insured member per month (PMPM); today the national average is about $5 PMPM. In some areas of the country where managed mental health care dominates the marketplace, mental health benefit costs have fallen below $3 PMPM (Ginsburg and Pickreign 1996; Levit et al. 1996a).

Looking to the future, it seems likely that, despite the very significant declines of the past decade, downward pressure on the utilization and costs of mental health care will continue and that payers and policymakers will look to managed care as the primary mechanism for managing costs. In this scenario, access to and reimbursement for much of the mental health and substance abuse care delivered in this country will remain under the control of a variety of managed care systems, including HMOs and mental health carve-out networks, as well as the newly emerging integrated delivery systems. So-called disease management firms specializing in the focused management of high-prevalence and/or costly illnesses (e.g., major depression or schizophrenia) will also take a share of the carve-out market in mental health and substance abuse care.

In areas of the country where managed care has already experienced significant market penetration (e.g., California, Minnesota, Oregon, Arizona), pressure to reduce utilization and costs of care may decrease as adverse patient outcomes related to the rationing of care become more evident to the public and the courts, as well as to legislators and regulatory agencies. As a result, federal regulations governing self-insured entities, which have, thus far, shielded HMOs and MCOs from any liability stemming from benefit decisions that contribute to adverse patient outcomes, may be changed through legal and/or legislative interventions. At the same time, in parts of the country where utilization and costs are still perceived as too high, employers and purchasing alliances, encouraged by the success of managed care systems in reducing costs, will increasingly turn to HMOs and MCOs to manage their mental health and substance abuse benefits, at least in the short term.

State governments, charged with the responsibility of providing care for Medicaid recipients, will, in the absence of cost-effective alternatives, also turn to managed care as the preferred mechanism for controlling expenditures for mental health and substance abuse care. As a result, state departments of mental health, which have traditionally overseen and/or delivered care to severely ill public sector patients, will have to struggle to avoid being increasingly marginalized, as MCOs and their networks of private sector providers assume both the clinical and financial risk of caring for this patient population (Callahan et al. 1995).

Growth of Integrated Delivery Systems and Capitated Reimbursement

Over the next two decades, the rapid growth of integrated delivery systems, especially those owned and controlled by providers, will offer the opportunity for mental health and substance abuse care to be "carved into" the general health benefit. In such systems, however, access to mental health care will be controlled largely by primary care physicians functioning as both the managers of financial risk and the gatekeepers to care. In this context, the willingness of primary care physicians to fund mental health and substance abuse care, and the degree to which they will delegate responsibility for such care to mental health professionals (as opposed to doing it themselves), will depend on our field's ability to demonstrate the cost-effectiveness of an integrated, as opposed to a carve-out, model of mental health care. In so doing, we will have to demonstrate to our medical colleagues that patients with mental illness and/or substance use disorders are, in the aggregate, also heavy users of medical and surgical care (Frank 1981; Strain et al. 1991) and that timely and appropriate mental health care can improve overall clinical outcome and ultimately reduce health service utilization in these patients.

In an effort to align incentives between payers and providers, purchasers of care will increasingly contract with delivery systems where care is reimbursed on a capitated basis and providers receive a prospectively determined, fixed, annual (capitated) fee for each "covered life" they agree to care for. Under such capitated reimbursement arrangements, providers will have to assume the financial, as well as the clinical, risks of care delivery. Similarly, MCOs competing for state contracts to manage the mental health and substance abuse care of Medicaid recipients will have to agree to take on the risk of capitation, and they, in turn, will increasingly require that both individual and institutional providers share in some of this risk. Mechanisms for provider risk-sharing will include withholding a portion of the fee contingent upon the financial performance of the entire MCO network or requiring that providers accept contracts in which they agree to care for a designated population for a predetermined, subcapitated rate. Regardless of the form that prospective reimbursement takes, the financial incentives will be aligned to lower the costs of care delivery; at the same time, contract renewals will be dependent on delivering quality care. How these often conflicting agendas will play out in the care of patients remains to be determined.

Trend Toward Managed Medicare

The current legislative debate about how to reduce federal expenditures for Medicare will most likely end in a bipartisan compromise in which Congress and the executive branch will share the blame for a moderate reduction in Medicare spending. Regardless of government actions, however, over the next decade, Medicare, which has been the traditional stronghold of fee-for-service medicine, will be reshaped by market forces. By the turn of the century, it is estimated that one-fourth to one-third of Medicare recipients over age 65 will have relinquished their unmanaged indemnity plan for a more comprehensive, but tightly managed, package of general and mental health benefits, offered through HMOs and other Medicare risk contractors. A significant number of patients covered under the Social Security Disability Income (SSDI) provision of the Medicare program, of whom about 25% are disabled as a result of severe and persistent mental illness (Kennedy and Manderscheid 1992), will also join HMOs or become part of other health care systems in which care will be tightly managed (Prospective Payment Assessment Commission 1996). These market trends will increase pressure to reduce the use of mental health and substance abuse services, especially hospital-based care, by elderly and/or chronically ill patients. At the same time, the use of partial hospital, outpatient, and home care will increase, particularly in systems where capitation is the preferred method of reimbursement.

Clinicians Face the Future

As we enter the next century, mental health practitioners will continue to experience economic pressures. As managed care networks and integrated delivery systems proliferate and capitated reimbursement for mental health and substance abuse care becomes more prevalent, payment for all types of clinical services may fail to keep pace with inflation, or even drop in absolute terms. Thus, for many clinicians, maintaining current income levels will mean seeing more patients for briefer visits at lower fees. Many clinicians will seek to join integrated delivery systems (see above) where they will have the opportunity to share in capitated risk arrangements with primary care physicians and other specialists.

In response to these pressures, the trend toward group practice will accelerate, as clinicians pool their resources in an effort to become more efficient, reduce practice expenses, and develop leverage in negotiating more favorable contracts with managed care systems and other purchasers of care. Indeed, large, organized, multidisciplinary groups of clinicians may provide the most viable (and credible) alternative to MCOs and disease management companies in the competition to develop direct contracting arrangements with self-insured employers, purchasing alliances, and even state governments for the care of the mentally ill. For those wishing to practice outside the constraints of managed care and managed benefits, the opportunity for greater clinical autonomy and to personally provide a wider scope of services (including psychotherapy) to one's patients will have to be balanced against the economic uncertainties of a market dominated by managed care.

Though linkage with so-called provider-sponsored networks may allow clinicians to participate in contracts that eliminate the managed care third party, competing successfully for such contracts will require these networks to partner with hospitals, clinics, home care agencies, and providers of subacute and chronic care for the mentally ill. The competitive advantage will rest with vertically integrated, geographically dispersed, cost-effective networks of services in which both the costs and clinical outcomes of care are carefully monitored. Such networks will also need information systems and financial management capabilities, not only to assume the risks of capitated reimbursement, but to ensure that the patients they are responsible for receive appropriate and high-quality care. Clearly, the complex interplay of financial, clinical, and ethical considerations inherent in provider-sponsored networks will be one of the key areas of concern and controversy for the health care professions as we enter the next millennium (American Medical Association Council on Ethical and Judicial Affairs 1990; Mechanic and Schlesinger 1996; Pellegrino 1986).

Finally, in the absence of credible data on the cost-effectiveness of integrating care, psychiatrists will continue to find their professional roles narrowly defined, with the emphasis on acute crisis management and the medication management of severely ill patients. Although many psychiatrists believe that treatment outcome is improved when pharmacotherapy is combined with psychotherapy (broadly defined) and that such combined treatment is ultimately more cost-effective, well-controlled studies supporting this contention will be required before payers are equally convinced. The same debate will take place as HMOs, MCOs, and provider-sponsored networks assume the financial risk of care delivery. If psychiatrists are to avoid being marginalized, we must demonstrate the economic, as well as the clinical, value of matching patients to treaters with the most appropriate level of expertise and consolidating treatment responsibility whenever possible.

How Many Psychiatrists and Other Mental Health Professionals Will Be Needed?

As economic factors continue to affect how mental health care is delivered and by whom, estimates of the future need for psychiatrists and other mental health professionals will continue to be shaped by disparate views about how care should be delivered, interdisciplinary politics, and the cost-reduction agendas of payers, including the federal government. However, if current estimates by payers and policymakers about current and future workforce needs are accurate, some of us are already in significant oversupply. For example, in a world in which all mental health care is tightly managed, some feel that the need for psychiatrists will be about 4 per 100,000 people, compared with the present national level of approximately 13 per 100,000. This forecasted over-supply will be even more acute in certain urban areas (e.g., Boston, Washington, San Francisco), where the current supply of psychiatrists exceeds 20 per 100,000 people (Blackwell and Schmidt 1992).

Left unchallenged, managed care estimates of the need for psychiatrists will certainly influence the composition of provider networks, the staffing of mental health care facilities, and government decisions about federal funding for graduate medical education in psychiatry. The perception of oversupply will also influence the career decisions of medical students whose enthusiasm for psychiatry will depend, in part, on whether the field offers some degree of job security. Over the last decade, the number of United States medical graduates choosing psychiatric training has declined by about 50%, although the number of residency training slots has not (Sieries and Taylor 1995). Instead, training programs have increasingly turned to international medical graduates (IMGs) to fill the approximately 1,100 positions available in each of the 4 years of residency training. If government proposals to reduce or eliminate federal funding for the training of IMGs are adopted, some residency training programs will disappear.

Some have opined that training programs that depend in large measure on IMGs to fill their slots are of lesser quality, both from the standpoint of the training offered and the trainees themselves, but simply reducing the number of IMGs in psychiatry, or, for that matter, in other medical specialties, will mean that some patients, particularly those in poor and/or underserved areas, will not get the care they need. In addition, the underrepresentation of blacks, Hispanics, and other minority groups among United States medical students entering psychiatry will mean that culturally competent care for patients from these groups is and will continue to be more difficult to obtain. Thus, it is essential that a broad consensus be reached on the future need for psychiatrists and other mental health professionals that takes into account the unmet needs of certain groups of patients, the current maldistribution of providers, and the demonstrated efficacy of mental health care. The APA and other mental health organizations, in collaboration with consumer groups and policymakers, must present the case for developing and maintaining a workforce of skilled care-givers to serve current and future generations. Failure to do so will mean that patients—particularly those in underserved areas (including those in the penal system) as well as children, adolescents, and others—will continue to get short shrift from the United States health care system.

Impact of Economic Trends on Care Delivery

Shift in the Locus of Care

As pressure to contain costs has intensified, the locus of mental health and substance abuse care has shifted inexorably from inpatient to acute residential, partial hospital, and outpatient settings. The next decade will see greater reliance on distributed networks of outpatient providers, coupled with case management, home care, and mobile crisis services, as managed care and integrated delivery systems, responding to the financial incentives inherent in capitation, attempt to keep patients out of high-cost settings (i.e., hospitals). At the same time, in the absence of adequate community-based treatment and social supports, the trend toward shorter inpatient stays will result in increased hospital readmission rates for some patient groups, particularly those with severe and persistent mental illness.

Cloudy Future for Hospitals

Pressure to contain the costs of mental health and substance abuse care will intensify the competition among institutional providers (i.e., hospitals and clinics) and among integrated mental health delivery systems for local, regional, and national business. At the same time, stringent controls on the use of inpatient care will result in further reductions in hospital occupancy rates and bed capacity. As a result, inpatient care, which in 1990 accounted for approximately 75% of all the dollars spent for mental health and substance abuse treatment, may, by the turn of the century, account for less than 50% of such costs (Strumwasser et al. 1991).

The most acute economic pressure will be felt by freestanding psychiatric hospitals, whose ongoing operations require large capital investments in facilities and infrastructure. These institutions will increasingly find themselves at a competitive disadvantage in comparison to smaller, more nimble, and/or lower-cost, community-based clinics and group practices and other types of organized provider networks. For psychiatric units in general hospitals, the ability to share the infrastructure and overhead costs of a larger entity will confer a temporary economic advantage, but as general hospitals also experience declining occupancy rates and reduced levels of reimbursement, they too will need to reduce overhead and treatment costs to remain competitive. In both settings, as the clinical criteria for accessing inpatient care become more stringent, rising levels of patient acuity will increase staffing requirements at the same time that competition is necessitating a reduction in treatment costs. How this issue is dealt with by payers and caregivers will determine whether care in inpatient settings is safe and effective, or expedient, mediocre, and, in the long run, more costly to the overall care system.

In the absence of rational, and evenly applied, national policies, teaching hospitals, which have traditionally subsidized both research and graduate medical education, will face particularly difficult economic pressures. As care is increasingly managed and reimbursement moves toward common (and very low) rates for every level of care, these hospitals will no longer be able to shift the costs of supporting their academic mission onto indemnity-based payers or the federal government (in the form of Medicare reimbursement for clinical care or graduate medical education). This shift will require that teaching hospitals develop new revenue streams to support these activities (Epstein 1995; Goldman 1996) or that government policies be changed to address this issue.

To compete successfully in a marketplace dominated by managed care, like clinicians, many hospitals will seek to become part of vertically integrated, geographically distributed care networks linked by common information systems, contracting mechanisms, clinical protocols, and risk-sharing arrangements. Such linkages will also provide opportunities for rationalizing the distribution of clinical and support services across hospitals, thus reducing both clinical redundancy and overhead costs. Within these systems, freestanding psychiatric hospitals and specialty units within general hospitals may both serve local patient populations and function as regional referral centers for tertiary and quaternary care. In so doing, however, these hospitals will also need to develop a full range of alternatives to hospital-level care. Indeed, the extent to which hospitals are able to establish community-based clinics and provider networks will determine their ability to survive in an environment in which flexibility and diversification will be important attributes.

In summary, after dominating American medicine, including the mental health sector, for almost two centuries, hospitals, with their tradition-bound cultures, high overhead costs, and perceived, or actual, inefficiencies, will be increasingly viewed as costly liabilities by payers and emerging health care delivery systems. At the same time, the mentally ill will continue to need, and benefit from, sophisticated hospital-based care. The challenge for hospitals, now and in the next century, will be how to survive economically without eroding their ability to provide that care.

What About the Quality of Care?

It should be evident from all of the foregoing that the impact of cost containment on the quality of patient care is a matter of considerable debate. MCOs, HMOs, and employee benefits managers generally claim that, despite the sharp decrease in the relative proportion of total health care dollars spent on mental health treatment, the quality of care and patient satisfaction remain at acceptable levels (Sullivan et al. 1995). At the same time, the paucity of well-designed treatment outcome studies that measure much beyond the utilization and cost of services makes it difficult to assess the effect of managed care on broader outcome measures such as patients' functional adjustment and quality of life. In the managed care marketplace, pressure to reduce costs, deliver savings to purchasers, and generate profits will accentuate the need for continued vigilance and pressure on the part of patient advocacy groups, purchasers, and providers if reasonable standards of care are to be maintained.

As concern about the erosion of quality has mounted, some professional groups, including the APA, have begun to develop practice guidelines. Although some have decried the trend toward evidence-based practice guidelines and care paths as a move toward "cookbook" medicine, others see guidelines as providing some reasonable ground rules for clinical decision making, defining the standards of acceptable care, and improving clinical outcomes (Katon et al. 1995). In addition, standard-setting and accrediting bodies such as the Joint Commission on the Accreditation of Healthcare Organizations (JCAHO) and the National Committee on Quality Assurance (NCQA) have begun to abandon their tendency to focus on the processes of care and are moving toward requiring that the broader outcomes of care be measured using valid and reliable instruments. The time is ripe for provider organizations such as the APA, in collaboration with patient advocacy groups, to define the appropriate treatment goals for each level of care and site of service for specific patient populations and to work to ensure that these goals are incorporated into the assessment, monitoring, and accreditation standards for health care organizations.

Is There a Future for Psychotherapy?

Over the past two decades, significant advances in the fields of neurobiology, molecular genetics, imaging, and psychopharmacology have done much to enhance our understanding of how the brain works in health and disease and to improve the care of the mentally ill. At the same time, these advances have, to some extent, diminished the perceived importance of psychosocial and developmental factors in the etiology, clinical course, treatment, and long-term outcome of psychiatric patients. Nowhere has the impact of this trend been more evident than in the practice of, and reimbursement for, psychotherapy (Sledge 1994).

Though many practitioners are convinced of the efficacy of psychodynamic, cognitive-behavioral, and other forms of psychotherapy in appropriately selected patients, the extent to which any of these modalities are supported and reimbursed will depend on our field's ability to overcome the skepticism that employers and payers have about the efficacy of psychotherapy. Moreover, as "medically necessary" mental health care is more narrowly defined by managed systems of care, there is a (not so) covert expectation that the care of patients with "problems of living" (as opposed to severe mental illness) will be largely self-funded and not subsidized by insurance benefits. To counter these trends, providers of care will need to emphasize findings, from both basic and clinical research, that demonstrate the inextricable interplay between mind and brain. Over time, more of what we have traditionally classified as Axis II disorders may turn out to have biogenetic, as well as developmental and psychosocial, antecedents. Conversely, those disorders we now define as *brain diseases* will be found to be shaped by, and responsive to, treatment directed at developmental, behavioral, and psychosocial factors. In both instances, patients' adherence to—and benefit from—treatment will be enhanced by the application of specifically designed psychotherapies as a primary or adjunctive treatment for mentally ill patients.

Conclusion

In this chapter, I attempt to provide a brief overview of some of the economic forces that have reshaped, and will continue to reshape, the financing and delivery of mental health care. Though the challenges for both individual and institutional caregivers in this environment are daunting, the future is not as bleak as some would suggest. Patients and their families still want sophisticated and humane care, and legislators have recently become more cognizant of this simple fact. At the same time, there is growing recognition that the solution to rising health care costs does not lie in reducing patients' access to care, the number and quality of caregivers, or what we, as a society, expect from our health care system.

The next decade will offer opportunities for psychiatrists and other mental health professionals to educate, advocate, and even litigate on behalf of patients as well as themselves. Our effectiveness in these activities will depend on our ability to develop—among ourselves and with key allies—a consensus about our strategic goals and how to pursue them. Our effectiveness will also require a willingness to resolve cross-disciplinary squabbles over therapeutic territory, focus on what is best for patients, and demonstrate a willingness to objectively measure the quality of the care we deliver while responsibly controlling its cost. The APA and other organizations concerned about the care of patients can play a vital role in these efforts, and, in so doing, enhance the future prospects for our patients and for our field.

References

American Medical Association, Council on Ethical and Judicial Affairs: Financial incentives to limit care: financial implications for HMOs and IPAs, in Code of Medical Ethics: Reports of the Council on Ethical and Judicial Affairs of the American Medical Association, Vol I. Chicago, IL, American Medical Association 1990, pp 130–135,19

Blackwell B, Schmidt GL: The educational implications of managed mental health care. Hospital and Community Psychiatry 43:962–964, 1992

Callahan J, Shepard D, Beinecke RH, et al: Mental health/substance abuse treatment in managed care: the Massachusetts Medicaid experience. Health Aff 14:173–184, 1995

Cooper H: Cost controls impel psychiatric hospitals to establish more outpatient programs. Wall Street Journal, March 16, 1993, p 1

Dorwart RA, Schlesinger M, Davidson H, et al: A national survey of psychiatric hospitals. Am J Psychiatry 148:204–210, 1991

Epstein AM: U.S. teaching hospitals in the evolving health care system. JAMA 273:1203–1207, 1995

Frank RG: Cost-benefit analysis in mental health services: a review of the literature. Administration in Mental Health 8:161–176, 1981

Ginsburg PB, Pickreign JD: Tracking health care costs. Health Aff (Fall):140–149, 1996

Goldman L: The academic health care system: preserving the missions at the paradigm shifts. JAMA 273:1549–1552, 1996

Goldsmith HF, Manderscheid RW, Henderson MJ, et al: Projections of inpatient admissions to specialty mental health organizations 1990–2010. Hospital and Community Psychiatry 44:478–483, 1993

Hawaii psychiatrists again victorious over psychologists. Psychiatric News XXXI(9):1, 24, May 3, 1996

Iglehart JK: The American health care system: managed care. N Engl J Med 327:742–747, 1992

Interstudy: The competitive edge industry report. St. Paul, MN, Decision Resources, August 1996

Karel RB: NME suit winds down as record settlement reached. Psychiatric News XXIX(15):1, 24, August 5, 1994

Karel RB: Psychologists press harder to prescribe. Psychiatric News XXX(6):1, 25, March 17, 1995

Katon W, Von Korff M, Lin E, et al: Collaborative management to achieve treatment guidelines: impact on depression in primary care. JAMA 273:1026–1031, 1995

Kennedy C, Manderscheid RW: SSDI and SSI disability beneficiaries with mental disorders, in Mental Health, United States, 1992 (DHHS Publ No SMA 92–1942). Edited by Manderscheid RW, Sonnenschein MA. Washington, DC, Center for Mental Health Services and National Institute of Mental Health, 1992, pp 219–230

Kessler RC, McGonagle KA, Zhao S, et al: Lifetime and 12-month prevalence of DSM-III-R psychiatric disorders in the United States: results from the National Comorbidity Survey. Arch Gen Psychiatry 51:8–19, 1994

Levit KR, Lazenby HC, Cowan CA, et al: National health expenditures, 1990. Health Care Financing Review 13:29–54, 1991

Levit KR, Lazenby HC, Sivarajan L: Health care spending in 1994, slowest in decades. Health Aff (Fall):130–144, 1996a

Levit KR, Lazenby HC, Sivarajan L, et al: National health expenditures, 1994. Health Care Financing Review 17:205–242, 1996b

Mechanic D, Schlesinger M: The impact of managed care on patients' trust in medical care and their physicians. JAMA 275:1693–1697, 1996

National Advisory Mental Health Council: Health care reform for Americans with severe mental illnesses: report of the National Advisory Mental Health Council. Am J Psychiatry 150:1447–1448, 1993

Pellegrino ED: Rationing health care: the ethics of medical gatekeeping. J Contemp Health Law Policy 2:23–45, 1986

Prospective Payment Assessment Commission: Medicare and the American Health System: Report to the Congress. Washington, DC, Prospective Payment Assessment Commission, June 1996

Regier DA, Narrow WE, Rae DS, et al: The de facto U.S. mental and addictive disorders services system. Arch Gen Psychiatry 50:85–94, 1993

Rice DP, Kelman S, Miller LS, et al: The economic costs of alcohol and drug abuse and mental illness, 1985 (DHHS Publ No ADM 90–1694). Washington, DC, U.S. Department of Health and Human Services, 1990

Rice DP, Kelman S, Miller LS: The economic burden of mental illness. Hospital and Community Psychiatry 43:1227–1232, 1992

Rowland D, Hanson K: Medicaid: moving to managed care. Health Aff (Fall): 150–152, 1995

Sieries FS, Taylor MA: Decline of U.S. medical student career choice of psychiatry and what to do about it. Am J Psychiatry 152:1416–1426, 1995

Sledge WH: Psychotherapy in the United States: challenges and opportunities. Am J Psychiatry 151:1267–1270, 1994

Strain JJ, Lyons JS, Hammer JS, et al: Cost offset from a psychiatric consultation-liaison intervention with elderly hip fracture patients. Am J Psychiatry 148:1044–1049, 1991

Strumwasser I, Paranipe NV, Udnow M, et al: Appropriateness of psychiatric and substance abuse hospitalization. Med Care 29 (suppl):AS77–AS89, 1991

Sullivan G, Wells KB, Morgenstern H, et al: Identifying modifiable risk factors for rehospitalization: a case-control study of seriously mentally ill persons in Mississippi. Am J Psychiatry 152:1749–1756, 1995

CHAPTER 20

Psychiatry in the Twenty-First Century

New Beginnings

Melvin Sabshin, M.D.

T he last quarter-century has been characterized by significant changes in our psychiatric diagnostic system and in our treatments. In past publication (Sabshin 1990; Sabshin and Weissman 1996), I have described this period as influenced heavily by the interaction of new science and new economic pressures. This interaction has been especially powerful in the United States and Western Europe, but similar changes have occurred throughout the world. Certainly, in many countries, the economic pressures are not new, but the mix of new treatment possibilities and the lack of appropriate resources to support them are very much evident. Concurrent with these changes, psychiatry has gradually emerged from disparate ideological pressures within the field to a much greater reliance on empiricism. Biological psychiatry, including molecular biology, brain imaging, psychopharmacology, and other aspects of neuroscience, has achieved a great deal in this past quarter-century; social and psychological aspects of psychiatry, which, until the late twentieth century, lagged behind, have begun to demonstrate a comparable vitality.

This volume, which addresses the foundations of twenty-first-century psychiatry, offers a forum to focus on what is likely to occur in the next century. In this chapter, I generally follow the outline of this volume, and I engage in predicting a few new beginnings. Predictions of this sort help to increase awareness of current needs in our field and also to stimulate clarity in how and what we might advocate. Furthermore, I believe that it is extremely wise to use our imaginations even when we are faced with some difficult current realities. These realities are generally related to economic concerns. Growth in the world's economy has not yet led to increased resources for mental health care. Despite the major scientific advances of the last quarter-century, these economic concerns have led to a pessimism among many psychiatrists. Interestingly, there also was a period of pessimism in our field at the end of the nineteenth century. Pessimism in that era was fueled by limited knowledge as well as limited resources. Perhaps, as we further focus on diagnosis, we will develop a new syndrome called "end of the century pessimism."

The rapid ongoing increases in our knowledge of the complex workings of the brain, coupled with new understanding of genetic influences on behavior, will further facilitate our developing new pharmacological agents with significantly fewer side effects. Concurrent with these advances will be the development of biological markers that will enable us to identify individuals with potential predispositions to develop specific psychiatric disorders. It is hoped that biological markers will be developed to assist in identifying the individual's capacity to cope over the life cycle. These biological markers will relate both to genetic markers (genes) as well as to the products of the body's biological system and will include varied chemical markers or markers obtained from our enhanced functional brain imaging. The evolving neurosciences will also assist in our developing, sometime in the next century, an etiologically and pathogenetically based nosology.

As our knowledge of the brain is enhanced, so too is our understanding of psychological process. Behavior is now understood to evolve throughout the life cycle. This knowledge will create, in addition to biological markers of disorders, behavioral markers of disorders and will give us an enhanced capacity to make better predictions of behavior based on psychological data.

Concurrent with these advances in brain sciences and psychology, which will add to the power of our nosology, will be the development of expanded multiaxial diagnostic systems. Although current multiaxial systems are frequently difficult for clinicians to apply, we will be able early in the twenty-first century to develop many indices that will assist our identifying the level of disability of our patients. These indices, coupled with new axes that more effectively utilize the clinician's experience, will enhance the power of our diagnostic system to inform our selection of appropriate therapies.

As our knowledge of behavior expands both in its depth and breadth, our field will develop practice guidelines or parameters that will address most of our psychiatric disorders. These guidelines are the product of our research and clinical expertise in understanding specific disorders. They become the consensus treatment algorithm for patients suffering from these disorders. The expanded list of disorders for which we develop these guidelines is linked to the ongoing evolution of our diagnostic system and to the evolving power of our therapeutic skills. Although we have now developed a model nosology and a number of model practice guidelines, it is essential that we study how the guidelines work in actual practice in varied settings with practitioners with varied interests and training. In psychiatry, that means each country will ideally need to develop its own mechanism to study practice patterns among its psychiatrists. In the United States, we are developing a systematically selected network of diverse practitioners to learn how they implement our scientific advances. Embedded within this concept is some concern that current systems of assessing treatment are insufficiently reflective of modal practice. It is hoped that many psychiatric associations across the world will encourage the development of programs to assess modal practice. Perhaps the World Psychiatric Association can play an important role in this new effort. As the twenty-first century progresses with a sustained sharpening of our diagnostic capacities, coupled with a new understanding of etiology, new textbooks will appear that link nosology more explicitly to practice guidelines.

As we look ahead to the twenty-first century, no question is possibly more critical to the maintenance and enhancement of our field than a description of the core therapeutics that will enable us to utilize all of the scientific advances of the twentieth century. The last two decades of the twentieth century created major advances in our knowledge of the brain. These advances have created a rapidly evolving pharmacotherapy for our patients' disorders. No doubt, one of the core areas of practice is and will continue to be the use and further mastering of these and still newer pharmacological agents. Of less clarity for some of our colleagues in anticipation of the therapeutic armamentarium of the twenty-first-century psychiatrist is the solo use of psychotherapy—or, more correctly, the diverse psychotherapies. Each of our countries will answer how extensively psychiatrists will practice the psychotherapies alone based on local traditions, economic realities, and the existence of other mental health providers.

However, what the twenty-first century will uniquely bring regarding psychotherapy is the refinement of the combined use of psychotherapy and pharmacotherapy by psychiatrists (Gabbard and Goodwin 1996). For this refinement to proceed effectively, we will need more data. We will also need treatment outcome studies that compare treatment responses of patients to two models of combined treatment: first are patients treated by psychiatrists who serve as both psychotherapist and pharmacotherapist; and, second, are responses to treatment of patients treated where these functions are split between two psychiatrists or between a psychiatrist and a non-M.D. psychotherapist. Further, we will need to know the impact of sequencing of the use of medication and psychotherapy. It will be this unique capacity of the psychiatrist to provide this combined treatment that will maintain a special robustness to the discipline in both its practice and research.

Of course, to perform combined psychotherapy and pharmacotherapy, it will continue to be essential for psychiatrists to learn how to perform and provide psychotherapy. In countries where the health system does not support graduate psychiatrists providing this treatment, it will still be essential for psychiatric residents to learn and master these skills in order to learn how to perform combined therapy. It must be clear that combined psychotherapy and pharmacotherapy is not simply "talk" that facilitates the patient complying with his or her medication regimen. Psychotherapy may include this, but it also includes all of the complex engagements between psychotherapist and patient that have been found to be useful in dealing with life issues.

Besides a focus on issues of treatment of disorders, twenty-first-century psychiatry should address primary prevention. Coupling our enhanced knowledge of the evolution of humans over the life cycle with knowledge of varied markers, which inform us about the etiology of psychiatric disorders, will enable us to develop strategies to prevent the occurrence of some, if not all, psychiatric disorders. Primary prevention, a wish or fantasy of the past, should become a reality during the mid-twenty-first century.

Assisting our development of primary prevention strategies will be our enlarged understanding of adaptive behavior over the life cycle. In the twenty-first century, we will learn about adaptation, just as in the twentieth century we have focused on psychopathology. To assist our primary prevention activities, we will need to be able to better understand how and why many individuals successfully cope with specific biological, psychological, and social stresses. We will study the dynamic forces of adaptation and not simply study its converse, that is, maladaptation or pathology. A new language of coping will emerge by the middle of the twenty-first century. Among the many implications of this development is included understanding of the boundaries between health and disorders.

Further, we will learn of the diverse ways individuals adapt over time to major psychiatric disorders. For most of the twentieth century, individuals with schizophrenia were housed in institutions away from population centers. Today, they live in our communities. With medication and varied psychosocial treatments, we observe that patients with schizophrenia seem to have a different course than those early in this century. This enables us to develop a number of new treatment approaches and new beginnings for secondary prevention in the twenty-first century.

The new beginnings in psychiatry that I have described will occur in an era of major technological changes in how we communicate and how we deal with information. Informatics, the use of computers and complex information systems, will be an essential part of the psychiatrist's training and practice. Other technical advances will create settings so that some patients may not need to be in the psychiatrist's office for assessment and treatment. The long-distance telephone therapy sometimes used today may ultimately be viewed as an archaic predecessor to the virtual reality systems of the latter twenty-first century. These new technologies will, of course, not alleviate our ongoing need to learn the core of the psychobiology of behavior with an ongoing knowledge of social context, but they will alter, as the century progresses, how we translate this knowledge into therapies.

A major area of change in the twenty-first century will address our use of theory. The evolution and expansion of our knowledge base will lead to our reexamining our current atheoretical tendency. I believe that the atheoretical bias of today's psychiatrists will be perceived in the second quarter of the next century as having been a historical necessity—a necessity for correcting the overly extensive theoretical preoccupation in the third quarter of the twentieth century.

It is worth noting that in the late twentieth century some increased interest in psychiatric theory exists; for example, a new journal, *Philosophy, Psychiatry, and Psychology* has garnered adherents in both the United Kingdom and the United States. I believe, however, that the current atheoretical period will continue to predominate in the first quarter of the new century. Ultimately the current absence of theory will stultify psychiatry rather than protect it as it does today. The information explosion plus a need to reconceptualize diagnosis and treatment will help to stimulate interest in new theoretical systems leading to new testable hypotheses. I am also convinced that a theoretically rich psychiatry will assist in recruiting some very bright people into the field, complementing those who enter the field with other motivations.

Of special concern to our discipline is how we and our patients will be perceived in the twenty-first century. Stigma associated with mental illness will not be eradicated by the end of the twenty-first century, but I believe that its potency will be markedly reduced. This stigma is based on a number of roots, which include irrationality, antipsychiatry, and moral conflict. These attitudes, along with residual ignorance, unfortunately, will survive the twenty-first century. The brave new world and Utopia will not exist.

Nevertheless, some of today's stigma associated with mental illness is related less to prejudice per se than to our current incapacity to respond adequately to a number of fundamental questions regarding mental illness. By the mid-1990s, stigma was significantly reduced in the United States at least partially in response to our enhanced knowledge. The debates in the U.S. Senate in 1996 regarding adequate treatment resources for patients with mental illness did indeed reflect changes in attitude. Ongoing public education regarding what we know and what we don't know will be vital to continue this process; otherwise we risk that stigma will increase, fueled by unrealistic expectations of psychiatry. I anticipate the gradual decline of stigma associated with mental illness over the twenty-first century.

Psychiatric alliances with patients, their families, and citizens' groups will be increasingly prominent throughout the twenty-first century. These alliances will serve to further reduce stigma and will be most important as well in securing economic support for psychiatric service, research, and training. As psychiatry evolves as a vital discipline in the twenty-first century, it will continue to move closer to the mainstream of medicine. However, our many unanswered questions and the resultant remaining mysteries of the mind that also serve to reinforce stigma will continue to provide impediments to our increasing acceptance as a major medical specialty.

As the twentieth century ends and one takes full stock of our accomplishments, our field can move ahead on a foundation of solid scientific advances and accomplishments. We must, however, never lose our focus on the patients we treat and their complex needs.

References

Gabbard G, Goodwin F: Integrating biological and psychosocial perspectives, in American Psychiatric Press Review of Psychiatry, Vol 15. Edited by Dickstein L, Riba M, Oldham J. Washington, DC, American Psychiatric Press, 1996, pp 527–544

Sabshin M: Turning points in twentieth-century American psychiatry. Am J Psychiatry 147:1267–1274, 1990

Sabshin M, Weissman S: Forces and choices shaping American psychiatry in the 20th century, in American Psychiatric Press Review of Psychiatry, Vol 15. Edited by Dickstein L, Riba M, Oldham J. Washington, DC, American Psychiatric Press, 1996, pp 507–525

AFTERWORD

Sidney Weissman, M.D.
Senior Editor

We have now completed our journey and overview of Psychiatry in the New Millennium. In
the course of our journey, we have been assisted
in our task by numerous guides, frequently the academic leaders of our discipline. Our experience is not unlike that of a visitor to a foreign city where
tours are arranged with expert guides to demonstrate and inform us of its mu-
seums and unique points of interest. We leave such tours awed by what we
have observed but are humbled by how much we still do not know. We also
struggle to understand how the institutions we have visited relate to each
other, and we become painfully aware that we do not truly know the city's citizens, their history, and their culture. In considering our journey through the
subdisciplines of psychiatry and those external disciplines that inform psychiatry, I am concerned that we have not presented the interstitial tissues that
bind them into a vibrant discipline. Indeed, in reading some chapters, there at
times appears a latent impression that one element of our field might represent the entire field. Psychiatry in 2000 will be neither molecular biology nor
psychoanalysis nor social psychiatry; yet it will be informed by all three of
these disciplines as well as by others.

Some have confused the expansion of our knowledge of the brain—and of
one its visible operative activities, the mind—as an indicator that the definition of a psychiatrist has changed. *Psyche* is derived from the Greek word
meaning "mind," and psychiatrists are physicians who focus on treating disorders of the mind. It is or should be obvious that to treat disorders of the mind,
in fact, means to treat the brain. This is so because mind is but a function of
brain. Psychotherapy or psychoanalysis uses words or experiences to alter ele-

ments of brain functioning that are frequently observable only by future changes in an individual's behavior or self-experience. At this point in the history of our field, many of these changes cannot be detected in alterations of brain functioning by our current routes of brain study. Even in cases where changes in brain function *can* be observed, brain function alone does not inform us of the specific thought content in that individual.

As our knowledge of brain expands, the brain is being revealed to be a uniquely plastic organ. We are now learning from molecular biology how specific genetic loading and specific genotypes will expose certain individuals to vulnerabilities from unique stressors. Restated, knowing an individual's genotype will not predict that individual's behavior but will inform us of his or her vulnerabilities and potential actions. Similarly, knowledge of brain functioning from ongoing studies may inform us of certain vulnerabilities in an individual, but these alone cannot predict or inform us of the specific elements of that individual's behavior.

Indeed, as we use different sources of information or data to understand mind/brain, we realize that we need strikingly different abilities to interpret our newfound sources of knowledge. How, indeed, does the molecular biologist psychiatrist talk to the psychoanalyst psychiatrist? How, during the limited period of the psychiatric residency, does the resident learn to effectively communicate with anyone in the field? Because of the complexity of our field, for varied reasons, many respond with either biological or psychological reductionistic models of mind/brain function. Each of these reductionist models ignores input from other sciences that study human behavior. Instead, what is needed is an approach that both assures the learning and facilitates understanding of the unique but different forces that affect mind/brain. This approach must also teach how to prioritize and organize the different sources of information that inform us regarding behavior. At a time when some look for simplicity in organizing our knowledge, we must look for a theory that will assist us, regardless of its complexity. General systems theory as proposed by Ludwig Von Bertalanffy (1968) offers such an approach. Although available as a organizing approach for decades, it has strikingly been avoided. Indeed, George Engel's (1977) biopsychosocial model is but a derivation. We all know many who nod favorably to the importance of the biopsychosocial model, but in fact many or most of us ignore it. The reasons for our inability to effectively use the biopsychosocial model, a systems-driven approach, are varied. I submit that one reason is that we as psychiatrists are not effectively trained to master all of the subdisciplines required.

If one conceptualizes that in a 4-year psychiatric residency, 1 day every week was devoted full-time to academic pursuits, the accumulated time would be less than 1 academic year. Even if this time were focused on only one discipline, say molecular biology, it would be insufficient to earn a master's degree in that area. With the massive expansion of knowledge in all areas, our residencies offer little time to become conversant in the languages of the subdisciplines of psychiatry. For psychiatry to prosper, we must redesign our residency programs to ensure such competence in all areas that inform our field. If we fail, we will in the future be reduced to being technicians treating a few narrowly defined behavioral syndromes. In that case, a new discipline will need to be invented to carry on the work of psychiatry. On the other hand, psychiatry's success in mastering the new sources of knowledge while using systems theory to organize our understanding of mind/brain will lead to further advances in our understanding of the brain and the complex forces that shape behavior and will thereby secure psychiatry's future.

References

Von Bertalanffy L: General Systems Theory. New York, Braziller, 1968

Engel GL: The Need for a New Medical Model: A Challenge for Biomedicine. Science 196:179–136, 1977

Index

*Page numbers printed in **boldface** type refer to tables or figures.*